THE OPERON

Edited by

Jeffrey H. Miller
University of Geneva

William S. Reznikoff
University of Wisconsin

Cold Spring Harbor Laboratory
1978

COLD SPRING HARBOR
MONOGRAPH SERIES

The Bacteriophage Lambda
The Molecular Biology of Tumour Viruses
Ribosomes
RNA Phages
RNA Polymerase
The Operon
The Single-Stranded DNA Phages

THE OPERON

© 1978 by Cold Spring Harbor Laboratory

Printed in the United States of America
Book design by Emily Harste
Picture credits: Page ix (*middle*) G.S. Stent; (*bottom*) Esther Bubley

Library of Congress Cataloging in Publication Data
Main entry under title:

The Operon.

  (Cold Spring Harbor monograph series)
  Includes bibliographies and index.
  1. Operons. I. Miller, Jeffrey H.
II. Reznikoff, William S. III. Series.
QH450.2.O63   574.8'732   78-60439
ISBN 0-87969-124-7

Contents

Preface

Cold Spring Harbor Laboratory has been the site of two meetings on the lactose operon, the meeting organized by Jon Beckwith and David Zipser in September 1969 and the meeting we had the pleasure of organizing in July 1976. The first lactose operon meeting and its associated book served as a catalyst for an outpouring of molecular analyses of the *lac* operon. The second meeting presented the fruition of the studies, which are critically reviewed in the first half of this volume. We hope that these chapters will give students and scientists an up-to-date picture of the molecular basis of gene regulation in the *lac* system.

The second half of this volume presents analyses of other bacterial genetic regulatory systems. These chapters describe mechanisms which contrast markedly with that found in the *lac* operon. The examples presented will provide the reader with an overview of various alternative approaches to gene regulation.

We wish to express our gratitude to Jim Watson for making this entire venture possible and to thank the staff of the Cold Spring Harbor Laboratory meetings and publications offices for all of their help, especially Chris Nolan for her expert editing of the manuscript.

Tragically, Jacques Monod died on May 31, 1976, shortly before our meeting. His death was a profound loss to us all, for his studies were the origin of those described in this text. To those of us who had the honor of knowing him, he was a unique and stimulating personality. This book is dedicated to his memory.

Jeffrey H. Miller
William S. Reznikoff

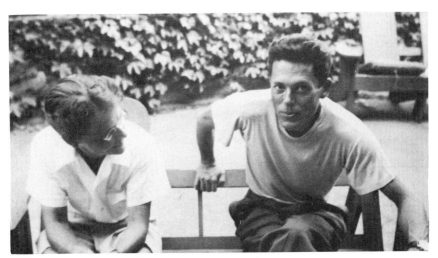

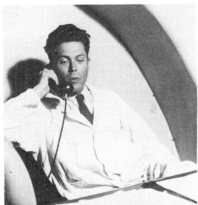

(Top) *At the Cold Spring Harbor Symposium in August 1947, Monod with Dr. Barbara McClintock.* (Middle) *This 1951 photo shows Monod working at his desk in the Pasteur Institute, Paris.* (Bottom) *Returning to Cold Spring Harbor to speak at the 1961 Symposium, Monod discusses the Jacob-Monod model of genetic regulation with Dr. Leo Szilard.*

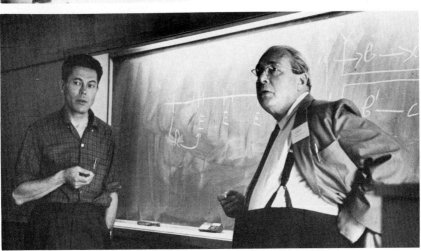

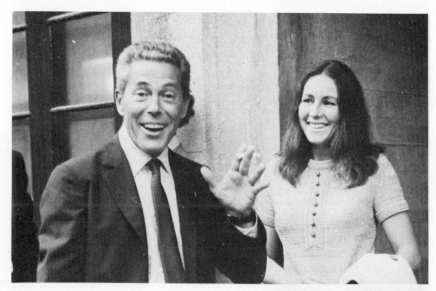

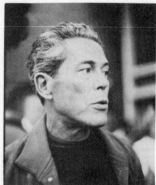

(Top) *Monod (with Dr. Suzanne Bourgeois) at the Lactose Operon Meeting held at Cold Spring Harbor in 1969.* (Middle) *A thoughtful Monod at the same meeting.* (Bottom) *In October 1969, Monod speaking before the Long Island Biological Association, at Cold Spring Harbor, on the occasion of its 50th Anniversary.*

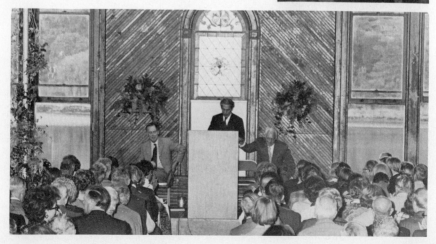

In Memoriam

Did I take on that awesome gift when death
parted my limp form from his protective
clasp?

Mechkonik

When I was asked to trace, in a personal way, the contributions of Jacques Monod to the origins of our present concept of induced enzyme synthesis, I chose to deal with the Monod of the pre-operon era of induced enzymes because it is a largely unknown chapter which is particularly illustrative of his creativity. This is appropriate because, in the last years of his life, Monod was intensely preoccupied with the creative process. He set the study of it as one of the goals of the Salk Institute which he helped found. In Jacques Monod, this process was characterized by taste, elegance, and parsimony.

In writing his own rather personalized curriculum vitae, Monod begins by saying:

> I was born in 1910 in Paris but in 1917 my parents moved to the south of France where I spent my youth. Consequently I consider myself more of a southerner than a Parisian. My father was a painter, a vocation rare in a Hugenot family dominated by doctors, pastors, civil servants and teachers. My mother was American, of Scotch descent, born in Milwaukee; another anomaly when one considers the mores of the French bourgeoisie at the end of the last century. I came to Paris in 1928 to begin my studies in the Faculté des Sciences.

Monod then recalls his debt to his teachers, André Lwoff, Boris Ephrussi, and Louis Rapkine. He tells us that in 1934 he was a Fellow of the Rockefeller Foundation at Caltech working with Thomas Hunt Morgan. In 1936 he returned to France, soon to be faced with the second world war—terrible years which he never mentions, leaving it as a blank in his curriculum vitae (during this time he was in the French Underground). After the liberation, in 1945, Monod joined André Lwoff's laboratory at the Pasteur Institute.

I met Monod in 1947 at a Cold Spring Harbor symposium. He presented a paper entitled "The Phenomenon of Enzymatic Adaptation and Its Bearings on Cellular Differentiation." He made the explicit point in his talk that we would have to understand enzymatic adaptation before we could understand differentiation, in particular, antibody synthesis.

1

This allusion, plus the enthusiastic support of my teacher, Alvin Pappenheimer, Jr., is what sent me packing for Paris.

In the winter of 1948 I began my postdoctoral work at the Pasteur Institute in Paris. We were housed in an attic. At one end was André Lwoff's closed laboratory and on the door was a cartoon showing the Duke of Wellington addressing his officers after the Battle of Waterloo. The caption read, "Tea cleared my head and left me with no misapprehensions." At the other end of the attic was the laboratory which Jacques Monod, Anna Maria Torriani, and I occupied. That year the Paris winter without heat was merciless. The glacial acetic acid remained frozen on the shelf until noon, at which time I had the distinct feeling that it was the heated discussion at the lunch table that thawed it out. Jacques was a choirmaster and during a good deal of that winter spent afternoons rehearsing the Bach Requiem he was to conduct that Christmas. On Sundays we practiced rock climbing at Fontainbleau. There were many things to decide about the direction of the work, but we simply could not settle down to any problem.

The most important preoccupation was that Monod, who symbolized reactionary Mendel-Morgan genetics, came specifically under vitriolic attack by French Marxist biologists who looked upon the very existence of adaptive enzymes as proof that the substrate induced a directed mutation or a permanent hereditary modification in the cell. This position had a certain respectability, for Sir Cyril Hinshelwood was defending the same point. Even J. B. S. Haldane felt constrained to write only apologetic essays in defense of genetics. We spent one Thursday evening of every month at the meeting of the Mitchurin-Lysenko Society, at the Sorbonne, superficially debating the facts of genetics, but in reality what concerned us was the meaning of the scientific method. For Jacques Monod, who was "engagé" in the Sartre sense, the debates were ugly and degrading and they stomped on his sense of elegance and parsimony. He was moved to make his life's goal a crusade against antiscientific, religious metaphysics whether it be from Church or State. The last time we strolled together on the beach at Torrey Pines, in 1974, he was bitter. "The battle against such ignorance will never be won," he said. "All that one can do is die without calling a priest to the bedside."

In the spring of 1949, we settled down to work. I remember that I felt like Alice in Wonderland when Monod identified three key characteristics of adaptive enzymes for study:

1. The response to a given substrate was specific for that substrate, i.e., the phenomenon was adaptive. The consequences of the existence of systems which paradoxically seem to have a purpose yet arise blindly by variation and selection were a constant theme in his thinking, culminating in his book *Chance and Necessity*.

2. The ability to metabolize a new substrate appeared as an autocatalytic function of time. This had led to the plasmagene hypothesis of Spiegelman in which a gene produced a cytoplasmic self-replicating unit which in turn synthesized the adaptive enzyme.
3. Substrates competed for each other in the induction of given enzymes. This was the striking "diauxie" phenomenon where an organism faced with two growth substrates metabolized one or the other preferentially. Today we call this *catabolite repression*. There was competition between substrates for the attention of the cell. For Monod, this implied competition for precursor subunit molecules.

Given what we now know, it seems remarkable that these three facts could have provided a solid basis for us to begin because they were so misleading. Yet Monod singled them out as he brought exquisite taste to bear on complexity. Today we know that of all of the misleading truths at the time, only these three could have led to the creation of the modern field of regulatory biology.

The Monod concept to explain these three facts was the following. A group of genes coded for a pool of precursor subunits. These could be complemented in various combinations to make different enzymes. It was the directive influence of the substrate which caused an aggregation of some of the subunits to make the corresponding enzyme. Once seeded, the crystallization process was autocatalytic. If two substrates were involved, there was competition for subunits. In other words, a large number of induced enzymes could be constructed from combinations of a smaller number of subunits which preexisted the appearance of the substrate in the milieu.

The way to test this hypothesis was to show that all substrates as well as competitive inhibitors were inducers. The hypothesis limited the choice of systems for study. *Escherichia coli* had ideal growth properties as well as an emerging genetics analyzable by mating and viral transduction. It expressed an adaptive enzyme, β-galactosidase, which had a substrate whose analogs were reasonably easy to synthesize. In 1950 I went to Bell's laboratory in Cambridge, England, and later to Helferich's laboratory in Bonn, Germany, to make the compounds which were sent back to Paris to test. By 1951, four findings changed our entire perspective:

1. Excellent substrates were *not* necessarily inducers, e.g., orthonitrophenyl-β-D-galactoside.
2. Excellent nonmetabolizable competitive inhibitors were *not* inducers, e.g., phenyl-β-D-thiogalactoside.
3. Poor nonmetabolizable competitive inhibitors could be excellent inducers, e.g., methyl- or isopropyl-β-D-thiogalactosides.

4. Noncompetitive inhibitors could be excellent inducers, e.g., the α-galactoside, melibiose.

The realization that his hypothesis was false had already crossed Monod's mind when, on October 14, 1950, he sent a telegram to me in England concerning phenyl-β-D-thiogalactoside which I had last given him to test.

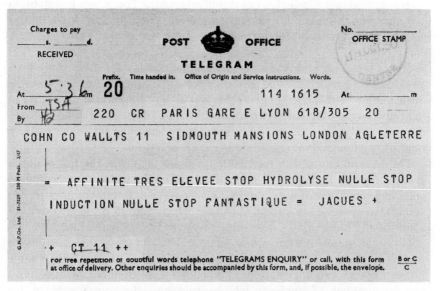

VERY HIGH AFFINITY STOP HYDROLYSIS NEGLIGIBLE STOP INDUCTION NEGLIGIBLE STOP FANTASTIC = JACQUES.

I show this telegram to illustrate the pleasure Jacques Monod derived in proving that his favorite idea was wrong; *fantastique* was the exact word. He was one of Karl Popper's greatest admirers and, like Popper, he insisted that scientific advance consisted in the falsification of hypotheses. I wish now that I could have realized that the Monod hypothesis on subunit complementation, which proved wrong for induced enzymes, would later prove correct for induced antibodies.

The existence of nonsubstrate inducers had a profound philosophical impact, for, like Ionesco, Monod had created a theater of the absurd. A bacterium growing on succinate was producing a useless enzyme, β-galactosidase, in response to a substance it could not metabolize. Monod, with great humor, invented the renowned Scottish philosopher, McGregor (his mother's maiden name), whom he quoted in all of his later writings. This time he attributed to McGregor the following quote: "Each of science's conquests is a victory of the absurd." The vitalist Hinshel-wood-Mitchourin-Lysenko position which irked him had been answered with experimental vengeance. For this reason he decided to drop the term "enzymatic adaptation" and use instead "induced enzyme synthesis," a term which was adopted eventually in an encyclical (*Nature 172*: 1096 [1953]) issued by the Adaptive Enzyme's College of Cardinals, Monod, Pollock, Spiegelman, and Stanier.

These four findings provoked Monod to toy with an idea which was very daring for 1951. The inducer had to be recognized by a stereochemically specific molecule which was *not* the induced enzyme itself. However, this idea left unexplained the autocatalytic nature of the response to lactose, a fact which now pointed strongly to a self-replicating gene product, the plasmagene, postulated by Spiegelman.

In 1951 Seymour Benzer, François Jacob, and Elie Wollman (returning from sabbatical leave) joined the laboratory. Jacob and Wollman viewed adaptive enzymes with great suspicion and by exploring elsewhere paved the way for the era of the operon. It was only in 1953, when Max Delbruck visited Paris and demanded accountability, that the suspicion was diffused and our endeavors became respectable. Seymour Benzer, on the other hand, nettled by Stanier's published statement that it could never be done, decided to tackle the question of the cause of the S-shaped autocatalytic induction curve. Using Monod's and Wollman's finding that certain *E. coli* bacteriophages could block enzyme induction, he followed the appearance of enzyme induced by lactose as the sole carbon source under conditions where only cells which contained enzyme could be lysed. It became obvious that the S-shaped curve was due to the heterogeneity of response of individuals in the population. A bacterium with one molecule of enzyme could metabolize lactose to make more enzyme and therefore had a great advantage. In other words, the postulated *E. coli* plasmagene turned out to be the bacterium itself. For Monod, the second paradox was resolved.

From these studies Monod now developed the concept of *gratuitous induction*. Under conditions where the carbon source and the inducer were separated, the heterogeneity and the S-shaped induction kinetics disappeared.

At this point Monod was ready to face his third basic fact, the competition between substrates. This implied competition for precursors which had led him to the subunit hypothesis that preformed subunits were shared between different enzymes. It became necessary that he know whether the enzyme was made de novo after induction or from preformed precursor subunits.

The answer required an isotope experiment in a laboratory that had never seen even the shadow of a Geiger counter. Fortunately he captured the interest of a Canadian physicist, Lou Siminovitch, who had been working with Louis Rapkine and André Lwoff since 1947. Siminovitch had discovered ^{35}S and proposed its use as a general protein marker. Siminovitch scrounged through the physics laboratories of Paris collecting junked parts which he checked off on his scribbled wiring diagram. He handed the precious do-it-yourself kit to Monod who, like a child with a tinker toy, put it together and made it work. At the Christmas party that year, I joshed Jacques in a skit which cast him as a bicycle repairman (*réparateur de vélos*).

David Hogness, now in the laboratory, began the experiment which required purification of very small amounts of β-galactosidase to greater than 95% purity. The only way to do this at the time was by immunologic methods. Six months later, Dave Hogness completed the definitive experiment, nervously counting each point on the tinker toy through the night, while Monod played his cello and I uncorked André Lwoff's best properly chilled Sancerre wine which he had carefully hidden in the cold room.

The result was clear. The enzyme was made from amino acids de novo after induction, at a maximum rate, virtually without lag.

This led Monod to formulate a new parameter which we christened as Monod's law, symbolized by $\Delta Z/\Delta B$ (the differential rate of synthesis), the basic unit of which was physiological time.

With hindsight it is easy to appreciate taste in science.

The three most important characteristics of induced enzyme synthesis formulated in 1949, misleading as they were, had led by 1953 to a clear definition of the problem, and Monod was prepared to pursue it virtually alone.

However, why we were so insufferably sure of ourselves is not clear to me. Given what we know today, one might say that we had not advanced very far. Justifiably annoyed by our arrogance, Martin Pollock produced a cartoon in 1953 which was upsetting to me but brought pleasure to Monod.

Pollock's cartoon shows Monod standing over a starry-eyed American (myself) symbolized by an outlandish tie, to whom he is saying, "Bravo my fine fellow! You have made remarkable observations—naturally without having done or understood anything—but nevertheless spectacular. Bravo! Continue the good work."

In the wastepaper basket are the papers of Pollock on penicillinase; on the wall is "Who killed cock robin (Sir Cyril Hinshelwood)?"; above that is Max Delbrück smiling approval; next to Max is plotted Monod's temperature as a function of Sol Spiegelman's publications (notice how normal it is after the Benzer experiment); Monod's law ($\Delta Z/\Delta B$) is inscribed on the French tricolor behind us; and on the left is Pollock's evaluation of our accomplishments: we had destroyed all existing so-called facts, replacing them with nothing he was willing to believe

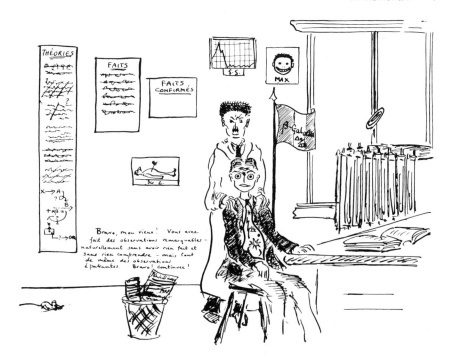

(*Faits confirmés*), and we had produced nothing but wild theories. This is how Pollock saw us in 1953. (He had a personal piece of advice for me—symbolized by the mouse in the left corner—which did not escape my notice: Go back to the study of antibody synthesis in mice! In fact, long before molecular biology could influence immunology, Pollock proposed as the key, the study of the clonal distribution of antibodies [1 cell–1 antibody].)

Today, I understand Monod's reaction of pleasure because such understanding could only have been the consequence of profound friendship.

Just before the modern era of the operon, one striking fact that we had generated had been ignored. With George Cohen and Germaine Stanier, Monod had shown that the end product of a biosynthetic pathway, in this case tryptophan and methionine, repressed the *synthesis* of the corresponding enzymes on that pathway. Not only was function inhibited as Novick and Szilard had shown, but constitutive enzyme synthesis itself was also repressed by its end product—a remarkable energy-saving device.

In his Nobel lecture, Monod muses about this:

> I had learned like any schoolboy that two negatives are equivalent to a positive statement. Mel Cohn and I debated this logical

possibility which we called the "theory of double bluff" recalling the subtle analysis of poker by Edgar Allan Poe. How blind I was not to take this hypothesis seriously sooner above all since several years earlier we had discovered that tryptophan inhibits the synthesis of tryptophan synthetase. I had always hoped that the regulation of constitutive and inducible systems would be explained by a similar mechanism. Why not suppose that induction could be effected by an anti-repressor rather than by repression of an anti-inducer? This was precisely the thesis which Leo Szilard proposed to us in a seminar. The preliminary results of the injection experiment (PaJaMo experiment) confirmed Leo Szilard's penetrating intuition and my doubts about "the theory of double bluff" were removed.

In a parallel world next door to us, Elie Wollman and François Jacob were creating the basis for genetic analyses which was soon to merge with induced enzymes to reveal what we know today as operon theory.

I did not participate in the merger which began in 1956 after I left Paris. This period is modern operon history: the discovery of the permease and transacetylase; the PaJaMa experiment; operator constitutive and promoter mutations, coordinate induction, polarity, and that remarkable insight, messenger RNA—all part of the 1961 Jacob-Monod Cold Spring Harbor paper. It was another great classic written like Monod's 1947 Cold Spring Harbor paper in that simple and direct Anatole France style. It took only one more concept formulated in 1965, that of allosteric interactions, to round out the story of regulation at the physiological level.

The key to the power of these Monod theories (1947, 1961, or 1965) was simply that they were physiological-level theories capable of reductionism, that is, they were capable of an analysis at the level of chemistry. They were truly theories of molecular biology, and this was the basis of their elegance and their parsimony.

Monod and I never finished our 1974 discussion on the Torrey Pines Beach. What was the next problem of regulation to be? Monod was concerned with the universality of the elements used in the regulation of the *lac* operon. Was there a limited number of elements which required minor rearrangements or was the number going to be large? Did we have to search for new generalizing rules on how they had to be organized? Were there any new laws which would come from the wiring diagrams, the logic of the circuitry? Were both positive and negative regulation fundamental to the integrated organism or could individuals have been constructed using only one switch or the other?

I believe that Jacques Monod had one of the most creative minds of our time, but not because he was a leader of righteous causes, a creator of molecular biology, or a founder and director of institutes of learning. He had one of the most creative minds simply because he thought deeply, ascetically, and in a Socratic way about how knowledge is acquired, and it is this process that he insisted should be the only basis for a system of ethical and aesthetic values.

Melvin Cohn
The Salk Institute

lac: The Genetic System

Reprinted in modified form from Beckwith 1970

Jonathan R. Beckwith
Department of Bacteriology and Immunology
Harvard Medical School
Boston, Massachusetts

INTRODUCTION

This chapter deals with the methods and tools used for genetic analysis of the *lac*[1] operon. The specific problems which arise in the genetic analysis of this system are, in many cases, similar to those encountered in other genetic regulatory units. Therefore, the solutions to these problems can provide a methodology applicable to at least certain of these other systems. The generality of the techniques and approach will be evaluated in this chapter. A more direct application of these techniques derives from the existence of strains in which the *lac* genes are fused to other bacterial operons, such as the *trp* and *purE* operons (Beckwith et al. 1966; Jacob et al. 1965). Since, in such strains, the *lac* genes are now part of the other operon, nearly all the methodology used for analysis of *lac* can be used for that operon (see Bassford et al., this volume).

HISTORICAL

Most of the major concepts of operon structure, expression, and regulation have come out of the work on the *lac* operon of *Escherichia coli*. That *lac* has generated so many of these ideas is due to several factors: (1) The happy coincidence of Monod and Jacob working in the same institute, thus affording a collaboration between two creative minds in the fields of bacterial physiology and regulation and bacterial genetics. The interplay of these fields has been of obvious importance to the rapid progress in understanding the mechanisms of genetic control. (2) The intuition of Monod, Jacob, and coworkers in formulating substantially correct models on the basis of their genetic and physiological studies. These models had the attractive features of providing strong predictions and of being rather easily testable (see Jacob [1966] and Monod [1966]—Nobel prize speeches—for some details and historical background). (3) Certain convenient aspects of the chemistry, physiology, and genetics of lactose metabolism in *E. coli*. These factors make it a

[1]See Table 1 and Figure 1 for abbreviations.

particularly profitable system to analyze. For instance, a large number of easily prepared β-galactosides have permitted (a) a simple enzyme assay, (b) induction with gratuitous inducers, and (c) use of chromogenic noninducing substrates such as XG to distinguish constitutive from inducible strains (see section on galactosides). Other systems, such as the arabinose operon (Englesberg et al. 1969), are more difficult to analyze since the enzyme substrates are unsubstituted monosaccharides and no hydrolytic enzymes occur in the pathway.

The discovery of bacterial conjugation by Lederberg and Tatum (1946a,b) and the refinement of this technique by Wollman et al. (1956) permitted an early genetic analysis of the genes determining lactose metabolism. Lederberg and his coworkers were the first to isolate and map crudely a series of lac^- mutations by the F^+ mating system then available (Lederberg et al. 1951; Lederberg 1952). Most of these mutations mapped in a single locus, defining the region now known as the lac locus. The subsequent isolation of Hfr donor strains, which in mating experiments donate chromosomal markers in an oriented fashion to the female, allowed a finer analysis of this region. Since the model for operon structure is based on the organization and linkage of these genes, recombination studies determining the nature of this organization were critical. Furthermore, the knowledge of the steps involved in bacterial conjugation allowed the famous "PaJaMa" (Pardee et al. 1959) experiments and zygotic induction experiments (Jacob and Wollman 1956), in which the properties of temporary merozygotes formed during conjugation led to the concept of the repressor.

A critical aspect of the analysis of operons and their regulation is the study of the interaction in the same cell of different alleles of regulatory genes and controlling elements. Since E. coli is a haploid organism, such analysis initially was impossible. Even with the discovery of sex in bacteria, the only means available for examining such diploids using the conjugation system was study of temporary merozygotes. However, at about the same time as the PaJaMa experiment was being done, a new and very important tool for the analysis of lac operon control became available, the F'lac episome. From experiments of Adelberg and Burns (1960), it was suggested that sex factors, upon recombining out of the bacterial chromosome, might occasionally carry adjacent chromosomal regions. Fortunately, since an Hfr was available which transferred lac as a terminal marker closely linked to the sex factor, Jacob and Adelberg (1959) found it relatively easy to isolate an F' episome which carried lac and no other known bacterial markers (Fig. 1). Since such episomes can be maintained in a cell independent of the bacterial chromosome, it was now possible to construct relatively stable merozygotes for accurate complementation studies.

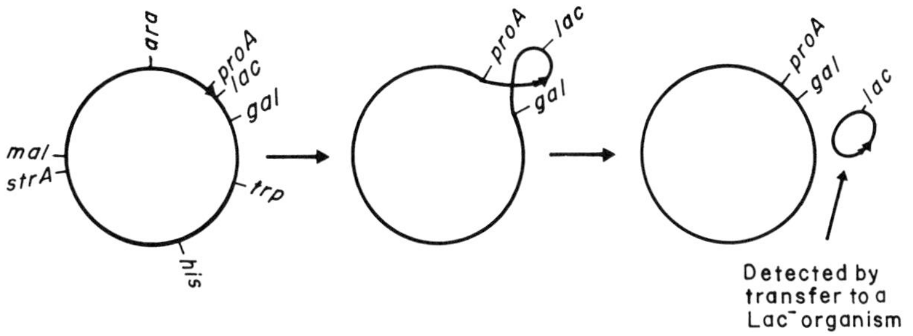

Figure 1 The origin of an F'*lac* episome. The arrow represents the origin and direction of transfer of the bacterial chromosome by this Hfr. Abbreviations used here, in subsequent figures, and in the text are as follows: *proA, proC, trp, his*—requirements for proline (two different loci), tryptophan, histidine, respectively; *ara, lac, gal, mal, mel*—inability to ferment arabinose, lactose, galactose, maltose, melibiose, respectively; *str, tonB, chlD*—sensitivity to streptomycin, bacteriophage T1, chlorate, respectively; *attλ, att80*—sites of insertion of temperate phages λ and φ80, respectively; *I, P, O, Z, Y, A*—repressor, promoter, operator, and structural genes for β-galactosidase permease, and thiogalactoside transacetylase.

φ80*lac* AND λ*lac*

The specialized transducing phages λ and φ80 have played an important role in studies of certain *E. coli* operons. However, the number of loci that could be transduced by such phages has been limited to those located close to the sites of insertion of the phage DNA in the bacterial chromosome (Signer 1966). In 1964, while working in the laboratory of Jacob at the Pasteur Institute, I isolated, by chance, a strain in which the *lac* genes had been transposed from their normal position on the chromosome to a position close to the attachment site for φ80 (*att80*) (Fig. 2A). Ethan Signer, working in the same lab, suggested that we try to get a φ80*lac* from the strain. We did (Beckwith and Signer 1966). This isolation and the subsequent isolation of a different φ80*lac* and of λ*lac* transducing phages have opened up several new approaches to the analysis of the *lac* region. Many of these will be described in detail in this chapter.

As a result of this piece of luck, we subsequently developed a technique for selecting for such happy transpositions, i.e., transpositions of genes to sites close to either *att80* or *attλ*. In the case of *att80*, this was done by selecting for insertion of an F'*lac* episome into the nearby locus (*tonB*) determining sensitivity to bacteriophage T1 (Fig. 2B) (Beckwith and Signer 1966; Beckwith et al. 1966). This insertion renders the locus inactive and makes the bacteria resistant to T1. In the case of *attλ*, this

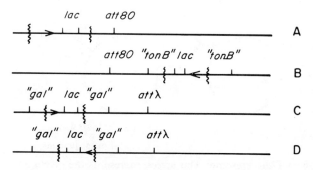

Figure 2 Transposition of the *lac* region close to phage attachment sites. Since the *lac* genes are inserted in the chromosome along with the sex factor, the strains are Hfr's with their origins of transfer indicated by arrows.

was done by selecting for insertion of the F'*lac* into the nearby *gal* operon (Fig. 2C,D) (J. R. Beckwith, unpubl.), using the technique for selection of Gal mutants described by Soffer (1962).

GALACTOSIDES USED IN *lac* ANALYSIS

A wide variety of naturally occurring and chemically prepared galactosides have been used in the analysis of *lac* operon regulation (Table 1). The sugars melibiose (Prestidge and Pardee 1965; Beckwith 1963), 6-O-α-D-galactopyranosyl-D-glucose, and raffinose (Schaefler 1967), α-D-galactopyranosyl-(1-6)-O-α-D-glucopyranosyl-(1-2)-β-D-fructofuranoside, both of which are α-galactosides, can be utilized as carbon sources by *E. coli* (at 42°C for melibiose) only if the *lac* permease, the *Y*-gene product, is functioning. Furthermore, although melibiose is an inducer of the *lac* region, raffinose is not and therefore requires constitutive *lac* expression for its metabolism. Since these α-galactosides are hydrolyzed not by β-galactosidase but by another enzyme or enzymes, they provide a means of assaying and selecting for *Y*-gene expression independent of *Z*-gene expression. One aspect of raffinose metabolism which is both a drawback and an advantage is that, even with constitutive levels of *lac* permease, *E. coli* K12 grows so slowly on this carbon source that sizable colonies are not formed on raffinose minimal agar for 10 to 14 days. Although this makes the use of raffinose rather frustrating for bacterial geneticists used to having answers in one or two days, it also makes it possible to select for higher-level permease producers from strains (such as those carrying promoter mutations) which make very low levels (Arditti et al. 1968).

One of the delights of working in the genetics of lactose metabolism is the spectrum of colors that we deal with. For *lac* indicator plates, we can use EMB agar where Lac[+] colonies have a green sheen, or MacConkey agar where Lac[+] colonies are deep red, or lactose tetrazolium agar where

Table 1 Galactosides

Galactoside	Substrate of β-galactosidase	Inducer	Chromogenic	Usefulness
Phenyl-β-D-galactoside (PG)	+	−	—	selection for constitutives
Orthonitrophenyl-β-D-galactoside (ONPG)	+	?	yellow	β-galactosidase assay
5-Bromo-4-chloro-3-indolyl-β-D-galactoside (XG)	+	−	blue	distinguishing *lac*-inducible from *lac*-constitutive bacteria
Melibiose	−	+	—	assaying for Y-gene function
Raffinose	−	−	—	selection for higher level *lac* expression or for constitutives
Isopropyl-β-D-thiogalactoside (IPTG)	−	+	—	one of the most effective gratuitous inducers
Orthonitrophenyl-β-D-thiogalactoside (TONPG)	−	?	—	selecting for *lac*⁻ mutations, particularly Y⁻
Methyl-β-D-thiogalactoside (TMG)	−	+	—	inducer; radioactive derivative used in permease assay
2-Nitrophenyl-β-D-fucoside (ONPF)	−	−	—	inhibitor of induction
Lactobionic acid	weak	−	—	for selecting constitutives or higher-level β-galactosidase producers

See Jacob and Monod (1961b) for description of many of these. Others are referred to in the text. Other references: XG—Horwitz et al. (1964); ONPF—Jayaraman et al. (1966); lactobionic acid—Langridge (1969).

Lac⁻ colonies are deep red (Ohlsson et al. 1968). The latter plates are useful for distinguishing leaky Lac mutants from wild-type. Then there is the yellow color of nitrophenol measured in the β-galactosidase assay (Pardee et al. 1959). For distinguishing constitutive from inducible strains, the nondiffusing blue color produced by the hydrolysis of 5-bromo-3-chloro-2-indolyl-β-D-galactoside (Davies and Jacob 1968) provides a sensitive test. This compound also is useful for observing different levels of *lac* operon expression among colonies on solid media containing the dye.

The fact that a product of the metabolism of the various galactosides is galactose itself gives rise to a valuable set of selective techniques. Certain mutations which block galactose metabolism confer sensitivity to galactose on the strains carrying them (Soffer 1962). Those cells which are Lac⁺ and which carry such mutations will therefore also be sensitive to lactose and other metabolizable galactosides. It then becomes possible to select for Lac⁻ bacteria in such strains by selecting mutants resistant to lactose (Malamy 1966).

A particularly useful application of the galactose-sensitive selection is in the mapping of the *I* gene and the operator. A difficult problem arises in recombination studies with mutations which affect regulatory genes or controlling elements in *lac* and, for that matter, in most systems. The phenotype of an *I*⁻ or *O^c* is still Lac⁺. One has to devise physiological conditions or strains in which the *lac*-constitutive character can be selected against. One technique for doing this is to construct *lac*-constitutive strains which are sensitive to galactose and to use the noninducing β-galactosidase substrate PG in the media to kill all constitutive derivatives (Davies and Jacob 1968). Another is to use the compound TONPG which is not an inducer, but, when transported into the cells by the *lac* permease, is lethal (Müller-Hill et al. 1968).

DIPLOID ANALYSIS

Both F'*lac* episomes and the *lac*-transducing phages, λ*lac* and φ80*lac*, can be used for diploid analysis of the *lac* region. Mutations in the *lac* region have been isolated which exhibit every conceivable type of behavior in complementation studies: recessive constitutivity (*I*⁻) (Jacob and Monod 1961a); dominant constitutivity (*I*⁻ᵈ) (Müller-Hill et al. 1968); cis-dominant constitutivity (*O^c*) (Jacob and Monod 1961a); dominant pleiotropic *lac*⁻ (*I^s*) (Willson et al. 1964); cis-dominant pleiotropic *lac*⁻ (polar mutants and *P*⁻) (Jacob and Monod 1961a; Scaife and Beckwith 1966). Thus, it is obviously important for any system that all mutations with apparent regulatory properties be thoroughly characterized in complementation studies before conclusions can be made about the structure affected.

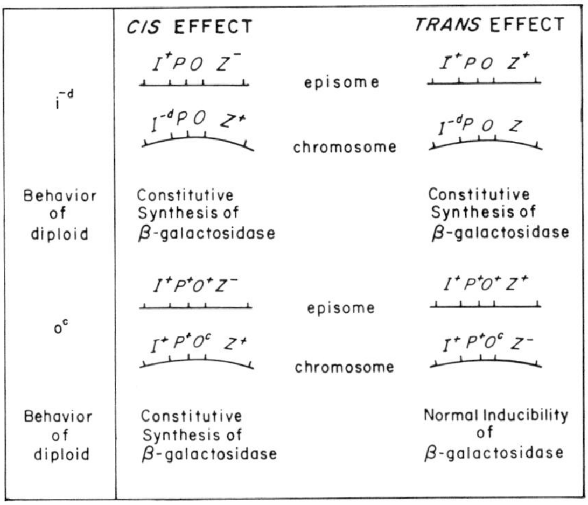

	CIS EFFECT		*TRANS* EFFECT
I^{-d}	$I^+ P\ O\ Z^-$ episome		$I^+ P\ O\ Z^+$
	$I^{-d}P\ O\ Z^+$ chromosome		$I^{-d}P\ O\ Z$
Behavior of diploid	Constitutive Synthesis of β-galactosidase		Constitutive Synthesis of β-galactosidase
O^c	$I^+ P^+ O\ Z^-$ episome		$I^+ P^+ O^+ Z^+$
	$I^+ P^+ O^c Z^+$ chromosome		$I^+ P^+ O^c Z^-$
Behavior of diploid	Constitutive Synthesis of β-galactosidase		Normal Inducibility of β-galactosidase

Figure 3 The use of *cis-trans* tests to distinguish I^{-d} constitutives from O^c constitutives. See Gilbert and Müller-Hill (1970) for explanation of I^{-d} mutations.

To distinguish between, for instance, an I^{-d} and an O^c mutation, a *cis-trans* test must be carried out (Fig. 3). It can be seen from the results of such a test that the I^{-d} mutation results in constitutivity for the gene located "in *trans*" on the episome as well as for the Z gene linked to it "in *cis*." In contrast, the O^c mutation only results in constitutivity for the Z gene linked to it "in *cis*."

It is now possible to isolate F' episomes carrying any *E. coli* gene. The accumulation of a large array of Hfr's with origins around the chromosome, the ability to select for Hfr's with their origins in predetermined places on the chromosome (Beckwith et al. 1966), and the simple technique of Low (1968) for isolating F' factors allow the collection of a series of F' factors which together cover nearly the entire chromosome. It is likely that transducing phages similar to λ*lac* and φ80*lac* can be isolated for almost any other gene. Gottesman and Beckwith (1969) described a technique for the isolation of φ80*ara* transducing phages which should be applicable in general to genes on the *E. coli* chromosome.

MAPPING OF THE *lac*-REGION 3-FACTOR CROSSES

A standard method for ordering markers in a small region is by reciprocal 3-factor crosses (Fig. 4) (Gross and Englesberg 1959). A good deal of the earlier mapping of the *lac* region which led to the order I-O-Z-Y was done in this way. In general, 3-factor crosses have proved fairly reliable. However, marker effects and high negative interference (Jacob and Wollman 1961), particularly in the case of closely linked mutations, can

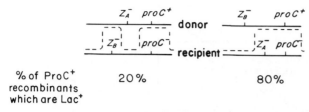

%of ProC⁺ recombinants which are Lac⁺: 20% ... 80%

Figure 4 A reciprocal 3-factor cross. Reciprocal 3-factor crosses are essential for conclusive mapping data. Ideally, this is done by Hfr crosses, selecting a marker distal to the *lac* region (e.g., $proC^+$ in the case of HfrH) and scoring, among recombinants for that marker, the frequency of Lac⁺ recombinants. If high negative interference does not make the data inconclusive, substantial differences in frequency should be observed between the two crosses. This is due to the requirement for a quadruple crossover in one case and not the other. This figure depicts a typical result.

result in serious mismapping. The problems can be seen, for instance, in the case of recombination between certain promoter mutations and a closely linked Z^- mutation (Fig. 5). The high negative interference is so great in these crosses that it is impossible to determine the order of the three markers *L8*, *L29*, and *U118*. I feel that a twofold difference in frequencies observed in reciprocal 3-factor crosses is not enough to give confidence of the order. Such confidence is particularly important in ordering markers in the promoter-operator region and in the adjoining regions of the *Z* and *I* genes. In these crucial regions which determine the initiation of transcription and translation and their control, any mapping data which is to lead either to new ideas about control mechanisms or to further experiments must be convincing.

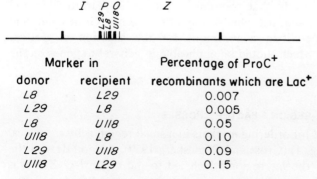

Marker in donor	recipient	Percentage of ProC⁺ recombinants which are Lac⁺
L8	L29	0.007
L29	L8	0.005
L8	U118	0.05
U118	L8	0.10
L29	U118	0.09
U118	L29	0.15

Figure 5 Results of reciprocal 3-factor crosses in the *lac* region. Crosses were carried out as described in Fig. 4 (Miller et al. 1968b).

DELETION MAPPING

A much more unambiguous method for mapping closely linked mutations is by recombination with deletions with ends in the region (Benzer 1959). Here, rather than comparing two recombination frequencies, a plus or minus answer is expected; the deletion either does or does not recombine with a particular mutation. For most genes or operons, the existence of a set of deletions useful for mapping depends on the chance finding of such deletions among mutations arising spontaneously or with various mutagens. Some of these deletions may be completely internal to the gene or operon (Malamy 1966). However, the most convenient way to carry out deletion mapping is to have a large collection of deletions which have one end outside the region under study. This would be a set of deletions beginning with one that removes only a marker or a few markers at one end of the gene cluster, and with succeeding deletions that cut farther and farther into the operon. Although other deletions can be used for mapping, because of the simplicity of analysis with these particular deletions, I shall call them "mapping deletions." A collection of such deletions forms what could be called a mapping kit. An example of ordering with mapping deletions in the *lac* operon is shown in Fig. 6. The unambiguous ordering results should be compared with those in Fig. 5 derived from 3-factor crosses.

There are several ways to specifically select mapping deletions with one end in the *lac* region. In one case, strains are used in which the *lac* region has been altered by mutation so that none of the structural genes are expressed. From such strains it is possible to select deletions which restore *Y*- and *A*-gene activities by fusing the operon to a nearby functioning gene or operon. Depending on the selection used, these deletions may end either in the *Z* gene or somewhere in the controlling-element region. One of the convenient aspects of galactoside metabolism

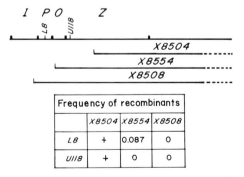

Figure 6 Deletion mapping of the *lac* region. Crosses and deletions are described in Ippen et al. (1968).

in *E. coli* K12 is that it is possible using melibiose to select for the functioning of the *lac*Y gene without a requirement for Z-gene activity. Strains which carry either I^s mutations or strong Z-gene polar mutations, and which are therefore phenotypically y⁻, are Mel⁻. Among Mel⁺ revertants selected from strains carrying these mutations, a certain proportion have restored permease activity as the result of fusion of *lac* to some other gene or operon (Fig. 7) (Beckwith 1964; Jacob et al. 1964; Schwartz and Beckwith 1969). In the case of the *lac* polar mutation, the deletion must cover at least the polar mutation site (Fig. 7A); with the I^s mutation, the deletion must result in insensitivity to *lac* repressor, since the selections are done in I^s/I^s diploid strains (Fig. 7B). Diploids are used to eliminate the very high background of I^s to I^- mutations.

This selection technique is obviously limited in its applications. First, even in *lac*, requirements of the selection may well eliminate certain types of deletions with ends in the controlling-element region. With regard to operons other than *lac*, a similar selective technique is necessary, i.e., the ability to select for the expression of a gene distal to the first gene of the operon. Although for most systems the structure of the operons and the particular enzymatic steps involved do not allow such selections, they are possible in the histidine operon (selection for growth on histidinol) (St. Pierre 1968) and possibly for tryptophan (selection for growth on anthranilic acid) (Margolin and Bauerle 1966).

A technique for selecting mapping deletions with more general applications derives from the ability to transpose *lac* and other genes to the *att80* site and to the *gal* locus. Closely linked to the *att80* site is the *tonB* locus, which has been used extensively as a deletion-selecting locus (Fig. 8). The gene or genes of the *tonB* locus determine the sensitivity of *E. coli* to the bacteriophages T1 and ϕ80 and to colicins V and B (Gratia 1964); Wang and Newton 1969a,b). Mutants resistant to the combination of ϕ80*vir* and colicins V and B, which occur only in this locus, are frequently the result of deletions of at least part of the locus. Many of these deletions extend into nearby unrelated genes. This property of

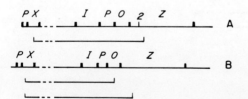

Figure 7 Deletions obtained as Mel⁺ revertants of a polar mutation (A) or I^s mutation (B). X represents a nearby unspecified gene with its own promoter, P. The marker, 2, is a strong *lac* polar mutation.

---

[2]These are now termed *tonB* mutations.

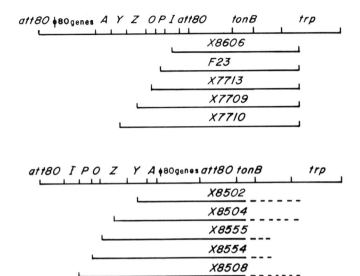

Figure 8 *TonB* mapping deletions of the *lac* region. The *X8500* series of deletions are described in Ippen et al. (1968) and Miller et al. (1968b). The others are discussed in the text.

mutations conferring T1 resistance $(T1')^2$ was first recognized as a means of selecting mapping deletions by Yanofsky, who used *tonB-trp⁻* deletions to map point mutations in the *trpA* gene (Yanofsky et al. 1964). Subsequently, Franklin et al. (1965) showed that in strains lysogenic for bacteriophage ϕ80, many *tonB* mutations are deletions that extend varying distances into the prophage map. Thus, when *lac* is incorporated in a ϕ80*lac* prophage, it is clear that many *tonB* mutations should be deletions which extend in the same way into the *lac* region (Fig. 8).

Strains lysogenic for ϕ80*lac* have been constructed with *lac* either in its usual orientation relative to other genes on the chromosome (ϕ80*lac*ᵢ) or in inverted orientation (ϕ80d*lac*ᵢᵢ) (Fig. 8). As a result, it is possible to isolate mapping deletions extending into either end of the *lac* region (Beckwith et al. 1966; Ippen et al. 1968; Miller et al. 1968b). Since, in order to detect *tonB-lac* deletions, the ϕ80*lac* lysogens must be haploid for the *lac* region, the particular strains used carry a complete deletion of the normally located *lac* region. When *tonB* mutations are selected from ϕ80d*lac*ᵢ and ϕ80d*lac*ᵢᵢ lysogens, the percentages of those with ends in the *lac* operon are 4% and 1.5%, respectively (Miller et al. 1970).

Several different techniques have been used for isolating *tonB-lac* deletions: (1) In strains lysogenic for ϕ80d*lac*⁺ᵢ or ϕ80d*lac*⁺ᵢᵢ, TonB mutants are selected on *lac* indicator plates. *Lac⁻* deletions are then screened by recombination tests to detect those in which the deletion does not remove the entire operon. Most of these are deletions which end in one of the structural genes, Z or Y (Beckwith et al. 1966; Miller et al. 1970). (2) If, instead of using a ϕ80dlac_I carrying a wild-type lac^+ region, a lac promoter mutation is recombined into the prophage, a new type of selection is possible. These strains on lac indicator plates score Lac⁻. A deletion which causes fusion of the lac controlling-element region to the trp operon will restore a Lac⁺ phenotype if the trp operon is being expressed at a high rate (Reznikoff et al. 1969; D. Mitchell and J. R. Beckwith, unpubl.). Thus, in such a strain carrying a lac promoter mutation in the prophage and a derepressed allele ($trpR^-$) of the trp regulatory gene, $tonB$ deletions have been selected with one end in the lac controlling-element region. These deletions occur at about 0.01% of the $tonB$ mutations (D. Mitchell et al., unpubl.). Finally, if in ϕ80dlac^+_I lysogens $tonB$ mutations are selected on solid media containing the indicator dye XG (see Table 1), deletions ending in the I gene are easily detected as deep blue colonies (Miller et al. 1968a). Using these different techniques, it has been possible to isolate $tonB$-lac deletions with ends in virtually every element of the lac region (Fig. 8). This provides a complete kit of mapping deletions. These deletions have been used to conclusively establish the order I-P-O-Z-Y-A (Miller et al. 1968b).

A second analogous system for isolating mapping deletions exists in strains where lac is transposed to the gal region. Shapiro and Adhya (1969) found that in strains lysogenic for certain λ derivatives, a selection can be devised to give mapping deletions of the gal operon. Furthermore, Adhya et al. (1968) showed that selection for chlorate resistance gives the same sort of deletions due to the existence of the $chlD$ locus between gal and $att\lambda$. Preliminary studies with strains in which lac is transposed to the gal region have yielded similar mapping deletions for lac (Fig. 9).

Finally, another class of mapping deletions can be obtained by isolating transducing phages which include only a portion of the lac region (Fig. 10). This type of transducing phage has been used extensively in the mapping of the gal operon with λdg phages. However, the types of deletions of lac which can be obtained in this way are limited (Beckwith

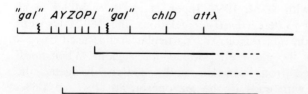

Figure 9 Deletions of lac transposed to the gal region. Using a selection involving a heat-inducible λ lysogen (Shapiro and Adhya 1969), we selected deletions cutting into the I gene and possibly into Z (Shapiro et al. 1969; Ippen et al. 1971).

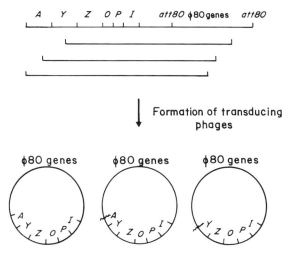

Figure 10 Origin of φ80*lac* transducing phages carrying *lac* deletions.

et al. 1966). The isolation of a terminal deletion of the *lac* operon by this technique indicated that the enzyme thiogalactoside transacetylase is not essential for lactose metabolism (Fox et al. 1966).

Since the techniques used for obtaining these transpositions of the *lac* region can be extended to other bacterial genes, most of these methods of deletion selection should be applicable to other operons. In many cases, this type of system could greatly simplify mapping problems.

One qualification of deletion mapping should be considered. Mapping deletions remove all genetic homology to one side of the mutation sites not included in the deletions. It is quite possible that mutations which lie close to the region covered by the deletion will be unable to recombine with that deletion because of the limited homology. So far no example of this has been found; in all deletions strains where by physiological tests we can demonstrate the existence of an element of the *lac* region, recombinants for the nearest marker can also be obtained. Although this problem is unlikely to generate errors in mapping order, it should be remembered if the deletions are to be used for other purposes.

A very useful method for increasing the sensitivity of the recombination techniques where low levels of recombination are expected is to measure frequencies in strains diploid for the *lac* region. If such strains carrying two different *lac* mutations are grown up to high density in liquid media, recombinants accumulate and the frequency of recombinants will be higher than in a transduction or Hfr × F⁻ cross (Ippen et al. 1968; Miller et al. 1968a,b). This technique has been used in mapping point mutations versus deletions.

OTHER USES OF *trp-lac* FUSION STRAINS

The properties of those deletions from $\phi80\text{d}lac_1$ lysogens which fuse
different elements of the *lac* region to the *trp* operon provide further
evidence for the structure of this region. *TonB* deletions which fuse the *I*
gene to the *trp* operon (Fig. 8, *X8606*) have no effect on the expression of
the *lac* operon except to render it constitutive. The *lac* operon is not put
under *trpR* control, and introduction of an I^+ gene on an F' episome
restores the normal inducible character (Miller et al. 1968a). Comparable
deletions which end in the *P* region either abolish or drastically lower *lac*
operon activity in $trpR^+$ derivatives, whereas the $trpR^-$ mutation causes
an increase in *lac* expression (Fig. 8, *F23*). A deletion which extends into
the operator region and recombines with no *O* or *P* mutations has no
effect on the structure of β-galactosidase made under tryptophan control
(Fig. 8, *X7713*) (Reznikoff and Beckwith 1969; Bhorjee et al. 1964).
Deletions ending in the *Z* gene result in *trpR* control of the *Y* and *A*
genes (Fig. 8, *X7709*). Finally, fusion deletions which end in the *Y* gene
exhibit control of transacetylase activity by the *trpR* gene (Fig. 8, *X7710*)
(Miller et al. 1970). In addition to providing a mapping system, the existence
of *trp-lac* fusions has opened up new approaches to other problems concerning *lac* operon expression and control. Some of these experiments are
covered in other chapters in Miller (1970). Again, all of these approaches
could be applicable to other *E. coli* operons and genes.

ESTIMATING DISTANCES IN THE *lac* OPERON

It is, of course, of great interest to know something about the size of such
regions as the operator and promoter. Recently, conclusive information
has come from a combination of genetic, biochemical, and physical
studies. We might ask whether the genetic mapping which has been done
in this region leads to any estimates of these distances.

There exist in the literature enough data to make it clear that any
estimates of true distances based on recombination frequencies could be
off by as much as an order of magnitude. This conclusion comes
particularly out of the work of Yanofsky and coworkers (Yanofsky et al.
1964; Drapeau et al. 1968) on the *trpA* gene and its product, the
tryptophan synthetase A protein, where it is possible to relate true
distances to recombination frequencies. The variation in the relationship
between recombination frequencies and true distances is probably due, in
part, to the types of effects seen by Herman (1968) and Zipser (1967).
Herman showed that the induction of *lac* expression can have an effect on
the frequency of recombination. We have also seen marker effects on
map distance (Miller et al. 1968b). Zipser found that recombination
frequencies between two very close mutations in the *Z* genes were much
lower than expected on the basis of other map distances in the *Z* gene.

CYCLIC AMP CONTROL

The *lac* operon is also controlled, together with several other operons, by a cyclic AMP (cAMP)-regulated system. A protein factor, CRP (originally termed CAP), activates these operons in the presence of cAMP and allows maximal levels of transcription. In the absence of CRP or cAMP, the levels of the *lac* enzymes are severely reduced. More detailed aspects of this system are reviewed by de Crombrugghe and Pastan (this volume) and by Reznikoff and Abelson (this volume).

POLARITY

Polar mutations are lesions in one gene which lower the amount of product synthesized by all of the distal genes of an operon. The only base-substitution mutations which have been shown to be polar create nonsense codons and result in chain termination. Zipser (1970) has reviewed some of the earlier models of polarity which invoked the so-called threading hypothesis (Martin et al. 1966), which postulates that ribosomes can only attach to mRNA near its 5′ end, or involved coupled mRNA and polypeptide synthesis which would lead to mRNA termination or breakdown upon chain termination. More recent developments in the field have been discussed by Adhya and Gottesman (1978) and point to the termination factor, rho, as causing polarity in gene expression by mediating premature transcription termination at discrete sites.

CONCLUDING REMARKS

Progress in the understanding of how genes work in bacteria has been heavily dependent on advances in bacterial genetics. The increasing sophistication of the methodology in this field has now made possible almost any conceivable manipulation of genes in *E. coli*. Although many of these manipulations at first seemed gratuitous (i.e., the isolation of $\phi80lac$ and subsequently λlac, who needs a second phage?), they all ultimately turned out to be useful.

There are still problems remaining in the *lac* operon which require precise genetic analysis. The portion of the *lac* region around the controlling sites includes the following interesting elements: an mRNA stop signal at the end of the *I* gene; the promoter site which may be relatively complex (see Miller 1970); the operator; and the translation-initiation signals at the beginning of *Z*. A careful mapping of mutations in these regions in conjunction with base-sequence analysis has already provided information about which sequences are important for the interaction of proteins with DNA.

ACKNOWLEDGMENTS
This work was supported by a career development award and a grant from the National Institutes of Health (GM-9027) and by grants from the National Science Foundation (GB-8247), the American Cancer Society, and the Jane Coffin Childs Memorial Fund for Medical Research.

APPENDIX

The following are references for published maps of the regions indicated:

I and *O*: Davies and Jacob (1968); Ippen et al. (1968); Miller et al. (1968a,b); Smith and Saddler (1974); Pfahl et al. (1974); Schmeissner et al. (1977a,b); Miller (this volume).

Z: Jacob and Monod (1961a,b); Jacob and Wollman (1961); Newton et al. (1965); Malamy (1966); Cook and Lederberg (1962); Schwartz and Beckwith (1969); Ullmann et al. (1968); Michels and Zipser (1969).

Y: Jacob and Monod (1961a,b); Jacob and Wollman (1961); Malamy (1966); Beckwith and Signer (1966); Hobson et al. (1977).

REFERENCES

Adelberg, E. A. and S. N. Burns. 1960. Genetic variation in the sex factor of *Escherichia coli*. *J. Bacteriol.* **79**:321.

Adhya, S. and M. Gottesman. 1978. Control of transcription termination. *Annu. Rev. Biochem.* (in press).

Adhya, S., P. Cleary, and A. Campbell. 1968. A deletion analysis of prophage λ and adjacent genetic region. *Proc. Natl. Acad. Sci.* **61**:956.

Arditti, R. R., J. G. Scaife, and J. R. Beckwith. 1968. The nature of mutants in the *lac* promoter region. *J. Mol. Biol.* **38**:421.

Beckwith, J. R. 1963. Restoration of operon activity by suppressors. *Biochim. Biophys. Acta* **76**:162.

———. 1964. A deletion analysis of the *lac* operator region in *Escherichia coli. J. Mol. Biol.* **8**:427.

———. 1970. *Lac*: The genetic system. In *The lactose operon* (ed. J. R. Beckwith and D. Zipser), p. 5. Cold Spring Harbor Laboratory, Cold Spring Harbor, New York.

Beckwith, J. R. and E. R. Signer. 1966. Transposition of the *lac* region of *E. coli*. I. Inversion of the *lac* operon and transduction of *lac* by φ80. *J. Mol. Biol.* **19**:254.

Beckwith, J. R., E. Signer, and W. Epstein. 1966. Transposition of the *lac* region. *Cold Spring Harbor Symp. Quant. Biol.* **23**:393.

Benzer, S. 1959. On the topology of the genetic fine structure. *Proc. Natl. Acad. Sci.* **45**:1607.

Bhorjee, J. S., A. V. Fowler, and I. Zabin. 1969. Biochemical evidence that the operator locus is distinct from the *z* gene in the *lac* operon of *Escherichia coli. J. Mol. Biol.* **43**:219.

Cook, A. and J. Lederberg. 1962. Recombination studies of lactose nonfermenting mutants of *Escherichia coli* K12. *Genetics* **47**:1335.

Davies, J. and F. Jacob. 1968. Genetic mapping of the regulator and operator genes of the *lac* operon. *J. Mol. Biol.* **36**:413.

Drapeau, G. R., W. J. Brammar, and C. Yanofsky. 1968. Amino acid replacements of the glutamic acid residue of position 48 in the tryptophan synthetase A protein of *Escherichia coli*. *J. Mol. Biol.* **35**:357.

Englesberg, E., D. Sheppard, C. Squires, and F. Meronk, Jr. 1969. An analysis of "revertants" of a deletion mutant in the *C* gene of the L-arabinose gene complex in *Escherichia coli* B/r: Isolation of initiation constitutive mutants (I^c). *J. Mol. Biol.* **43**:281.

Fox, C. F., J. R. Beckwith, W. Epstein, and E. R. Signer. 1966. Transposition of the *lac* region of *Escherichia coli*. II. On the role of thiogalactoside transacetylase in lactose metabolism. *J. Mol. Biol.* **19**:576.

Franklin, N. C., W. F. Dove, and C. Yanofsky. 1965. The linear insertion of a prophage into the chromosome of *E. coli* shown by deletion mapping. *Biochem. Biophys. Res. Commun.* **18**:910.

Gilbert, W. and B. Müller-Hill. 1970. The lactose repressor. In *The lactose operon* (ed. J. R. Beckwith and D. Zipser), p. 93. Cold Spring Harbor Laboratory, Cold Spring Harbor, New York.

Gottesman, S. and J. R. Beckwith. 1969. Directed transposition of the arabinose operon: A technique for the isolation of specialized transducing bacteriophages for any *Escherichia coli* gene. *J. Mol. Biol.* **44**:117.

Gratia, J. P. 1964. Résistance à la colicine chez *E. coli*. *Ann. Inst. Pasteur* **107**:132.

Gross, J. and E. Englesberg. 1959. Determination of the order of mutational sites governing L-arabinose utilization in *Escherichia coli* B/r by transduction with phage P1 bt. *Virology* **9**:314.

Herman, R. K. 1968. Effect of gene induction on frequency of intragenic recombination of chromosome and F-merogenote in *Escherichia coli* K12. *Genetics* **58**:55.

Hobson, A. C., D. Gho, and B. Müller-Hill. 1977. Isolation, genetic analysis, and characterization of *Escherichia coli* mutants with defects in the *lacY* gene. *J. Bacteriol.* **131**:830.

Horwitz, J. P., J. Chua, R. J. Curby, A. J. Tomson, M. A. DaRooge, B. E. Fisher, J. Mauricio, and I. Klundt. 1964. Substrates for cytochemical demonstration of enzyme activity. I. Some substituted 3-indolyl-β-D-glycopyranosides. *J. Med. Chem.* **7**:574.

Ippen, K., J. H. Miller, J. Scaife, and J. Beckwith. 1968. New controlling element in the *lac* operon of *E. coli*. *Nature* **217**:825.

Ippen, K., J. A. Shapiro, and J. R. Beckwith. 1971. Transposition of the *lac* region to the *gal* region of the *Escherichia coli* chromosome: Isolation of λ*lac* transducing bacteriophages. *J. Bacteriol.* **108**:5.

Jacob, F. 1966. Genetics of the bacterial cell. *Science* **152**:1470.

Jacob, F. and E. A. Adelberg. 1959. Transfer of genetic characters by incorporation into the sex factor of *Escherichia coli*. *C. R. Acad. Sci.* **249**:189.

Jacob, F. and J. Monod. 1961a. On the regulation of gene activity. *Cold Spring Harbor Symp. Quant. Biol.* **26**:193.

———. 1961b. Genetic regulatory mechanisms in the synthesis of proteins. *J. Mol. Biol.* **3**:318.

Jacob, F., A. Ullmann, and J. Monod. 1964. Le promoteur, élément génétique necéssaire à l'expression d'un opéron. *C. R. Acad. Sci.* **258**:3125.

――. 1965. Délétions fusionnant l'opéron lactose et un opéron purine chez *Escherichia coli. J. Mol. Biol.* **13**:704.

Jacob, F. and E. L. Wollman. 1956. Sur les processus de conjugaison chez *Escherichia coli.* I. l'induction par conjugaison ou induction zygotique. *Ann. Inst. Pasteur* **91**:486.

――. 1961. *Sexuality and the genetics of bacteria.* pp. 228–232, 273. Academic Press, London.

Jayaraman, K., B. Müller-Hill, and H. V. Rickenberg. 1966. Inhibition of the synthesis of β-galactosidase in *Escherichia coli* by 2-nitrophenyl-β-D-fucoside. *J. Mol. Biol.* **18**:339.

Langridge, J. 1969. Mutations conferring quantitative and qualitative increases in β-galactosidase activity in *Escherichia coli. Mol. Gen. Genet.* **105**:74.

Lederberg, E. M. 1952. Allelic relationships and reverse mutation in *Escherichia coli. Genetics* **37**:469.

Lederberg, J., E. M. Lederberg, N. D. Zinder, and E. R. Lively. 1951. Recombination analysis of bacterial heredity. *Cold Spring Harbor Symp. Quant. Biol.* **16**:413.

Lederberg, J. and E. L. Tatum. 1946a. Novel genotypes in mixed cultures of biochemical mutants of bacteria. *Cold Spring Harbor Symp. Quant. Biol.* **11**:113.

――. 1946b. Gene recombination in *E. coli. Nature* **158**:558.

Low, B. 1968. Formation of merodiploids in mating with a class of rec⁻ recipient strains of *Escherichia coli* K12. *Proc. Natl. Acad. Sci.* **60**:160.

Malamy, M. 1966. Frameshift mutations in the lactose operon of *E. coli. Cold Spring Harbor Symp. Quant. Biol.* **31**:189.

Margolin, P. and R. H. Bauerle. 1966. Determinants for regulation and initiation of expression of tryptophan genes. *Cold Spring Harbor Symp. Quant. Biol.* **31**:311.

Martin, R. G., D. F. Silbert, D. W. E. Smith, and H. J. Whitfield, Jr. 1966. Polarity in the Histidine Operon. *J. Mol. Biol.* **21**:357.

Michels, C. A. and D. Zipser. 1969. Mapping of polypeptide reinitiation sites within the β-galactosidase structural gene. *J. Mol. Biol.* **41**:341.

Miller, J. H. 1970. Transcription starts and stops in the *lac* operon. In *The lactose operon* (ed. J. R. Beckwith and D. Zipser), p. 173. Cold Spring Harbor Laboratory, Cold Spring Harbor, New York.

Miller, J. H., J. R. Beckwith, and B. Müller-Hill. 1968a. Direction of transcription transcription of a regulatory gene in *E. coli. Nature* **220**:1287.

Miller, J. H., K. Ippen, J. G. Scaife, and J. R. Beckwith. 1968b. The promoter-operator region of the *lac* operon of *Escherichia coli. J. Mol. Biol.* **38**:413.

Miller, J. H., W. S. Reznikoff, A. E. Silverstone, K. Ippen, E. R. Signer, and J. R. Beckwith. 1970. Fusions of the *lac* and *trp* regions of the *E. coli* chromosome. *J. Bacteriol.* **104**:1273.

Monod. J. 1966. From enzymatic adaptation to allosteric transitions. *Science* **154**:475.

Müller-Hill, B., L. Crapo, and W. Gilbert. 1968. Mutants that make more *lac* repressor. *Proc. Natl. Acad. Sci.* **59**:1259.

Newton, W. A., J. R. Beckwith, D. Zipser, and S. Brenner. 1965. Nonsense mutants and polarity in the *lac* operon of *Escherichia coli. J. Mol. Biol.* **14**:290.

Ohlsson, B. M., P. F. Strigini, and J. R. Beckwith. 1968. Allelic amber and ochre suppressors. *J. Mol. Biol.* **36**:209.

Pardee, A. B., F. Jacob, and J. Monod. 1959. The genetic control and cytoplasmic expression of inducibility in the synthesis of β-galactosidase of *E. coli. J. Mol. Biol.* **1**:165.

Pfahl, M., C. Stockter, and B. Gronenborn. 1974. Genetic analysis of the active sites of *lac* repressor. *Genetics* **76**:669.

Prestidge, L. S. and A. B. Pardee. 1965. A second permease for methyl-β-D-thiogalactoside in *Escherichia coli. Biochim. Biophys. Acta* **100**:591.

Reznikoff, W. S. and J. R. Beckwith. 1969. Genetic evidence that the operator locus is distinct from the *z* gene in the *lac* operon of *Escherichia coli. J. Mol. Biol.* **43**:215.

Reznikoff, W. S., J. H. Miller, J. G. Scaife, and J. R. Beckwith. 1969. A mechanism for repressor action. *J. Mol. Biol.* **43**:201.

St. Pierre, M. L. 1968. Mutations creating a new initiation point for expression of the histidine operon in *Salmonella typhimurium. J. Mol. Biol.* **35**:71.

Scaife, J. and J. R. Beckwith. 1966. Mutational alteration of the maximal level of *lac* operon expression. *Cold Spring Harbor Symp. Quant. Biol.* **31**:403.

Schaefler, S. 1967. Isolation of constitutive β-galactoside permease mutants in *Escherichia coli* by selection for raffinose fermentation. *Bacteriol. Proc.* **54**.

Schmeissner, U., D. Ganem, and J. H. Miller. 1977a. Genetic studies of the *lac* repressor. II. Fine structure deletion map of the *lacI* gene, and its correlation with the physical map. *J. Mol. Biol.* **109**:303.

———. 1977b. Revised gene-protein map for the *lacI* gene-*lac* repressor system. *J. Mol. Biol.* **117**:572.

Schwartz, D. O. and J. R. Beckwith. 1969. Mutagens which cause deletions in *Escherichia coli. Genetics* **61**:371.

Shapiro, J. A. and S. L. Adhya. 1969. The galactose operon of *E. coli* K12. II. A deletion analysis of operon structure and polarity. *Genetics* **62**:249.

Shapiro, J., L. MacHattie, L. Eron, G. Ihler, K. Ippen, J. Beckwith, R. Arditti, W. Reznikoff, and R. MacGillivray. 1969. The isolation of pure *lac* operon DNA. *Nature* **224**:768.

Signer, E. R. 1966. Interaction of prophages at the att80 site with the chromosome of *Escherichia coli. J. Mol. Biol.* **15**:243.

Smith, T. F. and J. R. Sadler. 1971. The nature of lactose operator constitutive mutations. *J. Mol. Biol.* **92**:93.

Soffer, R. L. 1962. Enzymatic expression of genetic units of function concerned with galactose metabolism in *Escherichia coli. J. Bacteriol.* **82**:471.

Ullmann, A., F. Jacob, and J. Monod. 1968. On the subunit structure of wild-type versus complemented β-galactosidase of *Escherichia coli. J. Mol. Biol.* **32**:1.

Wang, C. C. and A. Newton. 1969a. Iron transport in *Escherichia coli:* Relationship between chromium sensitivity and high iron requirement in mutants in *Escherichia coli. J. Bacteriol.* **98**:1135.

———. 1969b. Iron transport in *Escherichia coli:* Roles of energy dependent uptake and 2,3-dihydroxy benzoylserine. *J. Bacteriol* **98**:1142.

Willson, C., D. Perrin, M. Cohn, F. Jacob, and J. Monod. 1964. Non-inducible mutants of the regulator gene in the lactose system of *Escherichia coli*. *J. Mol. Biol.* **8**:582.

Wollman, E. L., F. Jacob, and W. Hayes. 1956. Conjugation and genetic recombination in *Escherichia coli*. *Cold Spring Harbor Symp. Quant. Biol.* **21**:141.

Yanofsky, C., B. C. Carlton, J. R. Guest, D. R. Helinski, and U. Henning. 1964. On the colinearity of gene structure and protein structure. *Proc. Natl. Acad. Sci.* **51**:266.

Zipser, D. 1967. Orientation of nonsense codons on the genetic map of the *lac* operon. *Science* **157**:1176.

Zipser, D. 1970. Polarity and translational punctuation. In *The lactose operon* (ed. J. R. Beckwith and D. Zipser), p. 221. Cold Spring Harbor Laboratory, Cold Spring Harbor, New York.

The *lacI* Gene: Its Role in *lac* Operon Control and Its Use as a Genetic System

Jeffrey H. Miller
Département de Biologie Moléculaire
Université de Genève
Genève, Switzerland

INTRODUCTION

One of the lasting contributions of the work of Jacob and Monod is that we can now envision the previously abstract notion of genetic control in terms of concrete, physical models. This is principally due to the conceptual breakthrough made during their studies of phage λ immunity and the enzymes concerned with lactose metabolism in *Escherichia coli* (Jacob and Monod 1961), namely, the idea that genes can be under the control of other "regulatory genes," and that regulation is carried out by an intermediate which is often the direct product of the regulatory gene itself.

A dominant theme in biology is that nature favors *selective* rather than *instructive* modes of development and control. This is evident not only for evolution and embryogenesis, but also for antibody synthesis and now gene control. For instance, rather than instructing a cell to acquire the capacity to synthesize a specific antibody molecule, a particular antigen is recognized, thereby selecting for the proliferation of cells in which this capacity preexisted. Jacob and Monod showed that, in a similar fashion, lactose does not dictate to cells how to synthesize an enzyme with the appropriate stereospecific properties; instead, recognition of lactose at the molecular level permits selection of enhanced expression of several of the many genes already present which are involved in the metabolism of different sugars.[1]

In the specific case of the *lac* operon, the product of the *I* gene, the *repressor*, was postulated to bind to a small region of the DNA, termed the *operator*, thus blocking synthesis of the *lac* enzymes (negative control). By also recognizing lactose and its analogs, the repressor could change its

---

[1]A more detailed discussion of the historical perspective of the operon model is given in the chapter by Cohn (this volume); see also the treatise by Jacob (1970) for a consideration of the history of heredity.

affinity for the operator and thus gene expression would occur at a high rate in the presence of the appropriate sugar. Subsequent experiments have verified this physical picture (Gilbert and Müller-Hill 1966, 1967, 1970; see Barkley and Bourgeois, this volume). In the nearly two decades since the elucidation of the operon model, similar methods and outlooks have been applied to scores of other operons (discussed elsewhere in this volume). In many cases completely different mechanisms have emerged (e.g., positive control in the *ara* operon of *E. coli*) (Lee, this volume). Even within the *lac* system itself, the discovery of the involvement of cyclic AMP in modulating the rate of transcription initiation (de Crombrugghe and Pastan, this volume) represents a new type of mechanism not explicity stated in the original model. Rather than contradicting the theories of Jacob and Monod, however, these findings actually give new dimensions to the central idea of control at the molecular level being exerted through intermediates encoded by regulatory genes.

HISTORICAL PERSPECTIVE

For students of biology, the original review by Jacob and Monod (1961) is recommended reading, not only because it is a chronicle of the experiments performed by the Pasteur Institute group which led to the concept of the operon, but also for its heuristic value as an example of how ideas and trains of thought are put together in a logical fashion to formulate a scientific theory. Some of these early experiments are summarized below.

Jacob and Monod used the lactose metabolism system of *E. coli* to attack the problem of enzyme adaption (Karstrom 1938), which had been observed in bacteria for many years (Duclaux 1899; Dienert 1900; Went 1901) and which was characterized by the appearance of a specific enzyme only in the presence of particular substrates. Initial studies had already established that such systems were mediated by specific genetic units (Monod and Audureau 1946), had demonstrated the inducible nature of β-galactosidase (Monod and Cohn 1952; Monod et al. 1952; Cohn 1957; Monod 1959), and had shown that a permease activity was also involved in lactose metabolism (Monod 1956; Rickenberg et al. 1956; Pardee 1957). The analysis of mutants indicated that each enzyme was encoded by a different gene. A transacetylase activity was also detected (Zabin et al. 1959), although at the time it was not clear whether this was part of the permease itself or was due to a separate protein. (Subsequent studies have revealed that these activities are encoded by different genes; the permease is the product of the *Y* gene, and transacetylase the product of the *A* gene [Zabin and Fowler, this volume].)

For the *lac* system, the induction phenomenon could be illustrated by the fact that in the presence of certain galactosides, cells produce 1000–10,000 times more β-galactosidase than when grown in the absence of such sugars (Monod and Cohn 1952; Cohen and Monod 1957; Jacob and Monod 1961). Immunological and isotopic methods showed that induction represented the de novo synthesis of enzyme molecules (Cohn and Torriani 1952; Monod and Cohn 1953; Rotman and Spiegelman 1954; Hogness et al. 1955), and kinetic studies established that these molecules could be detected as early as 3 minutes after addition of inducer (Monod et al. 1952; Herzenberg 1959; Pardee and Prestidge 1961). Moreover, the withdrawal of inducer brought about an abrupt halt in synthesis. These experiments were important because they argued against the activation by the inducer of a stable intermediate which accumulates in the cell (Monod 1956).

A detailed examination of the substrate specificity of induction provided further important clues as to the nature of the induction process. This work is summarized in Figure 1. Here the question was posed: What is the correlation between the catalytic center on the enzyme being induced and the molecular structure of the inducer? This was particularly relevant since, at the time, the notion was prevalent (see Cohn, this volume) that the inducer could *instruct* the formation of the catalytic center, in some way serving as a mold for the active site of the enzyme. It can be seen from Figure 1 that, although only galactosides serve as inducers, there is no correlation between the inducing capacity of a compound and its affinity for β-galactosidase (see, for instance, thiophenylgalactoside). Also, some strong inducers (e.g., IPTG) are not even substrates for the enzyme. These different stereospecificities for induction and binding to β-galactosidase clearly point to a controlling element which is distinct from the structural gene for β-galactosidase. Moreover, the quantitative correlation in the induction of β-galactosidase and transacetylase indicates that both enzymes are governed by the same controlling element.

The genetic analysis of this system permitted the definition of the *I* gene, linked to but distinct from the *Z* and *Y* loci, and controlling the inducibility of the *lac* enzymes. *I*⁻ mutations had a pleiotropic effect on the *lac* system. Mutants which were i⁻ synthesized maximal levels of β-galactosidase and transacetylase in the absence of inducer. The respective mutations mapped to one extremity of all known *Z* and *Y* mutations.

Although today the use of F′ factors which allow the formation of stable merodiploids is widespread, these were not available during the early stages of this work and other methods were sought to produce complementation tests. The introduction into F⁻ recipients of chromosomal fragments of Hfr strains carrying the *lac* region was a technique used to create transient heterozygotes for part of the

COMPOUND	CONCENTRATIONS	β-GALACTOSIDASE Induction value	V	$1/K_m$	GALACTOSIDE-TRANSACETYLASE Induct. value	V/K_m
β-D-thiogalactosides						
(isopropyl)	10^{-4} M	100	0	140	100	80
(methyl)	10^{-4} M	78	0	7	74	30
(methyl)	10^{-5} M	7.5	–	–	10	–
(phenyl)	10^{-3} M	<0.1	0	100	<1	100
(phenylethyl)	10^{-3} M	5	0	10,000	3	–
β-D-galactosides						
(lactose)	10^{-3} M	17	30	14	12	35
(phenyl)	10^{-3} M	15	100	100	11	–
α-D-galactoside						
(melibiose)	10^{-3} M	35	0	<0.1	37	<1
β-D-glucoside						
(phenyl)	10^{-3} M	<0.1	0	0	<1	50
(galactose)	10^{-3} M	<0.1	–	4	<1	<1
Methyl-β-D-thiogalactoside (10^{-4} M) phenyl-β-D-thiogalactoside (10^{-3} M)		52	–	–	63	–

Figure 1 Induction of galactosidase and galactoside-transacetylase by various galactosides. "Induction value" indicates specific activities developed by cultures of wild-type *E. coli* K12 grown on glycerol as a carbon source with each galactoside added at molar concentration stated. Values are given in percent of values obtained with isopropyl thiogalactoside at 10^{-4} M (actual units were about 7500 units of β-galactosidase and 300 units of galactoside-transacetylase per milligram of bacteria). Column *V* refers to maximal substrate activity of each compound with respect to galactosidase. Values are given in percent of activity obtained with phenylgalactoside. Column $1/K_m$ expresses affinity of each compound with respect to galactosidase. Values are given in percent of that observed with phenylgalactoside. For galactoside-transacetylase, only relative values V/K_m are given, since low affinity of this enzyme prevents independent determination of constants. (Adapted from Jacob and Monod 1961.)

chromosome (Wollman and Jacob 1955, 1959). In one classic experiment (Pardee et al. 1958, 1959), I^+ and Z^+ genes were transferred into I^-Z^- cells. Even in the absence of inducer, β-galactosidase synthesis starts immediately, gradually falling to the basal rate after 1 hour. The maximal rate can be restored by the addition of IPTG. This experiment had been interpreted to demonstrate the dominance of I^+ over I^-, the lag time in the establishment of repression reflecting the requirement to build up a sufficient level of a cytoplasmic product in order to convert the i⁻ cell to the i⁺ (inducible) state. Taken by itself, however, it does not strictly prove this, since one is not necessarily observing complementation in *trans*. In the absence of independent evidence (which was the situation at the time the experiment was published) showing that an i⁻z⁺ cell is converted to the i⁺ state by the introduction of I^+ genetic material, models involving a *cis* effect can still be entertained.[2] Although this could be achieved by the appropriate use of thermolabile i⁻ or z⁻ derivatives of the F⁻, the availability of stable merodiploids made this unnecessary. Experiments with the appropriate F′ factors (Jacob and Monod 1961) did establish a proper *trans* effect (see below) strengthening the interpretation of the kinetic effect.[3] More recently, versions of this experiment have been repeated using a mutation resulting in a tenfold greater synthesis of repressor (Müller-Hill et al. 1968). The higher rate of repressor synthesis eliminates the lag time in the establishment of repression.

The Hfr experiments of Pardee, Jacob, and Monod were also important because they appeared strikingly similar to the zygotic induction experiments of Jacob and Wollman (1954) (see below) in the λ system, and they led to the realization that the same type of control mechanism was operating in both cases.

The advent of episomes carrying the *lac* region (Jacob and Adelberg 1959) allowed cleaner complementation tests which verified that *I*, *Z*, and *Y* are independent cistrons, and showed that I^+ is dominant over I^- in the *trans* position[4] (Table 1). Therefore, the *Z* and *Y* genes are under the control of the *I* gene, and the control is mediated through the cytoplasm.

The work up to this point led to two general hypotheses which could explain these results: (1) The *I* gene determines the synthesis of a

---

[2]For instance, a *cis*-acting protein or even an RNA molecule which forms a loop structure and binds to the DNA just prior to the beginning of the *Z* gene, thus blocking transcription.

[3]Unfortunately, the apparent inability of the protein synthesis inhibitor 5-methyltryptophan to prevent this accumulation led to the incorrect conclusion that the repressor was not a protein.

[4]The later finding, discussed at length in subsequent sections, that some I^- alleles are partially dominant due to subunit mixing does not upset this result. Most of these require a high ratio of mutationally altered protein to wild-type repressor in order to exhibit this effect. Under normal conditions of complementation, with equal amounts of gene products being synthesized, dominant I^- mutations are very rare.

Table 1 Synthesis of galactosidase and galactoside-transacetylase by haploids and heterozygous diploids of regulator mutants

Strain	Genotype	Galactosidase		Galactosidase-transacetylase	
		noninduced	induced	noninduced	induced
1	$I^+Z^+Y^+$	<0.1	100	<1	100
2	$I3^-Z^+Y^+$	140	130	130	120
3	$I^+ZI^-Y^+/FI3^-Z^+Y^+$	<1	240	1	270
4	$I3^-ZI^-Y^+/FI^+Z^+Y^-$	<1	280	<1	120
5	$I3^-ZI^-Y^+/FI^-Z^+Y^+$	195	190	200	280
6	$\Delta(I,Z,Y)/FI^-Z^+Y^+$	130	150	150	170

Bacteria were grown in glycerol as a carbon source and induced, when stated, by IPTG at 10^{-4} M. Values are given as a percentage of those observed with induced wild type. Abstracted from Jacob and Monod (1961).

repressor. (2) The I gene codes for the structure of an enzyme which destroys an inducer produced by an independent pathway.[5]

A piece of evidence in support of the repressor model was the characterization of I^s mutations (Jacob and Monod 1961; Willson et al. 1964). Although mapping in the I gene, these mutations prevented the induction of the *lac* enzymes by lactose or IPTG. Moreover, they were dominant in *trans* to both an I^+Z^+ chromosome and an I^-Z^- chromosome (Table 2). The I^s mutation destroyed response to inducer, presumably by altering the stereospecific binding site. Therefore, even in the presence of IPTG, these molecules can still block *lac* enzyme synthesis. This would also explain their dominance, since the i^s repressor would be unaffected by wild-type repressor that was inactivated by inducer.[6] Moreover, experiments discussed below argued that i^s repressors are not overproduced and probably are not simply stronger repressors. A few reservations might be entertained at this point, however, since in a strict sense these results are also compatible with a model in which the I-gene product destroys an inducer, provided IPTG inactivates the I-gene product. In this case I^s mutations would also render the I-gene product insensitive to IPTG and

Table 2 Synthesis of β-galactosidase, galactoside permease, and galactoside-transacetylase by the wild type and by strains carrying different alleles of the regulator and operator loci

Genotype	Inducer	β-galactosidase (units/mg dry wt)	Galactosidase permease (μmolesTDG/mg dry wt)	Galactoside-transacetylase (units/mg dry wt)
$I^+Z^+Y^+$	none	<5	<1	<1
	IPTG 10^{-4} M	8700	30	580
$I^sZ^+Y^+$	none	10–20	~1	<1
	IPTG 10^{-2} M	10–20	~1	<1
$I^sZ^+Y^+/FI^+$	none	5		
	IPTG 10^{-3} M	8		
$I^sZ^+Y^+/FI^-$	none	8		
	IPTG 10^{-3} M	8		

Abstracted from Willson et al. (1964).

[5]It should be pointed out here that lactose itself is not the true inducer of the *lac* system, but rather a transgalactosidation product, which has been identified as allolactose (Jobe and Bourgeois 1972a). This conversion is mediated by the Z-gene product. Therefore, this type of mechanism already operates within the *lac* system during growth on certain galactosides. The question is whether an additional pathway exists for an independent inducer.

[6]In extraordinary situations, however, subunit mixing of wild-type and i^s repressors can upset this picture. See Gilbert and Müller-Hill (1970) for a discussion of this point.

its analogs. Everything else would follow in a similar fashion, including *trans* dominance over I^+. Also, the two I^s mutations first used in these studies were detected by screening Lac⁻ mutants for strains carrying dominant mutations. The two that were found mapped in the I gene. Since they were selected for dominance, this does not allow a statement as to what proportion of I^s mutations are *trans* dominant.[7] On the other hand, the essential point was the existence of these dominant mutations themselves, since their properties were precisely those expected of mutations altering the inducer-binding site. They clearly pointed to a direct interaction between the I-gene product and the inducer.

One limitation of genetic experiments is that they can never completely rule out more complicated alternative models except by negative evidence. Hypothesis 2 (above) is a more complicated model than the first model, since a system for the synthesis and action of the putative "true" inducer must be postulated. This predicts that certain Lac⁻ mutants will be due to mutations in this system. Since z⁻ mutants can still be induced by IPTG to make immunologically detectable altered β-galactosidase, these mutations would have to be distinct from Z^- mutations and should be recognizable as such. The failure to find mutations located outside this region which specifically produce the z⁻ phenotype represents the simplest argument against this alternative model, even though this type of argument has inherent limitations (see below). Since numerous enzyme systems are specifically inducible by their substrates or related compounds, to explain each of these effects by the second hypothesis would require an equal number of independent pathways, which seems highly unlikely.[8]

The Operator and the Operon

The specificity of interaction of the repressor with the *lac* system, which resulted in turning off enzyme synthesis, suggested a stereospecific complex with an element that Jacob and Monod termed the *operator*. They sought mutations in this recognition element which would render the operon constitutive even in the presence of active repressor. These mutations should be dominant in the *cis* position. By selecting for constitutivity in cells carrying two copies of the *lac* region, such mutants were found (Jacob et al. 1960b) and labeled o^c (for operator constitutive). As Table 3 indicates, strains carrying these mutations are capable of synthesizing maximal amounts of enzyme in the presence of IPTG, and

[7]As far as I know, all published I^s mutations were detected after selections for dominant mutations. However, the large set of I^s mutations described in a later section were not found in this manner (Miller and Schmeissner 1978). All of these are *trans* dominant to I^+.

[8]Other more complicated models postulate that the I product is an enzyme which itself synthesizes the repressor. However, these models run into the same problems.

Table 3 Synthesis of galactosidase, cross-reacting material, and galactoside-transacetylase by haploid and heterozygous diploid operator mutants

Genotype	Galactosidase		Cross-reacting material		Galactoside-transacetylase	
	noninduced	induced	noninduced	induced	noninduced	induced
O^+Z^+	<0.1	100	—	—	<1	100
O^+Z^+/FO^+Z1^-	<0.1	105	<1	310	—	—
O^cZ^+	25	95	—	—	15	110
$O^+Y^-/FO^cZ^+Y^+$	70	220	—	—	50	160
O^+Z^-/FO^cZ1^-	<0.1	90	30	180	—	—
$O^+Z1^-Y^+/FO^cZ^+Y^-$	90	250	<1	85	<1	220
$I^sO^+Z^+Y^+/FI^+O^cZ^+Y^+$	190	210	—	—	150	200

Abstracted from Jacob and Monod (1961).

synthesize 10–20% of these levels in the absence of inducer. The O^c mutations are dominant in the *cis* position,[9] as shown by lines 4 and 6 of Table 3. Mapping experiments pinpointed the operator locus between I and Z.

The data in Table 3 can also be used as an argument that the I^s mutation does not result in the overproduction of repressor, or is a more efficient repressor (simply binding more tightly to operator). In these cases one would expect better repression of o^c mutants (Willson et al. 1964). However, as line 7 of Table 3 indicates, this does not occur.

A large number of point mutations in the operator have now been detected (Smith and Sadler 1971), and the sequence change associated with each of eight different base substitutions has been determined (Gilbert et al. 1975; Barkley and Bourgeois, this volume). This work, together with other physical experiments (Gilbert et al. 1975, 1976), identifies the operator locus as a specific sequence of 17–25 nucleotides situated just before the structural Z gene (Barkley and Bourgeois, this volume). The O-Z-Y segment, now known to consist of the O-Z-Y-A segment,[10] constitutes a genetic unit of coordinate expression which Jacob and Monod termed the *operon* (Jacob et al. 1960b).

Temperate Phage

A parallel set of studies with the immunity system of the temperate phage λ also revealed a negative control element. Lysogenic cells are immune to superinfection by homologous phage, even though the phage DNA is injected into the cell (Bertani 1954; Jacob 1954). Complementation tests with stable merodiploids showed that the immune state is dominant in *trans* to the nonimmune state, thus implicating a cytoplasmic factor (Jacob et al. 1960a). Hfr crosses (Jacob and Wollman 1956) provided further evidence for a cytoplasmic repressor. When Hfr donors carrying λ injected their chromosomes into nonlysogenic recipients, the vegetative cycle was initiated. This effect, termed "zygotic induction," was not observed when lysogenic recipients were used or when nonlysogenic donors were mixed with lysogenic recipients.

As in the lactose system, an alternative explanation could be entertained in which the cytoplasmic factor destroys a metabolite required for phage multiplication. Since it was already known that different temperate phages had different patterns of immunity (Jacob and Campbell 1959), this would require postulating a different independent pathway for each known phage. The similarities with the lactose system were striking, and the genetic analysis of the C1 region of λ (responsible

[9]These complementation tests are diagramed by Beckwith (1970, and this volume).

[10]The subsequent definition of elements of the operon controlling transcription initiation is discussed by Reznikoff and Abelson (this volume).

for immunity), including the study of specific mutants, extended the analogy (Kaiser and Jacob 1957; Jacob and Campbell 1959). The establishment of a similar type of negative control operating in two otherwise unrelated systems provided the impetus to postulate repressor-operator interaction as a basic biological control mechanism.[11]

Characterization of the *lac* Repressor

Despite initial experiments indicating that repressor was synthesized during blockage of protein synthesis (Pardee and Prestidge 1961),[12] several genetic studies argued strongly that the *I*-gene product was indeed a protein. Horiuchi and Novick (1962, 1965) described an i⁻ mutant in which repression was thermolabile, the respective mutation mapping in the *I* gene. Sadler and Novick (1965) characterized extensively a strain which exhibited the iˢ phenotype at low temperature and the i⁻ character at high temperature. Kinetic studies indicated that repressor synthesis (but not repressor itself) was temperature-sensitive and argued for a multimeric nature of the *I*-gene product.[13] Partial stabilization of these thermolabile mutants by IPTG provided evidence for a direct interaction between repressor and inducer. Even more compelling was the discovery of suppressible nonsense mutations in the *I* gene (Bourgeois et al. 1965; Müller-Hill 1966), since the resulting amber (UAG) codons exert their effect by provoking polypeptide-chain termination during translation.

The decisive experiment, however, was provided by Gilbert and Müller-Hill, who isolated and purified the repressor by monitoring the binding of radioactive IPTG (for review, see Gilbert and Müller-Hill 1970). They demonstrated that the repressor is a protein consisting of four identical subunits, each with a molecular weight of approximately 38,000 (Beyreuther, this volume). Each molecule contains four IPTG-binding sites. In vitro, repressor binds to DNA containing the operator and comes off the DNA in the presence of IPTG (Gilbert and Müller-Hill 1966, 1967, 1970). Techniques developed by Bourgeois and coworkers (Barkley and Bourgeois, this volume) permitted the study of a wide range of interactions between repressor and both inducer and operator. More recently, the repressor has been shown to protect specific bases in the operator from methylating reagents (Gilbert et al. 1976).

These experiments were more than a simple verification of the operon model. They provided crucial proofs of the mechanism of repressor

[11]Further studies on phage λ are covered by Ptashne and Rosenberg et al. (both this volume).

[12]Subsequent experiments demonstrated the opposite effect (Barbour and Pardee 1966; Horiuchi and Ohshima 1966).

[13]The rapid restoration of the maximal rate of β-galactosidase synthesis following immediate removal of thermolabile *I*-gene product (by heating cultures) provided strong evidence that the repressor was the direct product of the *I* gene.

action which Jacob and Monod formulated. Virtually all genetic models ultimately require a direct biochemical experiment to eliminate alternative models. Although apparently unlikely, the possibility that the *I*-gene product destroys an inducer[14] could not be conclusively ruled out until Gilbert and Müller-Hill demonstrated physically that repressor bound to operator.

DEVELOPMENT OF THE GENETIC SYSTEM

Few systems have yielded as much combined genetic and physical data as the *lacI* gene-repressor system. This section covers the development of detailed genetic studies and considers mutations in the *I* gene from the standpoint of the types of altered repressors which result, supplementing earlier reviews on this topic (Müller-Hill 1975; Bourgeois and Pfahl 1976). (A subsequent section discusses *I* mutations with regard to the mutational events themselves.) We can outline some of the findings from this work at the outset. The repressor protein can be divided into at least two independent functional units or domains (see Beyreuther, and Weber and Geisler, both this volume; Müller-Hill 1975). One, consisting of approximately the amino-terminal 60 residues, is involved in DNA and operator binding, but not in inducer binding or aggregation (dimer and tetramer formation). The remainder of the protein contains the inducer-binding site and the regions important for aggregation. Mutationally altered repressors defective in each of these functions, as well as those displaying increased affinity for operator, have been characterized. A vast number of specific amino acid exchanges have been monitored, implicating certain residues as being important for different activities and also uncovering "silent" regions of the protein. The interdispersion of silent stretches with highly sensitive regions in the second half of the repressor may reflect aspects of the detailed secondary structure of the protein, possibly revealing the position of turns in the polypeptide chain.

Considerations for Deletion Mapping

An essential part of any detailed analysis is a fine-structure mapping system, since this allows the characterization of mutations according to their relative positions in the gene. Deletion maps are favored for this purpose because they provide a ready framework consisting of a set of

---

[14]As mentioned earlier, the main evidence against this possibility was the failure to detect *lac*⁻ mutations mapping outside the *lac* region. However, as detailed in this volume (see de Crombrugghe and Pastan), such mutations do exist, although they are not specific for the *lac* system, since other operons are affected. One of the relevant genes codes for adenyl cyclase, which actually synthesizes an internal inducer, cyclic AMP, which in turn activates another protein, the CRP factor. This type of mechanism is therefore in operation within the *lac* system itself, although not directly linked to the repressor-operator negative control system.

contiguous intervals based on qualitative yes-no tests, instead of requiring lengthy comparisons of quantitative data (see, e.g., Benzer 1961). Only when mutations are extremely close to a deletion endpoint does it become difficult to determine whether the mutation is covered by the deletion or not, since the rate of reversion can approach the rate of recombination. Together with a set of deletions, adequate techniques which permit the selection of i^+ recombinants are required.

Selective Methods

Since the principal physiological consequence of the i^+ phenotype is a very low level of expression of the *lac* enzymes in the absence of inducer, selections for i^+ recombinants or revertants from i^- cells are indirect, selecting against high levels of expression of *lac* permease or β-galactosidase. These procedures are hampered by the fact that unwanted secondary mutations can arise at frequencies high enough to obscure true recombinants.

There are two basic selective methods which have been employed to detect i^+ cells from i^- backgrounds. One involves the use of the compound orthonitrophenyl-β-D-thiogalactoside, TONPG (Gilbert and Müller-Hill 1966; Smith and Sadler 1971). In the presence of high enough levels of *lac* permease (the product of the Y gene), TONPG is sufficiently concentrated to inhibit growth. Inhibition is strongest when succinate or acetate is used as a carbon source (Smith and Sadler 1971). This selection does not operate in the presence of glucose. Both i^+ and y^- cells can form colonies on medium containing TONPG and succinate, and therefore some method has to be used to characterize the survivors. For this purpose, 5-bromo-4-chloro-3-indolyl-β D-galactosidase (Xgal) (see below) can be included in the selection plates themselves, since i^+ colonies are principally white and i^-y^- colonies are blue. Unfortunately, $i^-z^-y^-$ colonies (resulting from deletions or otherwise polar mutations) are also white, so the noninducibility of putative recombinants must be demonstrated in a further step.

A more widely used selection, first described by Davies and Jacob (1968), depends on the galactose sensitivity of *galE* strains (Fukasawa and Nikaido 1961; Malamy 1967) and the inability of phenyl-β-D-galactoside (Pgal) to induce the *lac* enzymes when glucose is used as a carbon source. β-Galactosidase cleaves Pgal, yielding galactose as one of the products. Therefore, in the presence of 0.05% Pgal, *galE* strains with high levels of β-galactosidase are killed and do not form colonies on glucose minimal medium. Cells which are i^+ do form colonies on this medium, as do spontaneous z^-, GalT$^-$, and GalK$^-$ mutants. These can be recognized by their failure to synthesize inducible β-galactosidase (in the case of z^- colonies) or by their constitutivity (in the case of GalT$^-$ or GalK$^-$

colonies). Cells which are i⁻z⁻ form white colonies on Xgal plates even in the presence of IPTG, whereas true i⁺z⁺ recombinants are white on Xgal medium, although they turn blue in the presence of IPTG. Both i⁻GalT⁻ and i⁻GalK⁻ cells form blue colonies on Xgal plates (Schmeissner et al. 1977a).

The *galE* method was first used in Hfr three-factor crosses between point mutations (Davies and Jacob 1968) and was subsequently adapted for use with a set of *tonB-lacI* deletion strains (see below) that were derived in a *galE⁺* background (Miller et al. 1970a). Episomes carrying point mutations were transferred from the respective deletion strains into a *recA⁻*, *galE⁻* "collector" strain after overnight growth (D. Ganem and J. H. Miller, unpubl.). Glucose minimal plates containing Pgal were used to detect recombination in the recipient background. Pfahl and coworkers employed this method to construct the initial deletion map of this region, separating 39 deletions into 19 groups (Pfahl 1972; Pfahl et al. 1974). An easier method eliminates the transfer step by utilizing *galE⁻* derivatives of the deletion strains. Overnight cultures are simply plated on the appropriate medium and surviving colonies are replicated onto Xgal plates with and without IPTG to identify i⁺ recombinants (Ganem 1972). This method has a high degree of resolution since 10^8 diploid cells from a population can be examined routinely. Its ease of application facilitates deletion mapping, and it has been employed for the original 39 *tonB-lacI* deletions (Ganem 1972; Ganem et al. 1973) and also for a larger set of over 400 deletions derived in a *galE⁻* background (Schmeissner et al. 1977a; see below).

A recently developed replica-plating method (Schmeissner et al. 1977a) permits rapid mapping of hundreds of mutations with only slightly less resolution than the liquid-culture methods. In this technique diploids are constructed by replica plating and then transferred first onto succinate + TONPG medium and then onto glucose + Pgal medium. After preliminary mapping by this procedure, more precise mapping can be carried out by the high-resolution method outlined above.

Selecting for i⁺ recombinants from iˢ cells is more straightforward, since many iˢ mutants cannot grow on lactose minimal medium, whereas i⁺ recombinants can. Several groups have employed this principle to map *I ˢ* mutations (Miller et al. 1968a,b; Pfahl 1972; Pfahl et al. 1974; Miller and Schmeissner 1978). Since i⁻ mutants also grow on lactose minimal medium, a subsequent step (such as replicating onto Xgal with and without IPTG) is required to distinguish between these colonies and the true i⁺ recombinants. A replica-plating technique involving transfer to succinate + TONPG (to eliminate i⁻ mutants) prior to replication onto lactose medium has also been reported (Miller and Schmeissner 1978).

Deletions in the *I* Region

In 1966 Beckwith and Signer described a set of strains in which the *lac* operon had been transposed to the *tonB-trp* region of the chromosome, as diagramed in Figure 2. This allowed the easy selection of mutants carrying deletions of the *tonB* locus which extend for varying lengths into the *lac* region. By mixing cultures of strains such as X7800 with lysates of φ80*vir* and ColV,B and plating survivors on Xgal + glucose plates, TonB mutants with constitutive levels of β-galactosidase can be isolated. Most of these have endpoints within the *I* gene (class I in Fig. 2). Originally, 39 deletions were detected in a *galE*⁺ background (Schmeissner et al. 1977a). Using the selective techniques described above, the 407 deletions were crossed against a large set of nonsense and missense mutations to produce a map containing 105 intervals (average interval length 10 nucleotides) (Schmeissner et al. 1977a,b). Because the distribution of most of the deletions appears to be random, many more intervals are assumed to be present (average length 2–3 nucleotides). This fine-structure deletion map allows a ready determination of the relative positions of mutations in the *I* gene. Moreover, a detailed correlation now exists between the genetic map and the physical map of the gene and protein, making possible the estimation of the position of a given mutation with a high degree of precision, often within a few nucleotides.

Correlation of the Genetic and Physical Maps

The exact physical positions of many mutations in the *lacI* gene are now known, which allows us in turn to mark the dimensions of many of the

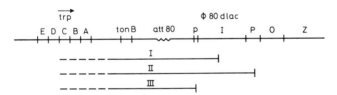

Figure 2 A schematic diagram of the *tonB-trp* region of the *E. coli* chromosome in strain X7800. The normal *lac* region of this strain has been deleted. A defective derivative of the phage φ80 carrying the *lac* region is integrated in the chromosome (Beckwith and Signer 1966). Deletions of the *tonB* locus can extend into the *trp* operon at one terminus and into the *lac* region at the other terminus. Three types of deletions which render the cell partially or fully constitutive for the *lac* enzymes are depicted. Type I deletions end within the structural gene; type II deletions end in the *lac* control region, fusing the *lac* operon to either the *trp* or another operon; type III deletions end within the *I* control region (Schmeissner et al. 1977a).

mutT

$$\begin{matrix} A & & C \\ | & \rightarrow & | \\ T & & G \end{matrix}$$ tyr = UAU or UAC

Figure 3   mutT-Induced transversion. The A:T→C:G transversion is stimulated by *mutT* (Cox and Yanofsky 1967) as is indicated here. The only mRNA codon which, as a result of this transversion, can be converted to UAG is UAU, one of the two tyrosine codons.

deletion intervals on the genetic map. These assignments were achieved by a variety of techniques. Initially, altered repressors resulting from a set of point mutations early in the gene were sequenced (Platt et al. 1972; Weber et al. 1972; Ganem et al. 1973; Files et al. 1974, 1975; Files and Weber 1978; Beyreuther, and Weber and Geisler, both this volume), permitting correlations of deletion intervals with portions of the physical map throughout the first 20% of the gene. Subsequently, I developed genetic techniques for correlating nonsense codons with specific points in the gene. Figures 3 through 5 provide an example of how this was accomplished (see also Miller et al. 1977). The mutator gene, *mutT*, specifically induces the A:T→C:G transversion (Cox and Yanofsky 1967), which will generate an amber (UAG) codon only from the UAU (tyrosine) triplet (Fig. 3). There are eight tyrosines in the repressor (Beyreuther et al. 1973), meaning that *mutT*-inducer amber mutations should occur in only a few specific places, corresponding to those tyrosines encoded by UAU instead of UAC (Fig. 4). In fact, when we collect a large number of independent amber mutations and compare those found in a *mutT* background with those appearing in a wild-type strain (Fig. 5), we can see that whereas 22 different UAG sites are represented in the latter collection, only six sites (one of which is defined by only a single occurrence) appear in a similar sample size for the *mutT*

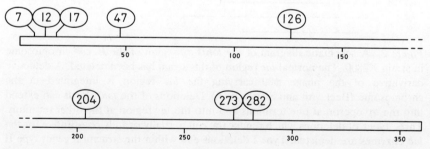

Figure 4 Tyrosines in the *lac* repressor. The positions of the eight tyrosine residues in the *lac* repressor (Beyreuther et al. 1973; Beyreuther, this volume) are shown. Some of these tyrosines are encoded by UAU and thus represent targets for the *mutT*-induced conversion to amber (UAG).

background. The repeated occurrences at five of these sites suggest that they are derived from *mutT*-induced events. Two of these are in the marked early region of the gene and could be correlated with the codons at positions 12 and 17, based on the peptide analysis of Su6-suppressed derivatives containing leucine at the amber-encoded position (Files et al. 1974). The three *mutT* amber "peaks" mapping past the codon for position 60 were then assigned to the respective codons for positions 126,

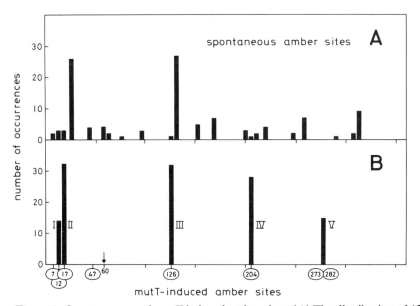

Figure 5 Spontaneous and *mutT*-induced amber sites. (*A*) The distribution of 130 spontaneous amber mutations is shown. Each peak represents one site. The number of independent occurrences at each site is indicated on the vertical scale, and the location in the gene is given from left to right on the horizontal scale (the genetic map). With one exception, each amber site is in a separate deletion group. (*B*) The same type of distribution for a collection of 120 *mutT*-induced amber mutations, which were selected in the identical manner as the mutations shown in *A*. Each amber site is in a separate deletion interval. The positions of the eight tyrosines in the protein are shown in the lower portion of *B*. Peak I maps in between the sequenced markers specifying positions 7 and 16 (see Fig. 6), and peak II maps in between the sequenced markers specifying positions 16 and 26 of the repressor. The assignment of these two peaks to the codons corresponding to tyrosines 12 and 17 has been verified by direct peptide analysis (Files et al. 1974). The amber mutation corresponding to position 7 is not present in the *mutT* collection, although it has been found spontaneously (see Fig. 6) (Files et al. 1974). The arrow indicates the position on the genetic map of the spontaneous amber mutation *I136*, which has been shown by protein sequencing to be derived from the codon specifying amino acid 60 (Ganem et al. 1973). The remaining *mutT* peaks are lined up over the corresponding tyrosine (see text) (Miller et al. 1977).

204, and either 273 or 282. This initial subdivision produced a new set of marked groups in the latter part of the emerging gene-protein map. We employed another specific mutagen, 2-aminopurine (Yanofsky et al. 1967; Osborn et al. 1967), to correlate amber and ochre mutations with tryptophan and glutamine codons. This marked the map in sufficient detail at this point to permit the assignment of other nonsense mutations by a number of genetic criteria involving analysis of suppression patterns, recombination tests, and mutagenic specificity (Coulondre and Miller 1977a).

Of the 90 different nonsense sites in the I gene, more than 80 have been assigned with a high degree of certainty to a specific codon. The gene-protein map resulting from the superimposition of this information onto the genetic deletion map is shown in Figure 6. Further protein and DNA sequencing has established several additional assignments (see legend to Fig. 6). Moreover, the elucidation of the full DNA sequence of the wild-type I gene (Farabaugh 1978; and see below) allows the verification of most of the remaining assignments due to the specific codon predictions involved (Coulondre and Miller 1977a; Miller et al. 1978b).

Constitutive Mutations: Selections for the i⁻ Phenotype

The most convenient selection for i⁻ cells employs the noninducing sugar Pgal. When it is used as the sole carbon source, i⁺ cells do not form colonies on minimal agar, provided appropriate precautions are taken to remove alternative carbon sources from the agar. This can be accomplished by applying a thin lawn of a strain deleted for the lac region and then incubating the plates for several hours before use (Smith and Sadler 1971). The use of strains carrying the up-promoter mutation $I^{q\,15}$ together with the lac down-promoter mutation $L8$ (Scaife and Beckwith 1967) provides a clean selection on Pgal without the need for "scavenger" strains (Miller et al. 1977). Operator-constitutive mutants also appear in this selection, but the presence of I^qL8 also greatly reduces the percentage of colonies with O^c mutations.

The 15-fold lower expression of the lac enzymes resulting from $L8$ (Scaife and Beckwith 1967) also allows the use of melibiose as a carbon source to select constitutive strains. At temperatures above 37°C, $E.\ coli$ requires the lac permease to transport this α-galactoside into the cell (Pardee 1957; Prestidge and Pardee 1965). Melibiose is a sufficiently weak inducer so that mutants with $L8$ do not build up high enough levels of permease to permit growth unless they are constitutive (Arditti et al. 1968). However, not all colonies appearing on melibiose minimal medium

[15]This mutation results in a tenfold increase in repressor synthesis (Müller-Hill et al. 1968). See section on I promoter region.

have mutations in the *lac* region, and subsequent testing on Xgal medium (see below) is usually required to verify the constitutive nature of the mutants. This method has been used to detect a variety of different nonsense, missense, and deletion mutations in the *I* gene (Ganem et al. 1973; Gho and Miller 1974).

A third procedure offers the opportunity to obtain i⁻ mutants by direct inspection, rather than by applying selective pressure. A large number of cells are plated on glucose medium containing the histochemical indicator Xgal. Colonies which are i⁻ appear blue, since constitutive β-galactosidase cleaves Xgal, releasing an indigo derivative (Horwitz et al. 1964; Davies and Jacob 1968; Beckwith 1970; Miller 1972). Blue specks from a lawn of as many as 100,000 cells can be identified with the aid of a magnifying lens, although 5000–10,000 cells per plate are more convenient to examine. This is of course more laborious than the direct selections, but it eliminates the bias inherent in any selective technique. Several collections of i⁻ mutants have been assembled by such direct screening (Müller-Hill 1975; Miller and Schmeissner 1978).

Mutations in the Early Portion of the *I* Gene: *I⁻ᵈ* Mutations

The original *I⁻* mutations described by Jacob and Monod were recessive to wildtype, meaning that heterodiploids of the type I^-/I^+ displayed the i⁺ (inducible) phenotype. Subsequent studies uncovered mutations with the opposite effect (Davies and Jacob 1968; Müller-Hill et al. 1968). These were initially thought to be O^c mutations, but appropriate tests demonstrated the *trans* nature of the partial dominance. The mutations, termed I^{-d}, were shown to map in the *I* gene (see below). One particular allele, *I24*, produces 50% constitutivity in combination with a second, I^+ gene. This is an exception, however, since most I^{-d} mutations produce weaker effects. In fact, mutations which display significant *trans* dominance are rare among *I⁻* mutations unless the I^q allele is used in combination with the I^{-d}. The I^q mutation results in a tenfold increased synthesis of repressor (Müller-Hill et al. 1968) due to an alteration in the *I* promoter (Calos 1978). When heterodiploids of the type $I^{q,-d}/I^+$ are used to test for *trans* dominance, a large percentage (30–50%) of missense mutations in the *I* gene score as I^{-d} due to the magnification of partial dominance resulting from the overproduction. Müller-Hill, Gilbert, and Davies originally suggested that the formation of mixed tetramers between i⁻ᵈ and i⁺ repressor subunits was responsible for the *trans* dominance. Work from several laboratories has shown this to be true and demonstrated that these mutations are a direct consequence of repressor structure.

A large number of I^{-d} mutations have been derived in strains carrying the I^q allele. All fully constitutive mutants selected for the i⁻ᵈ character

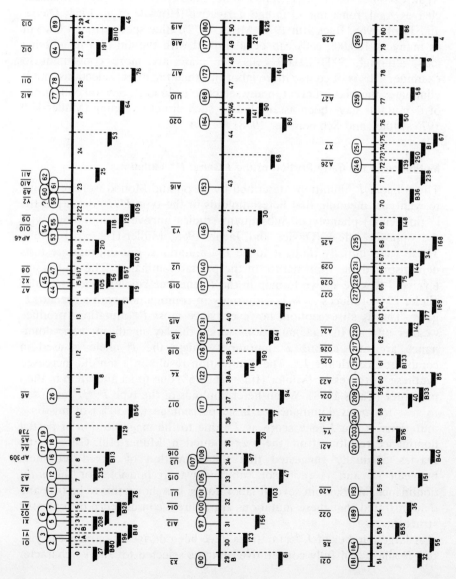

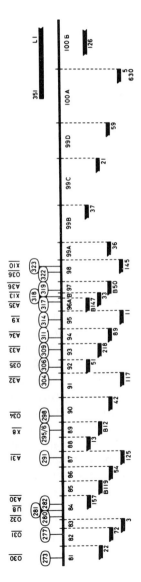

Figure 6 Gene-protein map of the *lacI* gene-repressor system. Each deletion interval shown in Figs. 5 and 6 of Schmeissner et al. (1977a) is depicted, together with the defining deletions. A set of mutations which have been correlated with specific codons in the gene is shown at the top of the diagram. The corresponding residue in the protein is indicated on the map below each allele number. For instance, in deletion interval 11, the mutation *A6* has been shown to alter the codon specifying residue 26 in the repressor. The correlations have been made by several different methods (Miller et al. 1977; Coulondre and Miller 1977a; Miller et al. 1978b). A number of markers have been determined by peptide analysis of altered repressor proteins for positions 5, 7, 12, 16, 17, 19, 26, 53, and 60 (Weber et al. 1975); for positions 61 and 62 (Files et al. 1975); for positions 201 and 220 (Sommer 1977); for position 3 (Schmitz et al. 1978); and additional markers by DNA sequencing (positions 311 and 351 [A. Maxam and W. Gilbert, unpubl.]; position 319 [Lillis 1977]; position 269 [Coulondre et al. 1978]). Because the entire nucleotide sequence of the *lacI* gene has been elucidated (Steege 1977; Farabaugh 1978), virtually all of the assigned markers appearing in the diagrams have been indirectly verified. (Reprinted, with permission, from Schmeissner et al. 1977b.) All reference numbers after position 153 are increased by 11 from those published previously, a -Gln- residue appears at position 231, and all numbers past position 219 are increased by 13 from those published previously (Miller et al. 1977; Schmeissner et al. 1977a) due to additional codons found in the *I* gene DNA (Farabaugh 1978).

51

carry mutations mapping in the portion of the gene that encodes the amino-terminal end (Adler et al. 1972; Pfahl et al. 1974; Müller-Hill 1975). In addition, when i⁻ mutants selected only for their constitutive character are analyzed, virtually all of the I^- missense mutations which map in the initial portion of the gene (encoding the first 60 residues of repressor) result in the i^{-d} phenotype (Schmitz et al. 1976; Miller and Schmeissner 1978). Even repressor fragments lacking parts of the amino-terminal end display the negative complementation characteristic of i^{-d} repressors (Weber and Geisler, this volume). Translational reinitiation following chain termination in vivo results in fragments lacking 41 or 61 amino-terminal residues which have i^{-d} activity (Platt et al. 1972; Ganem et al. 1973).

Repressors from i^{-d} strains have been isolated and have been shown to bind IPTG with normal affinities in many cases (Weber et al. 1972; Adler et al. 1972; Müller-Hill 1975; Beyreuther, this volume), but not to *lac* operator DNA (Adler et al. 1972; Müller-Hill 1975). This also includes reinitiation fragments generated in vivo lacking the first 41 and 61 residues, and fragments generated in vitro lacking the first 59 residues (Weber and Geisler, this volume). Moreover, a number of i^{-d} repressors have been shown to form tetramers by Sephadex column or sucrose gradient analysis (Müller-Hill et al. 1975; Weber et al. 1975; Schmitz et al. 1976; Miwa and Sadler 1977). Recent visualizations of hybrid tetramers between i^{-d} and wild-type subunits, and the observation that they display impaired DNA binding (Geisler and Weber 1976; Sadler and Tecklenburg 1976), demonstrate directly the molecular basis of *trans* dominance.

These facts have been taken to indicate that the amino-terminal end of repressor contains the predominant or sole determinants for DNA and operator binding (Adler et al. 1972). Several recent experiments confirm this suggestion. Hybrid molecules carrying only the amino-terminal region of the repressor have been produced by using deletions which fuse the *lacZ* gene to the *lacI* gene (Müller-Hill et al. 1976). Some of these molecules still bind to DNA. Moreover, the peptide containing only the first 59 residues of repressor has been isolated and has been shown to bind to DNA (Weber and Geisler, this volume) and even to protect the same bases in the *lac* operator as protected by the wild-type repressor (R. Ogata and W. Gilbert, unpubl.). These findings do not rule out a role in operator binding for the rest of the molecule, since the core part of the protein may hold amino-terminal regions in a favored conformation or may even contribute some contacts with the DNA. It is evident, however, that a significant part, if not all, of the recognition elements of repressor for operator resides in the initial portion of the protein. Moreover, it is also clear that both the IPTG-binding site and the determinants for dimer and tetramer formation do not reside in the first 59–61 residues; fragments lacking this entire region still form tetramers—and even mixed tetramers with wild-type subunits—and bind IPTG normally. *Trans* dominance follows directly from these two aspects of repressor structure, since I^- mutations in this region result in repressors which can no longer bind DNA but can still form mixed aggregates. (Virtually no alteration of this region appears to destroy the aggregation properties of repressor.) Thus, all of the missense mutations mapping in the first portion of the gene derived from a series of different mutagens result in i^{-d} repressors (Miller and Schmeissner 1978). Were a given amino acid replacement to produce a defect which altered both activities, hybrid repressors could not form and the respective mutation would be recessive and difficult to recognize.

Miwa and Sadler (1977) have analyzed a set of N'-methyl-N'-nitro-N-nitrosoguanidine (NG)-induced i^{-d} mutants, many of which do not have fully constitutive levels. All strongly constitutive i^{-d} mutants in their collection result from mutations mapping in the first segment of the gene, although moderately constitutive i^{-d} mutants were found in which the respective mutation mapped somewhat later. These authors point out that some amino acid exchanges may remove only one contact between repressor and operator and result in partial constitutivity without loss of aggregation. The weak i^{-d} constitutive effects they describe for some mutants could be examples of this. However, very weak effects of this type are difficult to interpret, and physical studies are required to determine whether additional contacts with the operator occur past the amino-terminal end.

The distribution of I^- mutational sites in the early region of the map, as derived from one extensive investigation (Miller and Schmeissner 1978), is shown in the top panel of Figure 7 (see also Pfahl et al. 1974; Bourgeois and Pfahl 1976). Specific amino acid replacements have been identified in a number of cases (Beyreuther, and Weber and Geisler, both this volume; and see below), although no obvious pattern of exchanges exists. There are numerous mutational sites in the portion of the gene corresponding to the first 60–70 residues, relative to, for instance, the portion encoding the subsequent 90–100 amino acids. This is in accord with experiments citing the importance of this region in DNA binding. Particularly noteworthy is the high density of sites in two regions, corresponding approximately to residues 15–34 and 50–59. Interestingly enough, one (Adler et al. 1972) or both of these stretches (Gursky et al. 1977) have been implicated in models for repressor-operator recognition based on theoretical considerations (see also Müller-Hill 1975).

Mutations Affecting Aggregation

Several lines of evidence argue that, whereas repressor monomers cannot bind operator sufficiently to be detected in vitro or to allow repression in

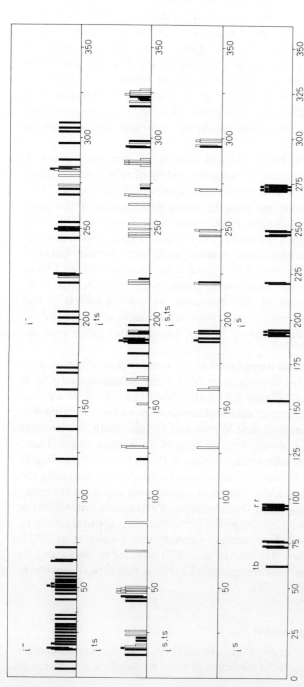

Figure 7 The distribution of mutational sites in the *I* gene. The top panel shows the sites resulting in the i⁻ phenotype, and the second panel depicts those detected by the resulting temperature-sensitive repression (iᵗˢ). The third and fourth panels give the sites leading to the iˢ·ᵗˢ phenotype and the iˢ phenotype, respectively. The horizontal scale gives the position of the corresponding residue in the protein. Virtually all sites which map past the initial portion of the gene (encoding the first 60 residues) and which cause the iᵗˢ phenotype also produce some type of iˢ or iⁿ character (see text), even though these effects are often very weak. Each bar represents a single missense mutation site, regardless of the number of recurrences at that site. These data were produced by analyzing over 1000 independent mutations. Open bars in the top panel indicate repressor with defective aggregation properties, but normal inducer binding. Open bars in the middle panels depict weaker effects for the selected property (weaker ts effects in panel 2, and weaker iˢ effects in panel 3). Repressors which bind operator more tightly are indicated by tb. (Reprinted, with permission, from Miller and Schmeissner 1978.)

vivo, multimers containing two wild-type repressor subunits can bind, provided the dimers are in the appropriate orientation (Kania and Brown 1976; Geisler and Weber 1976). Therefore, I^- mutations which prevent dimer formation will result in the i^- phenotype, as will at least some of those which block the dimer-to-tetramer-association step. We can screen for altered repressor aggregation among i^- mutants which retain IPTG-binding activity, since we can follow this activity on a sucrose gradient. Figure 8 shows the IPTG-binding activity of representatives of more than 700 i^- mutants (Schmitz et al. 1976). Virtually all of the mutations mapping in the beginning of the gene lead to repressors which still retain inducer binding, as expected from the above discussion. These repressors still form tetramers. Most of the repressors resulting from mutations mapping past this point cannot be detected in cellular extracts by IPTG-binding tests. Either these molecules are present in reduced amounts, or else the IPTG-binding activity is sufficiently impaired to hamper detection by these methods. Studies with immunological assays are required in order to analyze these mutants further.

Mutations mapping in two distinct clusters can be identified, however, which do affect aggregation. Sucrose gradient studies of partially purified

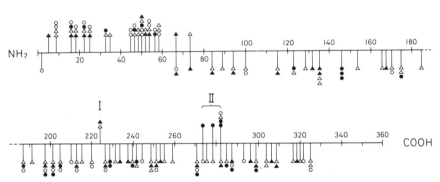

Figure 8 Missense substitutions in the *lac* repressor. Each vertical line represents a set of mutants resulting from mutations in a specific deletion group or subgroup. (●) Mutants isolated in the presence of *mutT*; (○) mutants from 2-aminopurine treatment; (△) mutants from ultraviolet-light treatment; (▲) mutants from 4-nitroquinoline-1-oxide treatment, which have been screened biochemically for IPTG-binding activity. All mutants carrying mutations above the line have partial or full IPTG-binding activity. Mutants below the line have less than 5% of wild-type activity. The distances are given in terms of amino acids of the *lac* repressor protein and have been determined to a degree of accuracy of approximately five amino acids. Although several small deletions and insertions may be present, the vast majority of these mutations are missense mutations. (Updated from Schmitz et al. [1976]; mutations shown to affect initiation, to cause unsuppressed nonsense codons, or to result from large insertions have been removed.)

repressors resulting from mutations from each of these two late clusters (Fig. 8) demonstrate that tetramer formation is defective, since the IPTG-binding activity is found as a mixture of monomers and dimers (Schmitz et al. 1976). One of these regions extends from tyrosine 273 to tyrosine 282 and contains numerous charged residues. The replacement of tyrosine 282 by either serine or glutamine can be shown to specifically cause this mutant phenotype (see below). The other region is near residue 224.

The repressor resulting from the *L1* deletion is missing nine residues from the carboxyl-terminal end (W. Gilbert, D. States, and A. Maxam, unpubl.) and is found principally as a dimer in solution (Miller et al. 1970b), suggesting that this region is involved in the dimer-tetramer equilibrium. The *L1* repressor retains partial operator-binding activity in vivo, particularly when overproduced (to compensate for in vivo proteolytic degradation) (Platt et al. 1970), indicating that these dimers are in the appropriate orientation. Other mutations affecting this region of the protein should be analyzed; they would result in a partial i⁻ phenotype, particularly in an I^q background, and might be difficult to detect.

I^s Mutations

The i^s phenotype is defined by the inability of lactose or suitable analogs to induce the *lac* operon in vivo. The severity of the effect differs according to the particular mutation involved. Usually, only effects sufficient to prevent growth on lactose are considered. We can envision three types of changes in the repressor which prevent the induction of the *lac* enzymes by lactose or IPTG: weakened affinity for inducer, increased affinity for operator, and impaired ability to undergo the appropriate allosteric change required for induction. Mutations affecting each of these properties have been described and located on the gene-protein map.

The best selections for i^s mutants are modifications of the Pgal-suicide procedure used for selecting i^+ recombinants, with the inclusion of IPTG at different concentrations in the medium (Pfahl et al. 1974; Miller and Schmeissner 1978). In addition to the original I^s mutations described by Willson et al. (1964), numerous I^s mutations were detected after treatment with NG and mapped by Pfahl and coworkers (Pfahl 1972; Pfahl et al. 1974; Gho, as described in Müller-Hill 1975). None of the mutations were located in the beginning of the gene, although several groups clustered just after the region encoding the first 60 residues, and protein sequencing has established that substitutions at residues 74 and 75 are responsible for two of the respective mutants (Beyreuther, this volume). A particularly large cluster was evident in the middle of the gene, although this is in part a reflection of NG-induced hotspots.

To overcome the problems arising from mutagenic specificity and genetic hotspots (Benzer 1961; Coulondre and Miller 1977b), we have used a variety of mutagens to induce different types of I^s mutations (Miller and Schmeissner 1978) and have mapped these on the correlated gene-protein map, taking care to distinguish different mutational sites. Figure 7 (bottom panel) depicts these results. As found for NG-induced mutations, the first portion of the map contains no I^s mutations which are detected by the Pgal-suicide selection. This follows from the fact that removal of this region does not interfere with IPTG binding (Weber and Geisler, this volume). Repressors which display increased operator binding and which cause an i^s phenotype can result from lesions affecting this part of the protein, but these are relatively rare among I^s mutations. More striking is the tight clustering seen in the second part of the protein. I^s mutations map close together in stretches surrounding residues 193–194, 220, 248, and 273. Many of these mutations severely impair induction, even by 10^{-1} M IPTG, suggesting that these regions are either part of the inducer-binding site or are involved in maintaining its conformation. Studies with suppressed derivatives have even identified some of the specific residues in these stretches (Miller et al. 1978a; and see below).

Bourgeois and coworkers (Jobe et al. 1972; Barkley and Bourgeois, this volume) have examined several i^s repressors in vitro. All of these show significantly reduced affinities for IPTG, sufficient to explain their i^s phenotype in vivo. However, several i^s repressors with amino acid replacements between residues 70 and 100 also display altered allosteric effects, implicating this part of the protein as being involved in conveying the conformational change subsequent to inducer binding. Several repressors from this group also exhibit slight increases in affinity for operator.

Repressors in which only the allosteric effect is altered have not been observed without concomitant secondary effects. One type of repressor with altered allosteric properties—the i^{rc} repressor (Myers and Sadler 1971)—binds IPTG with high affinity and is in fact stabilized by inducer binding. Apparently the repressor is frozen in the DNA-binding conformation, since increasing amounts of inducer result in increasing repression in vivo; the induction profile is thus the reverse of the normal curve. In the absence of increased DNA binding (see the following section), the reverse curve is evidence for an altered allosteric response. This mutation maps in the general region between residues 80 and 120 (Pfahl et al. 1974; Müller-Hill 1975). Several additional mutations conferring similar or identical properties have been reported (Miller and Schmeissner 1978) and mapped more precisely, being within or extremely close to the region spanning residues 95–100 (see Fig. 7). (A broader series of altered repressors exhibiting partial stabilization in vivo upon inducer binding is considered later.)

Tight-Binding Mutants

A number of studies have centered on repressors which bind operator and DNA more tightly than wild-type repressor. The first repressor found to be in this category results from the I^r mutation *X86* (Chamness and Willson 1970; Jobe and Bourgeois 1972b), which causes a serine-to-leucine change at position 61 in the polypeptide chain (Files and Weber 1978). Strains carrying *X86* are partly constitutive, although low inducer concentrations increase repression, prompting the term "i^r repressor" (for reverse). The X86 repressor binds operator 50-fold more tightly than wild-type repressor (Jobe and Bourgeois 1972b) and also shows a greatly increased affinity for DNA not containing the *lac* operator (Pfahl 1976). Theoretical considerations predict that tight-binding repressors may result in i^r curves (von Hippel et al. 1974), and Pfahl (1976) has proposed an explanation for the induction curves of X86 based on the increased affinity for DNA. As DNA is synthesized in a growing cell population, the slower dissociation rate from nonoperator sites impedes the association of the X86 repressor with the *lac* operator. Therefore, the stronger the binding to DNA, the greater the "kinetic trap" for the repressor. (The failure to induce fully at high inducer concentrations results from the partial affinity for operator by the IPTG-saturated repressor.) This idea is supported by in vitro experiments (Pfahl 1976).

In agreement with this theory are the results from a second tight-binding repressor, I12, which carries a tyrosine-for-proline substitution at position 3 (Schmitz et al. 1978). This repressor is similar to X86 both in increased DNA and operator binding and in the in vivo induction curves. When these two mutations are combined to produce a doubly altered repressor, even stronger tight-binding effects are seen, with affinity for operator increasing 10,000-fold with respect to wild-type repressor (Schmitz et al. 1978). In vivo these cells are nearly fully constitutive, repression increasing with increasing IPTG concentration. Even 10^{-1} M IPTG fails to induce, since the mutational alterations compensate for the 1000–10,000 reduction in affinity of the IPTG-repressor complex for the operator (Barkley and Bourgeois, this volume). This effect can also be shown by in vitro experiments. The increased binding is at least partly sequence-specific, and the doubly altered repressor has been used to analyze pseudo-operators in the DNA (A. Schmitz and D. Galas, unpubl.).

Additional mutations have been reported which result in tight-binding repressors and which also map in the early part of the gene (Betz and Sadler 1976). Again, i^r curves result from the increased binding. Some of these repressors have been characterized extensively with respect to inducer binding and repressor-operator interaction (Betz and Sadler 1976).

Temperature Effects

The analysis of temperature-sensitive mutants is hampered by the fact that many strains display small or intermediate temperature effects. Figure 7 (middle panels) shows the distribution of the respective mutational sites throughout the gene, as determined from one set of studies (Miller and Schmeissner 1978). Virtually all of the temperature-sensitive mutations mapping past the initial 15–20% of the gene result in strains which are not normally inducible at low temperature, displaying some type of i^s, i^r, or i^{rc} character. Some of these mutations invariably have secondary effects which damage inducer binding. Many sites, however, represent a broader class of mutations that produce repressors in which the thermal instability (on either the subunit or aggregate level) is partially overcome by inducer binding. The stabilization may in fact occur during the aggregation process itself. At higher inducer concentrations, induction overcomes stabilization, which accounts for the i^r nature of some of the resulting curves. Many proteins are stabilized against thermolability by substrate binding (M. Levitt, pers. comm.). For the *lac* repressor, this is supported by the finding that, in a number of temperature-sensitive mutants, the binding of either anti-inducer (ONPF) or inducer (IPTG) can overcome the effects of high temperature. The failure of IPTG to stabilize any of the repressors altered in the first 60 residues is further evidence for the independence of this region of the protein from the remaining core. In the latter part of the gene-protein map, the $I^{s,ts}$ sites cluster in the same regions as the I^s sites. Possible interpretations of this are considered below.

The Use of Suppressed Nonsense Mutations to Generate Altered Repressors

The set of correlated nonsense mutations referred to above (Miller et al. 1977, 1978b; Coulondre and Miller 1977a) offers a unique opportunity to generate a family of altered *lac* repressor molecules by the use of nonsense suppressors. At each position in the protein specified by an amber codon, five different residues can be inserted by characterized suppressors: serine, glutamine, tyrosine, leucine, and lysine (Gorini 1970). In addition, lysine, glutamine, and tyrosine can be inserted in response to the ochre codon, and tryptophan at UGA sites. Since ochre codons can be converted to amber codons, this permits the exchange of 3–5 residues at each of the 90 positions corresponding to a nonsense site. Because the wild-type amino acid is known in virtually every case, this produces a set of over 300 altered repressors with known sequence changes. Figure 9 shows the residues in the repressor which can be replaced by this technique.

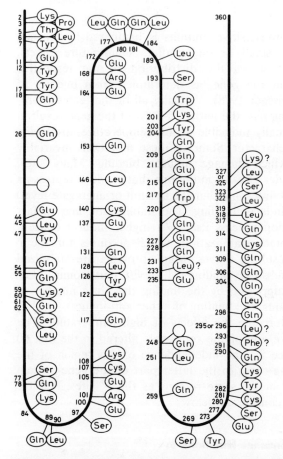

Figure 9 Substitution sites in the repressor. The 90 substitution sites in the *lac* repressor which result from nonsense mutations in the *lacI* gene are shown. In each case the wild-type amino acid is given.

This type of study offers several advantages over the conventional analysis of missense mutations. As pointed out above, specific amino acid replacements can be identified without having to sequence every altered protein. Moreover, at each site under study, a hierarchy of amino acid exchanges can be compared. Very rare substitutions are subject to investigation. For instance, some replacements achieved by this method would require two or even three base changes if produced by direct mutagenesis. Also, selection for different phenotypes is not required, since each amber mutation is detected by screening only for the i⁻ character of the resulting polypeptide fragment in an Su⁻ strain. Therefore, replacements leading to no measurable change in repressor activities are also amenable to analysis, permitting the determination of "silent" regions in the protein.

We have monitored the activities of the resulting altered molecules and have tabulated these data quantitatively (Miller et al. 1978b). Figure 10 and Table 4 summarize some of the essential findings (see Miller et al.

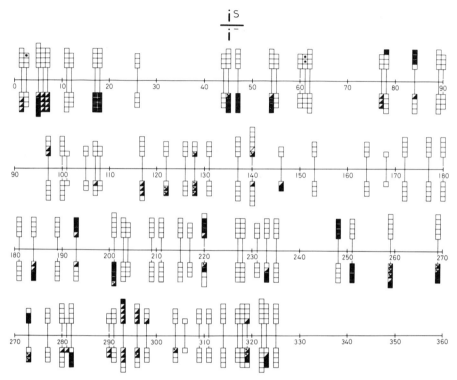

Figure 10 Effects of amino acid replacements in the *lac* repressor. At each position corresponding to a known residue, between one and six substitutions have been scored. These are indicated by a set of boxes. The i^s phenotype is considered above the horizontal line, which corresponds to the length of the protein. Replacements which do not result in an i^s repressor are represented by open boxes above the line. Amino acid exchanges producing i^s repressors are depicted by filled-in boxes. Boxes that are half-filled represent weak i^s effects, and those with a dot in the unfilled portion indicate temperature-sensitive i^s proteins. For example, five different substitutions at residue 220 result in three i^s proteins, one weak i^s protein, and one protein which is not i^s. The asterisks at positions 3 and 61 indicate partial i^s character due to repressors which bind operator more tightly than wild type. The i^- phenotype is considered in a similar manner below the line. Filled-in boxes represent molecules which cannot repress in vivo. Half-filled boxes indicate weak i^- effects, and a dot depicts temperature-sensitivity. Open boxes indicate replacements which do not affect the ability to bind operator.

Table 4 Effect of amino acid replacements in the *lac* repressor

Position	Wild-type residue	Su1 Ser	Su2 Gln	Su3 Tyr	Su6 Leu	SuB Gln	SuC Tyr	Su5 Lys	Su9 Trp
2	Lys	+	+	+	+			+	
3	Pro					+	s*	+	
5	Thr	±	−	−	−			−	
6	Leu	+	+	+	+			−	
7	Tyr	±	±	+	±			∓	
11	Glu	+	+	+	+			∓	
12	Tyr	+	+	+	+			∓	
17	Tyr	−	−	+	∓			−	
18	Gln	−	+	−	−				
26	Gln	+	+	+	+			−	
44	Glu	+	+	+	+			∓	
45	Leu	−	−	∓	+			−	
47	Tyr	−	−	+	−			−	
54	Gln	∓	+	−	−			∓	
55	Gln	+	+	+	+				
60	Gln	+	+	+	+			−	
61	Ser	+	+	s*	s*			∓	
62	Leu	+	+	+	+			+	
77	Ser	+	∓	±	±			−	
78	Gln	+	+	+	+			s	
84	Lys	s	∓	s	s			±	
89	Gln	+	+	+	+			+	
90	Leu	+	+	+	+			∓	
97	Ser	+	s	+	+			s	
100	Glu	+	+	+	+			−	
101	Arg								+
105	Glu					+	+	−	
107	Cys								+/s
108	Lys					+	+	+	
117	Gln	+	+	±	±			∓	
122	Leu	ts/+	ts	+	+			−	
126	Tyr	+	+	+	+			−	
128	Leu	∓	±	s/+	+			−	
131	Gln	+	+	+	+			∓	
137	Glu	+	+	+	+	+	−	−	
140	Cys	+	+	+	+			±	s/+
146	Leu					−	∓	−	
153	Gln	+	+	+	+			−	
164	Glu					+	+	±	
168	Arg								+
172	Glu	+	+	+	+			−	
177	Leu	+	+	+	+			−	
180	Gln	+	+	+	+			+	
181	Gln	+	+	+	+			+	
184	Leu	−	−	±	+			−	
189	Leu					+	+	+	+

Table 4   (Continued)

Position	Wild-type residue	Su1 Ser	Su2 Gln	Su3 Tyr	Su6 Leu	SuB Gln	SuC Tyr	Su5 Lys	Su9 Trp
193	Ser	+	s	s	s			∓/s	
201	Trp	−	−	ts	−			−	∓**
203	Lys	+	+	+	+			+	
204	Tyr	+	+	+	+			−	
209	Gln	+	+	+	+			+	
211	Gln	+	+	+	+			±	
215	Glu	+	+	+	+	∓	∓	−	
217	Glu					+	+	+	
220	Trp	s	s/ts	s	s			−	+
221–226	?	∓	−	+	+			−	
227	Gln	+	+	+	+			±	
228	Gln	+	+	+	+			+	
231	Gln					+	+	−	
233?	Leu?	−	∓	+	+			−	
235	Glu	+	+	+	+			∓	
243–251	?	+	+	−	s/+			−	
248	Gln	s	+	s	s			s	
251	Leu	−	−	−	+			−	
259	Glu	∓	∓	∓	±			−	
269	Ser	+	ts	−	−			−	
273	Tyr	s	s/r	+	+			−	
277	Glu					+	+	+	
280	Ser	+	+	+	+	∓	−	−	∓
281	Cys								∓
282	Tyr	−	−	+	+			−	
290	Lys					−	∓	−	
291	Gln	+	+	+	+			−	
293	Phe?	+/s	s	s	+/s			s	
295/6	Leu	±	+/s	+/s	+			∓/s	
298	Gln	+	+	+/s	+			±	
304	Leu	+	ts	+	+			−	
306	Gln					+	+	−	
309	Gln	+	+	+	+			−	
311	Gln	+	+	+	+			∓	
314	Lys	+	+	+	+			−	
317	Gln	+	+	+	+			∓	
318	Leu	+	+	+	+			±	
319	Leu	±	±	s	+			−	
322	Ser	+	+	+	+			+	+
323	Leu	−	−	+	+			−	
325/7?	Lys?	+	+	+	+			∓	

The results of indicator plate tests and β-galactosidase assays are summarized. In general, for the i⁻ phenotype, a + indicates more than 300-fold inducibility, ± indicates between 20 and 100, ∓ indicates between 5 and 20, and − indicates less than 5. Tight-binding mutants at positions 3 and 61 are indicated by s*, and ** indicates poor suppression by Su9 at this particular site.

[1978b] for a more detailed analysis of these results). In the amino-terminal end of the protein, this work complements the peptide analysis of repressors resulting from missense substitutions (Beyreuther, and Weber and Geisler, both this volume). It shows, for instance, that whereas tyrosines 17 and 47, and to a lesser extent tyrosine 7, are essential for operator binding, tyrosine 12 can be replaced by a variety of amino acids without noticeably damaging repression in vivo. Substitution of tyrosine for proline at position 3 results in a tight-binding repressor which would be extremely difficult to obtain otherwise, since three base changes would be needed to convert the CCA codon to UAU or UAC (Steege 1977; Schmitz et al. 1978). On the other hand, glutamine or lysine at this position does not increase operator binding relative to wild type.

Beyreuther (this volume) and coworkers have established that exchanges at positions 74 and 75 lead to i^s repressors. Suppressed nonsense mutations allow us to now identify certain replacements at positions 78, 84, 97, 193, 220, 248, 273, and probably 293 and 296, among others, as also resulting in i^s repressors of various strengths. Temperature-sensitive proteins (i.e., serine to glutamine at position 269), temperature-sensitive mutants with i^r curves in vivo (i.e., tyrosine to glutamine at position 273), and mutants failing to make tetramers (tyrosine to serine or glutamine at position 282) also appear readily in this analysis.

In general, the effects of the substitutions are in good agreement with the findings of Perutz and coworkers (Perutz and Lehmann 1968) for the hemoglobin system concerning the nature of the residue being replaced. Polar residues (43–44 of the 53 tested in the *lac* repressor) can usually be replaced by both polar and nonpolar amino acids, whereas nonpolar residues are generally sensitive to substitution by polar residues (only 13 of 32 nonpolar residues can be replaced by at least one of the three polar residues tested). Overall, many amino acid substitutions in the repressor are effectively neutral. Of the 302 replacements scored, 58% do not result in a detectable change in repression in vivo or in the response to inducers.

By directing the substitution of specific residues in the repressor, nonsense suppression can greatly aid spectroscopic studies. Changes in fluorescence after tryptophan substitution (Sommer et al. 1976) have been monitored, as has the ^{19}F NMR spectrum of 3-fluorotyrosine containing repressor after specific tyrosine substitution (Lu et al. 1976; P. Lu, M. Jarena, and R. Friedman, unpubl.).

Some aspects of repressor structure are already revealed by considering the results from suppressed derivatives together with missense substitution data in the second part of the protein (Fig. 7). Mutations resulting in i^s proteins cluster in small regions separated by distinct spaces. Moreover, $I^{s,ts}$ and even certain I^- mutations cluster in the same regions. Figure 11 superimposes the data from the suppressed nonsense and missense mutation studies for the i^s character. This comparison is striking in that it shows how the two methods of obtaining altered proteins complement each other (Miller 1978). Through the use of suppressed derivatives, we can demonstrate that the spaces between the sensitive regions of the protein are indeed significant and reflect some aspect of the protein structure itself rather than being an artifact at the genetic level. Over 100 different amino acid replacements have been made in the stretches between the clusters, and none of these result in i^s repressors. The near regularity (25–29 residues) between the tight grouping of sensitive residues is also striking. It has been suggested (F. Crick, pers. comm.) that the clusters might represent turns in the polypeptide chain between regions of regular secondary structure (such as β-sheets), since these turns often form the active sites of proteins, as in the case of immunoglobulins (Davies et al. 1975). Replacements in these regions are more likely to cause a significant change in ligand-binding properties than substitutions in a region which is part of an extensive β-sheet but does not play a direct role in the conformation of the binding site. These speculations are in accord with predictions of the secondary structure of these regions made from a consideration of the amino acid sequence (Chou et al. 1974; Bourgeois et al. 1978; M. Levitt, pers. comm.), although the knowledge of the three-dimensional structure of repressor is clearly required to test this hypothesis.

The *I* Control Region

Chemical analysis at both the RNA level (Steege 1977) and the DNA level (Calos 1978) has elucidated the nucleotide sequence of the *I* control region (Fig. 12). The *I* promoter appears to have homologies with other promoters in the −28 to −38 region (the similarities here are weak) and the −7 to −12 region (Calos 1978; Reznikoff and Abelson, this volume). A leader sequence of 28 bases precedes the GUG start codon on the mRNA (Steege 1977).

Several mutations in the *I* promoter have been characterized. Müller-Hill and coworkers detected the first up-promoter mutation described in any system. Termed *I*^{q}, this mutation results in a tenfold increased synthesis of repressor (Müller-Hill et al. 1968). Sequence studies show that *I*^{q} represents a single base change at −35 in the *I* promoter (Calos 1978), slightly increasing the homology of this stretch of nucleotides with the −35 region of other strong promoters (see also Fig. 12). A second step mutation derived from *I*^{q}, termed *I*^{sq} (Miller et al. 1970a), directs the synthesis of 50 times more repressor than wild type. However, this mutation is unstable, which limits its use in biochemical preparations. Müller-Hill and coworkers have described a stable, nitrosoguanidine-induced mutant which synthesizes 50- to 100-fold more repressor than wild type (Müller-Hill et al. 1975). These overproducing mutations,

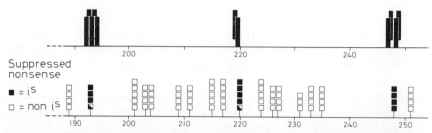

Figure 11 Amino acid replacements causing the i[s] phenotype. The combined results of studies of missense mutations and suppressed nonsense mutations in the *lacI* gene are shown. The missense mutation sites (see Fig. 7) that map in the second half of the gene and generate i[s] repressors are shown at the top of the diagram. The horizontal axis represents the length of the corresponding repressor protein. The cluster of sites at the far right arises from the i[s,ts] and i[ts] selection and represents weaker i[s] effects than do the other clusters. The bottom part of the diagram summarizes results from the study shown in Fig. 10. Each replacement made in this portion of the protein is indicated by a box. Filled-in boxes indicate i[s] proteins, and partially filled-in boxes indicate i[s] proteins with somewhat weaker effects. Open boxes depict replacements which do not produce the i[s] phenotype. In a few cases these replacements do result in i[-] proteins, which can be deduced by referring to Fig. 10.

when crossed onto heat-inducible, lysis-deficient prophage, permit the accumulation of large amounts of repressor (1–5% of the soluble cell protein following prophage induction) and greatly facilitate the biochemical analysis of repressors (Beyreuther, this volume).

Several lesions which destroy promoter function have also been analyzed. The mutation *UJ177* removes four bases from the important homology region between −7 and −12 in the promoter, resulting in at least a 100-fold reduction in repressor synthesis (M. Calos and J. H. Miller, unpubl.). The deletion *B116* removes all of the *I* promoter, leaving

```
                                        pppGGAAGAGAGUCAAUUCAGGGUGGUGAAUGUGAAACCAGUAACG
                                                         met.............
 -50       -40        -30       -20       -10            10        20        30        40
GACACCATCGAATGGCGCAAAACCTTTCGCGGTATGGCATGATAGCGCCCGGAAGAGAGTCAATTCAGGGTGGTGAATGTGAAACCAGTAACG
CTGTGGTAGCTTACCGCGTTTTGGAAAGCGCCATACCGTACTATCGCGGGCCTTCTCTCAGTTAAGTCCCACCACTTACACTTTGGTCATTGC
             ↓                                  Δ UJ177
        I[q]  T
             A
```

Figure 12 The *I* control region. The nucleotide sequence including the *I* promoter region and the *I* leader region is shown (Steege 1977; Calos 1978). The base change resulting from the I[q] mutation is shown (Calos 1978). This alteration results in a tenfold increase in repressor synthesis. The four bases deleted by mutation *UJ177* (M. P. Calos and J. H. Miller, unpubl.) are also indicated.

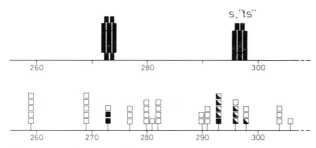

Figure 11   (Continued)

the entire leader sequence intact (Sommer et al. 1978). In this case the *I* message is fused to the *trp* attenuator region (Platt, this volume). The B116 repressor, containing 16 additional amino acids encoded by the *trp* leader and the *I* leader, is now synthesized under *trp* control. (For a description of a broad class of chimeric repressors in which β-galactosidase is fused to *lac* repressor, see Müller-Hill and Kania [1974], Müller-Hill et al. [1977], and Bassford et al. [this volume].)

Translation Initiation and Reinitiation

Figure 13 depicts the first part of the *I* mRNA together with the corresponding protein sequence (Steege 1977). The possible initiation codons are underlined. It is interesting to note that, although there are three GUG codons in phase near the beginning of the structural part of the message, only the last is used for initiation in the wild type. Steege (1977) has reported that this GUG is preceded by the most substantial complementarity to the 3′ end of the *E. coli* 16S rRNA. This seems to be the case for the selection of other initiator codons in bacterial and phage ribosome binding sites (Shine and Dalgarno 1974; Steitz et al. 1977). In accordance with this is the recent finding of base-substitution mutations which alter the initiation codon (K. Talmidge, U. Schmeissner, and J. H. Miller, unpubl.). No repressor or altered repressor is detected in these strains (less than 5%), showing that even in the absence of the preferred GUG triplet the other nearby GUG codons cannot initiate.

The elucidation of the mRNA sequence for this part of the gene allows the analysis of translation reinitiation following chain termination at nonsense sites. Reinitiation can be directed by the GUG codon at position 23, the AUG codon at position 42, and the UUG codon at position 62 (Weber and Geisler, this volume). Possible explanations for the selection of these codons in terms of complementary pairing with 16S rRNA and the predicted secondary structure of the mRNA are considered by Steege (1977).

pppG.GAA.GAG.AGU.CAA.UUC.AGG.AGG.GUG.GUG.AAU.GUG.GUG.AAA.CAA.GUA.ACG.UUA.UAC.GAU.GUC.GCA.GAG.UAU.
    Met-Lys-Pro-Val-Thr-Leu-Tyr-Asp-Val-Ala-Glu-Tyr-

GCC.GGU-GUC.UCU.UAU.CAG.ACC.GUU.UCC.CGC.GUG.GUG.AAC.CAG.GCC.AGC.CAC.GUU.UCU.GCG.AAA.ACG.CGG.GAA.
Ala-Gly-Val-Ser-Tyr-Gln-Thr-Val-Ser-Arg-Val-Val-Asn-Gln-Ala-Ser-His-Val-Ser-Ala-Lys-Thr-Arg-Glu-

AAA.GUG.GAA.GCG.GCG.AUG.GCG.GAG.CUG.AAU.UAC.AUU.CCC.AAC.CGC.GUG.GCA.CAA.CAA.CUG.GCG.GGC.AAA.CAG.UCG.UUG.
Lys-Val-Glu-Ala-Ala-Met-Ala-Glu-Leu-Asn-Tyr-Ile-Pro-Asn-Arg-Val-Ala-Gln-Gln-Leu-Ala-Gly-**Lys**-Gln-Ser-Leu-

Figure 13 The *I* message. The first part of the *lacI* mRNA (Steege 1977) is shown, together with the corresponding protein sequence. The GUG, AUG, and UUG codons are underlined. Reinitiation of translation has been detected at the codons at positions 23, 42, and 62 (Weber and Geisler, this volume). (Several ambiguities in the mRNA sequence were removed by consideration of the DNA sequence; see discussion by Steege [1977].)

USES OF THE *lacI* SYSTEM

The intensive genetic and physicochemical investigations of the *lacI* region have resulted in a system which now makes it possible to rapidly analyze at the DNA sequence level many different genetic phenomena. The elements of the system are as follows: (1) Small plasmid derivatives of pMB9 carrying the *I* region have been constructed and characterized (Calos 1978), facilitating the preparation of sufficient quantities of DNA to allow sequence analysis. (2) The wild-type *I* gene sequence is known (Farabaugh 1978). This is depicted in Figure 14. (3) The genetic system outlined in the preceding section permits rapid detection and mapping of many different types of mutations. (4) Mutations in the *I* gene can be crossed onto the small plasmids by genetic techniques (in vivo recombination). Therefore, many different mutations are subject to analysis. This system has already been employed to elucidate the sequence basis for genetic hotspots, deletion formation, and integration points for insertion elements and transposons. Some of these initial results are outlined below.

Hotspots

Genetic "hotspots" have intrigued molecular biologists ever since Benzer (1961) first described them in the *rII* region of phage T4 and suggested that some aspect of the surrounding base sequence made certain sites more mutable than others. Figure 15 shows the distribution of 140 spontaneous mutations in the *lacI* gene. Both point mutations and deletions are evident, although the spectrum is dominated by two hotspots which map together in the middle of the gene (these two sites are distinguishable by reversion tests). The DNA altered by examples of the "hot" mutations has been sequenced (Farabaugh et al. 1978), as indicated in Figure 16.

In the wild-type gene, the sequence CTGG is repeated three times in tandem. Both hotspots are generated by the addition or deletion of one unit of four bases from this sequence. Mutants carrying the fourth repeating unit are unstable, reverting to wild type at a high rate (around 10^{-5}–10^{-4}). However, mutants which have lost four bases from the wild type, leaving only two repeats, cannot reacquire an additional unit at a detectable rate. We can rationalize these results in terms of a model proposed by Streisinger and coworkers (Streisinger et al. 1966) to explain the prevalence of certain types of frameshifts. "Slipped mispairing" following single-strand breakage is invoked as a mechanism for stabilizing intermediates in frameshift formulation. Thus, repeating units which allow the most mispairing will be favored sites for frameshift formation; whether deletions or additions occur depends on which strand (template or growing) slips. The CTGG repeat in the *I* gene allows the largest

```
                                          10
                         CGGGAAGAGAGTCAATTCAGGGTGGTGAAT
                         GCCCTTTCTCTCAGTTAAGTCCCACCACTTA
                         HPAII        MboII
                                                              40
NH2
METLYSPROVALTHRLEUTYRASPVALALAGLUTYRALAGLYVALALASERTYRYRGLNTHRRVALSERARGVALVALASNGLNALASERHISVALSERARGLALYSTHRRARGGLULYSVALGLUALA

GTGAAACAGTAACGTTATACGATGTGCGAGAGTATGCCGGTGTCTCTTATCAGACCGTTTCCCGCGTGGTGAACCAGGCAGCCACGTTTCTCGCGAAAAGTGGAAGCG
CACTTTGGTCATTGCAATATGCTACAGCGTCTCATACGGCCACAGAGAATAGTCTGGCAAAGGGCGCACCACTTGGTCGGTCGGTGCAAAGAGCGCTTTTGCACCTTCGC
                                               HPAII                                        HAEIII
                                                                                                            80
ALAMETALAGLULEUALASNTYRILELEUPROGLNSERARGVALALAGLNLNLEUALAGLYLYSGLNSERLEULEUGLUILEGLQLYVALALATHRSERSERLEUVALALALEUHISALAPROSERGLNLNILEVAL
150
GCGATGGCGGAGCTGAATTACATTCCCGGCCAAAACGTGCGGGCAAACAGTGCGTTTGCTGCTGATTGGCGTTGCTGCCTGCCACCGCGGCTGCCAAATTGTC
CGCTACCGCCTCGACTTAATGTAAGGGTTGGCCGACCGTGTTGTTGTCAGCAAACGACTAACCGCAACGGTGAGGTCAGACCGGCGGCGGCCAGCGTTTAAACAG
ALUI                                                                          HAEIII
                                                                                                           120
ALAALAILELYSSERARGALAASPGLNLEUGLYYALASERVALVALVALSERMETVALALGLUARGSERGLYVALGLUALACYSYSLYSALALAVALHISASNLEULEULEUALAGLNLNARGVALSER
300                                      350
GGGCGGATTAAATCTCGCGCCGATCGGGTGGTGTGTTCATGGTAGAACGAAGCGGCGTCGAGCCTGTAAAGCGGCGGTGCACAATTCTCTCGCCGCAACCGTCAGT
CGCCGCCTAATTTAGAGCGCGGCTAGTTGACCCACGGTGACCATCTTGCTTCGCCGCAGTTCGGCGCACGTGTTAGAAGAGCGGCGTTGCGCAGTCA
                     TAQI                                    MBOII
                                                                                                           160
GLYLEUILEILEASNTYRRPROLEUVASPASPGLNASPALAILEALAVALALALASPALAALACYSTYRHISASNVALPROGLNALALEUPHEELEUVALASPVALSERERASPASPGLNTHRRPROILEGLNSERILEILE
                                         450                                   500
GGGCTGATCATTAATAACTATCCGCTGGAATGACCAGGATGCCATTGCTGTGGAAGTCGCCTGCGACTATCTTCGGCCGTATTTCTTGATGTCTGACCAGACACCATCAAACAGTATTATT
CCCGACTAGTAATTGATTAGGCGACCTTTACTGGTCCTACGGTAACGACACTTACAGCGGACGTGAATAAAGAAACTACAGAGACTGGTCTGTGGTAGTTGTCATAATAA
                  ALUI                                                    HPAII
                                                                                                           200
PHESERHISGLUASPGLYTHRRARGGLEUGLYVALALGLUHISLEUVALALAALALEUGLYHISSERGLNGLNILEALAALEULEUEUALAGLYPROLEUSERSERVALSERALAARGLEUVALARGLEUVALALAGLY
170                                     180                                   190
```

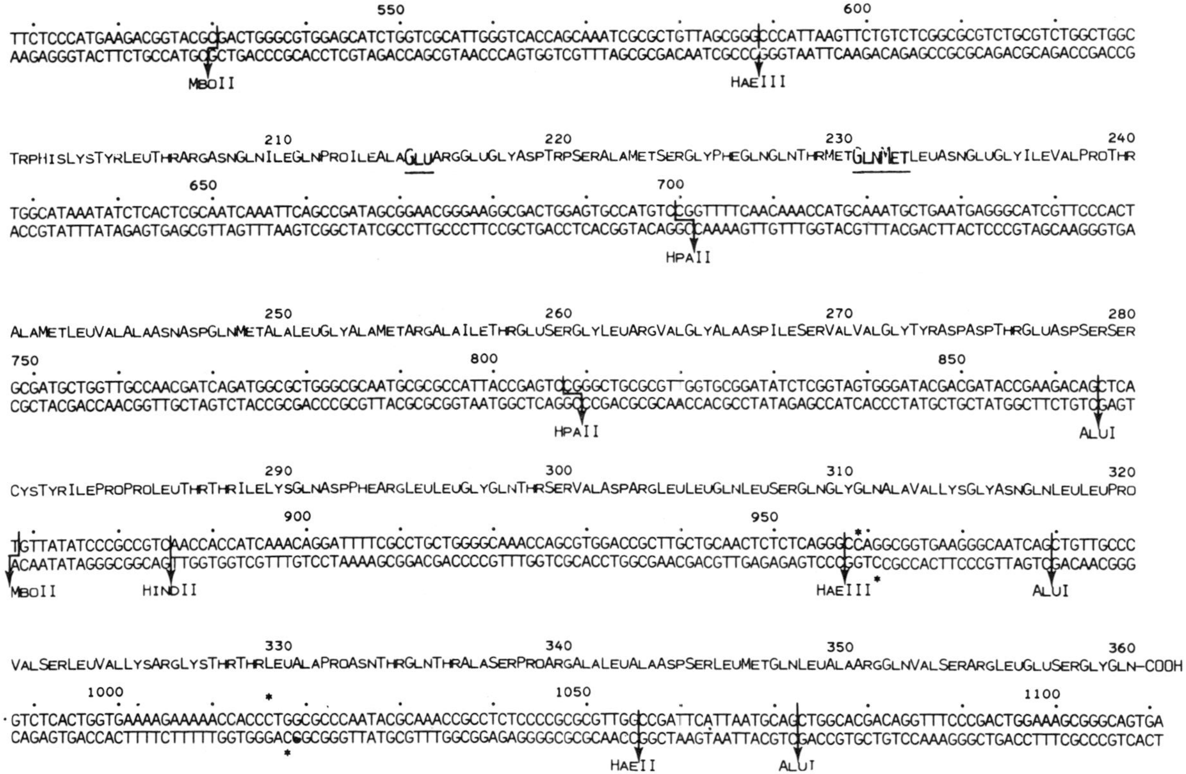

Figure 14 The *lacI* sequence. The DNA sequence of the *I* gene is shown together with the corresponding protein sequence. (Reprinted, with permission, from Farabaugh 1978.)

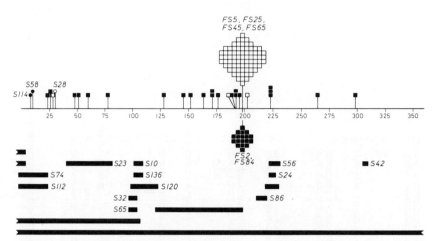

Figure 15 The distribution of 140 spontaneous mutations in the *lacI* gene. Each mutation is of independent origin and resulted in the i⁻ phenotype. A single occurrence of an apparent point mutation is represented by a square. (■) Mutations with very low or undetectable reversion rates; (□) mutations which are unstable, reverting at frequencies of 10^{-5} or greater. Deletions are shown below the line, which represents the length of the gene given in terms of the position of the corresponding residue in the *lac* repressor. All mutations were mapped against the deletions used to divide the gene into over 100 marked sections (Schmeissner et al. 1977a,b). The allele numbers are given in cases where the mutational change has been sequenced. *S114* and *S58* are insertions of the transposable element IS*1* (Calos et al. 1978b). *S28* is an unstable duplication of 88 base pairs (Calos et al. 1978a). The other sequenced mutations are described in the text and in Farabaugh et al. (1978). One suppressible nonsense mutation was found in this particular collection.

mispairing (nine bases) of any such sequence in the gene (Galas 1978), which is consistent with it being the hottest mutational site (at least for frameshifts of this type). Identification of the enzymes involved and a comparison with hotspots in other systems are important topics for further studies.

Deletions

Twelve of the deletions from the collection shown in Figure 15 have been analyzed by DNA sequencing (Farabaugh et al. 1978). Seven of these

5'-G T C T G G C T G G C T G G C T G G C-3'

FS5, 25, 45, 65

wild-type   G T C T G G C T G G C T G G C

FS2 | FS84

G T C T G G C T G G C

Figure 16 Sequence change resulting from the two mutational hotspots. Four examples of the larger hotspot and two examples of the second hotspot were analyzed by DNA sequencing (Farabaugh et al. 1978).

S74, S112

75 bases

T C A A T T C A G G | G T G G T G A A | T G T G A A A C C -------- C G C | G T G G T G A A | C C A G G --

SITE (no. of b.p.)	SEQUENCE REPEAT	BASES DELETED	OCCURRENCES	
20 to 95	GTGGTGAA	75	2	*S74, S112*
146 to 269	GCGGCGAT	123	1	*S23*
331 to 351	AAGCGGCG	20	2	*S10, S136*
316 to 338	GTCGA	22	2	*S32, S65*
694 to 707	CA	13	1	*S24*
694 to 719	CA	25	1	*S56*
943 to 956	G	13	1	*S42*
322 to 393	None	71	1	*S120*
658 to 685	None	27	1	*S86*

Figure 17 Sequence change resulting from deletions in the *I* gene. The sequence analysis of 12 deletions in the *lacI* gene is summarized. Many deletions occur between repeated sequences, as shown for *S74* and *S112*. Both of these mutations represent independent occurrences of the identical deletion of 75 nucleotides. The deletion removes one copy of the repeated sequence GTGGTGAA and can be pictured in either one of the two ways shown. (See Farabaugh et al. [1978] for further details.) (Only the repeats of 5 bases or greater are considered significant here.)

occur between repeated sequences (Fig. 17). Moreover, in three cases the identical deletion has been found twice, indicating that these are hotspots for deletion formation (considering the small number of deletions appearing in this collection). It is conceivable that these events are simply extreme examples of frameshifts occurring by some type of slippage mechanism. On the other hand, it is possible that an independent mechanism using different enzymes is involved. The largest deletion from the sequenced set removes 123 base pairs. It is of interest to ask whether significantly larger deletions also predominate at repeated stretches of nucleotides.

Insertions and Duplications

Examination of the altered DNA resulting from each of the mutations in Figure 15 (excluding the deletions and frameshift hotspots) has revealed three cases in which additions of greater than 50 bases had occurred. One of these represents a perfect tandem duplication of 88 base pairs in the *I* gene (Calos et al. 1978a). The other two are examples of the transposable element IS*1*. The junctures of *lacI* and IS*1* DNA have been sequenced in each case (Calos et al. 1978b). As shown in Figure 18, the insertion of IS*1* into the *I* gene generates a direct repeat of nine bases, one copy of which

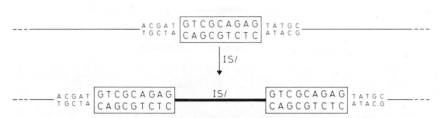

Figure 18 Molecular consequences of IS*1* integration. The insertion of IS*1* into the *lacI* gene generates a direct repeat of nine base pairs which is seen at either end of the inserted element. One copy of the nine bases preexisted in the wild-type gene prior to integration (Calos et al. 1978b).

was already present in the gene.[16] Recent studies with the transposon Tn*9* (which contains the genetic determinants for chloramphenicol resistance flanked by two IS*1* elements) (Rosner and Gottesman 1977; MacHattie and Jackowski 1977; Chow and Bukhari 1977) demonstrate the facility of using this system. Numerous transpositions of Tn*9* into the *I* region have been detected and the junctures at the integration points have been sequenced in three cases (Johnsrud et al. 1978), again revealing the existence of a 9-base repeat. These studies suggest that the repeat is generated during the process of insertion itself, since the repeated sequence is different in each of the three cases which have been analyzed, even though the Tn*9*s originated from the same point.

Base-substitution Hotspots

The set of correlated nonsense sites (Coulondre and Miller 1977a) permits the rapid characterization of base-substitution mutations (Coulondre and Miller 1977b), since we can classify each nonsense site according to the specific transition or transversion required to generate it from wild type. This is diagramed in Figure 19 for amber sites in the *I* gene. Figure 20 shows the amber mutations found in a collection of spontaneous i⁻ mutants. Of immediate interest are the two hotspots in panel A, which result from G:C→A:T transitions. Inspection of the DNA sequence shows that these sites are part of a CCAGG pentanucleotide (Coulondre et al. 1978), the second C on each strand being converted to 5-methyl-cytosine in *E. coli* K12 (Gold et al. 1966; Farabaugh 1978). It is precisely the second C which is involved in the C→T transition that generates the amber mutation at these positions. Eleven of the remaining sites generating an amber mutation by a similar C→T transition are not part of such a sequence. Subsequent experiments (Coulondre et al. 1978) have

---

[16]Similar findings have been reported by Grindley (1978) for IS*1* insertions in *gal*; IS*2* in lambda also generates a repeated sequence (Rosenberg et al., this volume).

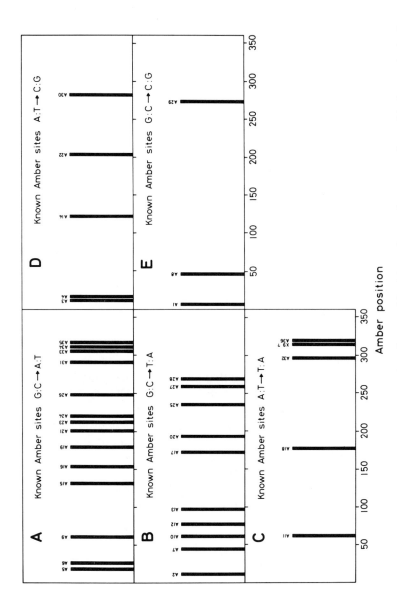

Figure 19 Known amber sites. The amber sites used in this study are shown together with the particular base substitution required to generate each site. The bars depict sites, and the allele numbers correspond to those given in the tables of Coulondre et al. (1977a,b) and Miller et al. (1978b). The horizontal axis represents the gene-protein map expressed in amino acid position.

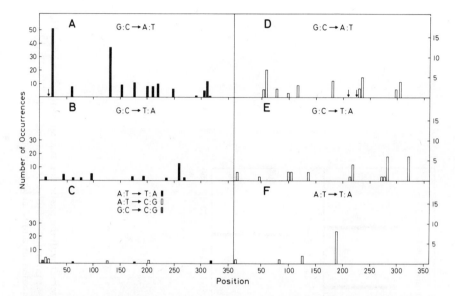

Figure 20 The distribution of 222 spontaneous amber mutations (panels *A, B,* and *C*) and 76 spontaneous ochre mutations (panels *D, E,* and *F*) is shown. The mutations are of independent origin and have been characterized previously (Miller et al. 1977; Coulondre et al. 1977a,b). Although the ochre scale has been magnified to permit a direct comparison of amber and ochre mutations (to compensate for the difference in sample size), hotspots can be detected with a greater degree of assurance by considering the amber and ochre distributions as separate groups. The arrows in panels *A* and *D* indicate transition sites not found in this collection. (Only half of the spontaneous collection was assayed for the missing site, *A5.*) Transversion sites not represented in this collection can be recognized by consulting Fig. 19.

shown the following: (1) An additional CCAGG sequence introduced into the *I* gene results in a new hotspot at that point in the gene. (2) The use of an *E. coli* B strain which does not methylate the CCAGG sequence eliminates the hotspots.

The above results demonstrate that 5-methylcytosine is responsible for the observed transition hotspots. An attractive hypothesis involves the enzyme uracil-DNA glycosidase (Lindahl et al. 1977), which excises uracil from DNA. Spontaneous deamination of cytosine to uracil is normally corrected by this enzyme, which recognizes the uracil moeity; deamination of 5-methylcytosine results in thymine (5-methyluracil), which is not recognized. Therefore, a higher percentage of G:T mispairs remain in comparison to G:U mispairs, resulting in a relative hotspot. Experiments using mutants lacking uracil-DNA glycosidase support this hypothesis (B. Duncan and J. H. Miller, unpubl.).

Mutagenic Specificity

We have used the nonsense-mutation system to analyze the specificities of several mutagens (Coulondre and Miller 1977b). Figures 21 through 24 summarize the results for 4-nitroquinoline-1-oxide (NQO), ultraviolet light (UV), ethylmethanesulfonate (EMS), and N'-methyl-N'-nitro-N-nitrosoguanidine (NG). It can be seen that NQO favors transitions and transversions at G:C base pairs (transitions being highly favored), whereas UV is not as specific (see legend to Fig. 22). EMS and NG induce virtually exclusively G:C→A:T transitions, transversions being stimulated only at very low relative rates. (NG does generate A:T→G:C transitions at about 1–5% the frequency of G:C→A:T transitions.)

NQO AMBER SITES

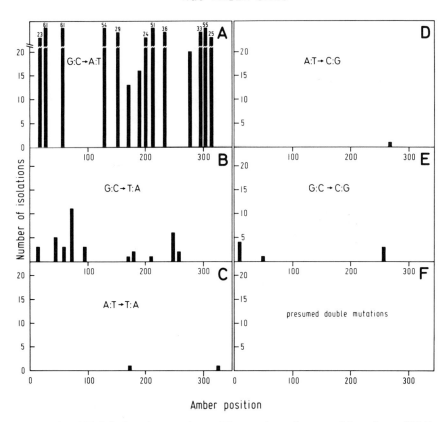

Figure 21 NQO-induced mutations. The amber sites resulting from NQO treatment are shown. The height of each bar represents the number of independent occurrences. (Reprinted, with permission, from Coulondre and Miller 1977b.)

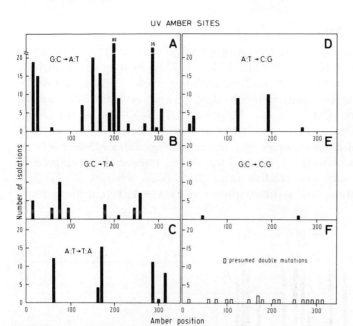

Figure 22 UV-induced mutations. The amber sites derived by UV are shown. (Reprinted, with permission, from Coulondre and Miller 1977b.)

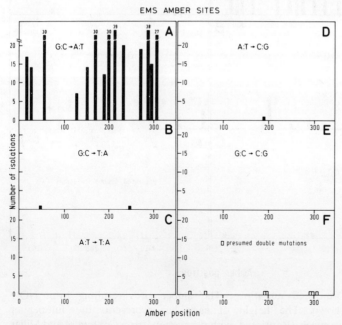

Figure 23 EMS-induced mutations. The amber sites derived by EMS are shown. (Reprinted, with permission, from Coulondre and Miller 1977b.)

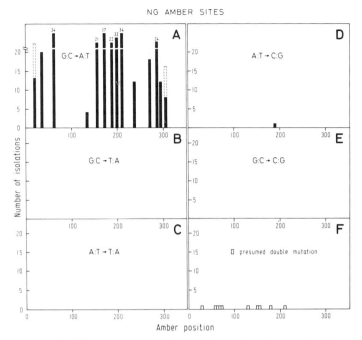

Figure 24 NG-induced mutations. The amber sites derived by NG are shown. (Reprinted, with permission, from Coulondre and Miller 1977b.)

Figure 25 displays the different hotspots seen among both amber and ochre sites for each of the mutagens used, together with spontaneous and 2-aminopurine (2AP)-induced nonsense mutations. It can be seen that the position of the hotspots varies according to the mutagen (compare UV with 2AP). The frequencies of occurrence of each mutation have been analyzed with respect to the surrounding base sequence (Coulondre et al. 1978).

ACKNOWLEDGMENTS

I would like to thank my coworkers Don Ganem, Terry Platt, Jim Files, Klaus Weber, Christine Coulondre, Ursula Schmeissner, Albert Schmitz, Hans Sommer, Ponzy Lu, David Galas, Birgitta Friedli, Murielle Hofer, Michèle Calos, Lorraine Johnsrud, and Phil Farabaugh, who participated in various stages of the work reviewed here. I am indebted to Walter Gilbert, James D. Watson, Sydney Brenner, and Francis Crick for providing support and encouragement during the past several years, and to Walter Gilbert for providing laboratory space. I was supported by a grant from the Swiss National Fund (F.N. 3.179.77).

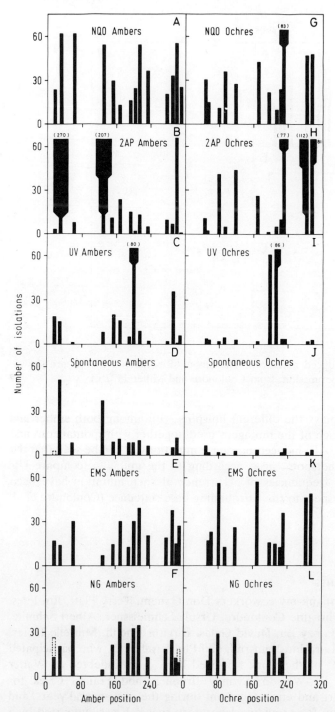

Figure 25   (See legend on facing page.)

REFERENCES

Adler, K., K. Beyreuther, E. Fanning, N. Geisler, B. Gronenborn, A. Klemm, B. Müller-Hill, M. Pfahl, and A. Schmitz. 1972. How *lac* repressor binds to DNA. *Nature* **237**:322.

Arditti, R., J. G. Scaife, and J. R. Beckwith. 1968. The nature of mutants in the *lac* promoter region. (Letter to the editor.) *J. Mol. Biol.* **38**:421.

Barbour, S. D. and A. B. Pardee. 1966. The establishment of β-galactosidase repression in the mating system of *Escherichia coli* K12. *J. Mol. Biol.* **20**:505.

Beckwith, J. R. 1970. Lac: The genetic system. In *The lactose operon* (ed. J. R. Beckwith and D. Zipser), p. 5. Cold Spring Harbor Laboratory, Cold Spring Harbor, New York.

Beckwith, J. R. and E. R. Signer. 1966. Transposition of the *lac* region of *E. coli*. I. Inversion of the *lac* operon and transduction of *lac* by φ80. *J. Mol. Biol.* **19**:254.

Benzer, S. 1961. On the topography of the genetic fine structure. *Proc. Natl. Acad. Sci.* **47**:403.

Bertani, G. 1954. Lysogenic versus lytic cycle of phage multiplication. *Cold Spring Harbor Symp. Quant. Biol.* **18**:65.

Betz, J. L. and J. R. Sadler. 1976. Tight-binding repressors of the lactose operon. *J. Mol. Biol.* **105**:293.

Beyreuther, K., K. Adler, N. Geisler, and A. Klemm. 1973. The amino-acid sequence of *lac* repressor. *Proc. Natl. Acad. Sci.* **70**:3576.

Bourgeois, S. and M. Pfahl. 1976. Repressors. *Adv. Protein Chem.* **30**:1.

Bourgeois, S., M. Cohn, and L. E. Orgel. 1965. Suppression of and complementation among mutants of the regulatory gene of the lactose operon of *Escherichia coli*. *J. Mol. Biol.* **14**:300.

Bourgeois, S., R. L. Jernigan, S. C. Szu, E. A. Kabat, and T. T. Wu. 1978. Composite predictions of secondary structures of *lac* repressor. *Biopolymers* (in press).

Figure 25 Genetic hotspots. The distribution of 3738 mutations arising from the G:C→A:T transition is shown. The number of independent occurrences at each site is indicated by the bar height. One amber mutation and one ochre mutation from each mutagenized culture were analyzed. Therefore, hotspots can be directly identified by considering the frequency of induction of an amber site relative to the other amber sites, and of an ochre site relative to the other ochre sites. Wide areas, instead of bar heights, indicate numbers of occurrences greater than 60. For instance, one of the 2AP-induced amber sites was detected 270 times in this collection, as indicated at the left side of *B*. To consider amber and ochre mutations together, the relative frequency of each type of mutation and the respective sample sizes must be taken into account to produce a normalization factor. For instance, to compare spontaneous ochre sites directly with the spontaneous amber sites, the ochre bar heights must be multiplied by a factor of 3. For EMS- and NG-induced mutations, the ochre bar heights should be multiplied by factors of 2.3 and 1.9, respectively. For 2AP-, NQO-, and UV-induced ochres, the relevant factors are 0.9, 0.6, and 0.7, respectively.

82   J. H. Miller

Calos, M. 1978. DNA sequence for a low-level promoter of the *lac* repressor gene and an "up" promoter mutation. *Nature* **274**:762.

Calos, M., D. Galas, and J. H. Miller. 1978a. DNA sequence change resulting from an intragenic duplication. *J. Mol. Biol.* (in press).

Calos, M., L. Johnsrud, and J. H. Miller. 1978b. DNA sequence at the integration sites of the insertion element IS*1*. *Cell* **13**:411.

Chamness, G. C. and C. W. Willson. 1970. An unusual *lac* repressor mutant. *J. Mol. Biol.* **53**:561.

Chou, P. Y., A. J. Adler, and G. D. Fasman. 1974. Conformational prediction and circular dichroism studies on the *lac* repressor. *J. Mol. Biol.* **96**:29.

Chow, L. T. and A. I. Bukhari. 1977. Bacteriophage Mu genome: Structural studies on Mu DNA and Mu mutants carrying insertions. In *DNA insertion elements, plasmids, and episomes* (ed. A. I. Bukhari et al.), p. 295. Cold Spring Harbor Laboratory, Cold Spring Harbor, New York.

Cohen, G. N. and J. Monod. 1957. Bacterial permeases. *Bacteriol. Rev.* **21**:169.

Cohn, M. 1957. Contributions of studies on the β-galactosidase of *E. coli* to our understanding of enzyme synthesis. *Bacteriol. Rev.* **21**:140.

Cohn, M. and A. M. Torriani. 1952. Immunochemical studies with the β-galactosidase and structurally related proteins of *Escherichia coli*. *J. Immunol.* **69**:471.

Coulondre, C. and J. H. Miller. 1977a. Genetic studies of the *lac* repressor. III. Additional correlation of mutational sites with specific amino acid residues. *J. Mol. Biol.* **117**:525.

———. 1977b. Genetic studies of the *lac* repressor. IV. Mutagenic specificity in the *lacI* gene of *Escherichia coli*. *J. Mol. Biol.* **117**:577.

Coulondre, C., J. H. Miller, P. J. Farabaugh, and W. Gilbert. 1978. Molecular basis of base substitution hotspots in *Escherichia coli*. *Nature* **274**:775.

Cox, E. C. and C. Yanofsky. 1967. Altered base ratios in the DNA of an *E. coli* mutator strain. *Proc. Natl. Acad. Sci.* **59**:1895.

Davies, D. R., E. A. Padlen, and D. M. Segal. 1975. Three-dimensional structure of immunoglobulin. *Annu. Rev. Biochem.* **44**:639.

Davies, J. and F. Jacob. 1968. Genetic mapping of the regulator and operator genes of the *lac* operon. *J. Mol. Biol.* **36**:413.

Dienert, F. 1900. *Ann. Inst. Pasteur* **14**:139.

Duclaux, E. 1899. *Traité de microbiologie*. Masson et Cie, Paris.

Farabaugh, P. J. 1978. Sequence of the *lacI* gene. *Nature* **274**:765.

Farabaugh, P. J., U. Schmeissner, M. Hofer, and J. H. Miller. 1978. Genetic studies of the *lac* repressor. VII. On the molecular nature of spontaneous hot spots in the *lacI* gene of *E. coli*. *J. Mol. Biol.* (in press).

Files, J. G. and K. Weber. 1978. Direct identification of the amino-acid changes in two mutant *lac* repressors. *J. Mol. Biol.* (in press).

Files, J. G., K. Weber, and J. H. Miller. 1974. Translational reinitiation: Reinitiation of *lac* repressor fragments at three internal sites early in the *lacI* gene of *Escherichia coli*. *Proc. Natl. Acad. Sci.* **71**:667.

Files, J. G., K. Weber, C. Coulondre, and J. H. Miller. 1975. Identification of the UUG codon as a translation initiation codon *in vivo*. *J. Mol. Biol.* **95**:327.

Fukasawa, T. and H. Nikaido. 1961. Galactose sensitive mutants of *Salmonella*. II. Bacteriolysis induced by galactose. *Biochim. Biophys. Acta* **48**:470.

Galas, D. 1978. An analysis of sequence repeats in the *lacI* gene of *E. coli*. *J. Mol. Biol.* (in press).

Ganem, D. 1972. "Genetic studies on *lac* repressor." Honors thesis, Harvard University, Cambridge, Massachusetts.

Ganem, D., J. H. Miller, J. G. Files, T. Platt, and K. Weber. 1973. Reinitiation of a *lac* repressor fragment at a codon other than AUG. *Proc. Natl. Acad. Sci.* **70:**3165.

Geisler, N. and K. Weber. 1976. Isolation of a set of hybrid *lac* repressors made *in vitro* between normal *lac* repressor and its homogeneous tryptic core. *Proc. Natl. Acad. Sci.* **73:**3103.

Gho, D. and J. H. Miller. 1974. Deletions fusing the *i* and *lac* regions of the chromosome in *E. coli. Mol. Gen. Genet.* **131:**137.

Gilbert, W. and B. Müller-Hill. 1966. Isolation of the *lac* repressor. *Proc. Natl. Acad. Sci.* **56:**1891.

———. 1967. The *lac* operator is DNA. *Proc. Natl. Acad. Sci.* **58:**2415.

———. 1970. The lactose repressor. In *The lactose operon* (ed. J. R. Beckwith and D. Zipser), p. 93. Cold Spring Harbor Laboratory, Cold Spring Harbor, New York.

Gilbert, W., A. Maxam, and A. Mirzabekov. 1976. Contacts between the *lac* repressor and DNA revealed by methylation. In *Control of ribosome synthesis* (ed. N. Kjeldgaard and O. Maaløe), p. 139. Munksgaard, Copenhagen.

Gilbert, W., J. Gralla, J. Majors, and A. Maxam. 1975. Lactose operator sequences and the action of *lac* repressor. In *Protein-ligand interactions* (ed. H. Sund and G. Blauer), p. 193. Walter de Gruyter, Berlin.

Gold, M., R. Gefter, R. Hausmann, and J. Hurwitz. 1966. In *Macrocmolecular metabolism*, p. 5. Little Brown, Boston.

Gorini, L. 1970. Informational suppression. *Annu. Rev. Genet.* **4:**107.

Grindley, N. D. F. 1978. IS*1* insertion generates duplication of a 9 base pair sequence at its target site. *Cell* **13:**419.

Gursky, G. V., V. G. Tumanyan, A. S. Zasedatelev, A. L. Zhuze, S. L. Grokhovsky, and B. P. Gottikh. 1977. A code controlling specific binding of proteins to double-helical DNA and RNA. In *Nucleic acid-protein recognition* (ed. H. J. Vogel), p. 189. Academic Press, New York.

Herzenberg, L. 1959. Studies on the induction of β-galactosidase in a cryptic strain of *E. coli. Biochim. Biophys. Acta* **31:**525.

Hogness, D. S., M. Cohn, and J. Monod. 1955. Studies on the induced synthesis of β-galactosidase in *E. coli*: The kinetics and mechanism of sulfur uptake. *Biochim. Biophys. Acta* **16:**99.

Horiuchi, T. and A. Novick. 1962. A thermolabile repression system. *Cold Spring Harbor Symp. Quant. Biol.* **26:**247.

———. 1965. Studies of a thermolabile repressor. *Biochim. Biophys. Acta* **108:**687.

Horiuchi, T. and Y. Oshima. 1966. Inhibition of repressor formation in the lactose system of *E. coli* by inhibitors of protein synthesis. *J. Mol. Biol.* **20:**517.

Horwitz, J. P., J. Chua, R. J. Curby, A. J. Tomson, M. A. DaRooge, B. E. Fisher, J. Mauricio, and I. Klundt. 1964. *J. Med. Chem.* **7:**574.

Jacob, F. 1954. *Les bactéries lysogènes et la notion de provirus. Monograpies de l'Institut Pasteur*. Masson et Cie, Paris.

———. 1960. *Genetic control of viral functions. Harvey Lect.* **54:**1.

———. 1970. *La logique du vivant: Une histoire de l'hérédité*. Editions Gallimard, Paris. (Eng. trans. *The logic of living systems: A history of heredity*. Allan Lane, Penguin Books, London; Pantheon Books and Vintage Books, New York.)

Jacob, F. and E. A. Adelberg. 1959. Transfert de caractères génétique par incorporation au facteur sexuel d'*Escherichia coli*. *C. R. Acad. Sci.* **249**:189.

Jacob, F. and A. Campbell. 1959. Sur le système de répression assurant l'immunité chez les bactéries lysogènes. *C. R. Acad. Sci.* **248**:3219.

Jacob, F. and J. Monod. 1961. Genetic regulatory mechanisms in the synthesis of proteins. *J. Mol. Biol.* **3**:318.

Jacob, F. and E. Wollman. 1954. Induction spontanée du dévelopement du bacteriophage λ au cours de la recombinaison génétique chez *Escherichia coli* K12. *C. R. Acad. Sci.* **239**:317.

―――. 1956. *Ann. Inst. Pasteur* **91**:486.

Jacob, F., P. Schaeffer, and E. L. Wollman. 1960a. Episomic elements in bacteria. In *Microbial genetics. Tenth Symposium of the Society for General Microbiology* (ed. W. Hayes et al.), vol. 10, p. 67. University Press, Cambridge, England.

Jacob, F., D. Perrin, C. Sanchez, and J. Monod. 1960b. L'opéron: Groupe de gènes à expression coordonnée par un opérateur. *C. R. Acad. Sci.* **250**:1727.

Jobe, A. and S. Bourgeois. 1972a. *Lac* repressor-operator interaction. VI. The natural inducer of the *lac* operon. *J. Mol. Biol.* **69**:397.

―――. 1972b. The *lac* repressor-operator interaction. VII. A repressor with unique binding properties: The X86 repressor. *J. Mol. Biol.* **72**:139.

Jobe, A., A. D. Riggs, and S. Bourgeois. 1972. *Lac* repressor-operator interaction. V. Characterization of super- and pseudo-wild-type repressors. *J. Mol. Biol.* **64**:181.

Johnsrud, L., M. P. Calos, and J. H. Miller. 1978. The distribution of Tn*9* insertions in the *lacI* gene of *E. coli* and the DNA sequence at the integration sites. *Cell* (in press).

Kaiser, A. D. and F. Jacob. 1957. Recombination between related temperate bacteriophages and the genetic control of immunity and prophage localization. *Virology* **4**:509.

Kania, J. and D. T. Brown. 1976. The functional repressor parts of a tetrameric *lac* repressor-β-galactosidase chimaera are organized as dimers. *Proc. Natl. Acad. Sci.* **73**:3529.

Karstrom, H. 1938. *Ergeb. Enzymforschung.* **7**:350.

Lillis, M. 1977. Sequence change in the DNA from the *lacI* gene arising from an amber mutation. *J. Mol. Biol.* **117**:568.

Lindahl, T., S. Ljungquist, W. Siegert, B. Nyberg, and B. Sperens. 1977. DNA-glycosidases. Properties of uracil-DNA glycosidase from *E. coli. J. Biol. Chem.* **252**:3286.

Lu, P., M. Jarema, K. Mosser, and W. E. Daniel, Jr. 1976. *lac* Repressor: 3-Fluorotyrosine substitution for nuclear magnetic resonance studies. *Proc. Natl. Acad. Sci.* **73**:3471.

MacHattie, L. A. and J. B. Jackowski. 1977. Physical structure and deletion effects of the chloramphenicol resistance element Tn*9* in phage lambda. In *DNA insertion elements, plasmids, and episomes* (ed. A. I. Bukhari et al.), p. 219. Cold Spring Harbor Laboratory, Cold Spring Harbor, New York.

Malamy, M. H. 1967. Frameshift mutations in the lactose operon of *E. Coli. Cold Spring Harbor Symp. Quant. Biol.* **31**:189.

Miller, J. H. 1972. *Experiments in molecular genetics.* Cold Spring Harbor Laboratory, Cold Spring Harbor, New York.

————. 1978. On the protein structure of the *lac* repressor as revealed by genetic experiments. *J. Mol. Biol.* (in press).

Miller, J. H. and U. Schmeissner. 1978. Genetic studies of the *lacI* gene. X. The analysis of missense mutations in the *lacI* gene of *E. coli. J. Mol. Biol.* (in press).

Miller, J. H., J. R. Beckwith, and B. Müller-Hill. 1968a. Direction of transcription of a regulatory gene in *E. coli. Nature* **220:** 1287.

Miller, J. H., C. Coulondre, and P. J. Farabaugh. 1978a. Correlation of nonsense sites in the *lacI* gene with specific codons in the nucleotide sequence. *Nature* **274:** 770.

Miller, J. H., D. Ganem, P. Lu, and A. Schmitz. 1977. Genetic studies of the *lac* repressor. I. Correlation of mutational sites with specific amino acid residues: Construction of a colinear gene-protein map. *J. Mol. Biol.* **109:** 275.

Miller, J. H., T. Platt, and K. Weber. 1970a. Strains with the promoter deletion *L1* synthesize an altered *lac* repressor. In *The lactose operon* (ed. J. R. Beckwith and D. Zipser), p. 343. Cold Spring Harbor Laboratory, Cold Spring Harbor, New York.

Miller, J. H., K. Ippen, J. G. Scaife, and J. R. Beckwith. 1968b. The promoter-operator region of the *lac* operon of *Escherichia coli. J. Mol. Biol.* **38:** 413.

Miller, J. H., C. Coulondre, M. Hofer, U. Schmeissner, H. Sommer, and A. Schmitz. 1978b. Genetic studies of the *lac* repressor. IX. The generation of altered proteins by the suppression of nonsense mutations. *J. Mol. Biol.* (in press).

Miller, J. H., W. S. Reznikoff, A. E. Silverstone, K. Ippen, E. R. Signer, and J. R. Beckwith. 1970b. Fusions of the *lac* and *trp* regions of the *E. coli* chromosome. *J. Bacteriol.* **104:** 1273.

Miwa, J. and J. R. Sadler. 1977. Characterization of i^{-d} repressor mutations of the lactose operon. *J. Mol. Biol.* **117:** 843.

Monod, J. 1956. Remarks on the mechanism of enzyme induction. In *Units of biological structure and function*, p. 7. Academic Press, New York.

————. 1959. Biosynthese eines enzyms. *Angew. Chem.* **71:** 685.

Monod, J. and A. Audureau. 1946. Mutation et adaption enzymatique chez *Escherichia coli*-mutabile. *Ann. Inst. Pasteur* **72:** 868.

Monod, J. and M. Cohn. 1952. La biosynthèse induite des enzymes (adaption enzymatique). *Adv. Enzymol.* **13:** 67.

————. 1953. In *Symposium on Microbial Metabolism. Sixth International Congress of Microbiology*, Rome, p. 42.

Monod, J., A. M. Pappenheim, Jr., and G. Cohen-Bazire. 1952. La cinétique de la biosynthèse de la β-galactosidase chez *E. coli* considérée comme fonction de la croissance. *Biochim. Biophys. Acta* **9:** 648.

Müller-Hill, B. 1966. Suppressible regulator constitutive mutants of the lactose system in *Escherichia coli. J. Mol. Biol.* **15:** 374.

————. 1975. *Lac* repressor and *lac* operator. *Prog. Biophys. Mol. Biol.* **30:** 227.

Müller-Hill, B. and J. Kania. 1974. *Lac* repressor can be fused to β-galactosidase. *Nature* **249:** 561.

Müller-Hill, B., L. Crapo, and W. Gilbert. 1968. Mutants that make more *lac* repressor. *Proc. Natl. Acad. Sci.* **59:** 1259.

Müller-Hill, B., G. Heidecker, and J. Kania. 1976. Repressor-galactosidase-chimaeras. In *Structure: function relationships of proteins. Proceedings of the Third John Innes Symposium* (ed. R. Markham and R. W. Horne), p. 167. Elsevier/North-Holland, Amsterdam.

Müller-Hill, B., B. Gronenborn, J. Kania, M. Schlotmann, and K. Beyreuther. 1977. Similarities between *lac* repressor and *lambda* repressor. In *Nucleic acid-protein recognition* (ed. H. J. Vogel), p. 219. Academic Press, New York.

Müller-Hill, B., T. Fanning, N. Geisler, D. Gho, J. Kania, P. Kathmann, H. Meissner, M. Schlotmann, A. Schmitz, I. Triesch, and K. Beyreuther. 1975. The active sites of *lac* repressor. In *Protein-ligand interactions* (ed. H. Sund and G. Blauer), p. 211. Walter de Gruyter, Berlin.

Myers, G. L. and J. R. Sadler. 1971. Mutational inversion of control of the lactose operon of *E. coli. J. Mol. Biol.* **58**:1.

Osborn, M., S. Person, S. Phillips, and F. Funk. 1967. A determination of mutagen specificity in bacteria using nonsense mutants of bacteriophage T4. *J. Mol. Biol.* **26**:437.

Pardee, A. B. 1957. An inducible mechanism for accumulation of melibiose in *Escherichia coli. J. Bacteriol.* **73**:376.

Pardee, A. B. and L. S. Prestidge. 1961. The initial kinetics of enzyme induction. *Biochim. Biophys. Acta* **49**:77.

Pardee, A. B., F. Jacob, and J. Monod. 1958. Sur l'expression et le rôle d'allèles inductible et constitutif dans la synthèse de la β-galactosidase chez des zygotes d'*Escherichia coli. C. R. Acad. Sci.* **246**:3125.

———.1959. The genetic control and cytoplasmic expression of inducibility in the synthesis of β-galactosidase of *E. coli. J. Mol. Biol.* **1**:165.

Perutz, M. F. and H. Lehmann. 1968. Molecular pathology of human haemoglobin. *Nature* **219**:902.

Pfahl, M. 1972. Genetic map of the lactose repressor gene (*i*) of *Escherichia coli. Genetics* **72**:393.

———. 1976. *Lac* repressor-operator interaction: Analysis of the X86 repressor mutant. *J. Mol. Biol.* **106**:857.

Pfahl, M., C. Stockter, and B. Gronenborn. 1974. Genetic analysis of the active sites of *lac* repressor. *Genetics* **76**:669.

Platt, T., J. H. Miller, and K. Weber. 1970. *In vivo* degradation of mutant *lac* repressor. *Nature* **228**:1154.

Platt, T., K. Weber, D. Ganem, and J. H. Miller. 1972. Translational restarts: AUG reinitiation of a *lac* repressor fragment. *Proc. Natl. Acad. Sci.* **69**:897.

Prestidge, L. S. and A. B. Pardee. 1965. A second permease for methyl-β-D-thiogalactoside in *Escherichia coli. Biochim. Biophys. Acta* **100**:591.

Rickenberg, H. V., G. N. Cohen, G. Buttin, and J. Monod. 1956. La galactoside-perméase d'*Escherichia coli. Ann. Inst. Pasteur* **91**:829.

Rosner, J. L. and M. M. Gottesman. 1977. Transposition and deletion of Tn9: A transposable element carrying the gene for chloramphenicol resistance. In *DNA insertion elements, plasmids, and episomes* (ed. A. I. Bukhari et al.), p. 213. Cold Spring Harbor Laboratory, Cold Spring Harbor, New York.

Rotman, B. and S. Spiegelman. 1954. On the origin of the carbon in the induced synthesis β-galactosidase in *Escherichia coli. J. Bacteriol.* **68**:419.

Sadler, J. R. and A. Novick. 1965. The properties of repressor and the kinetics of its action. *J. Mol. Biol.* **12**:305.

Sadler, J. R. and M. Tecklenburg. 1976. Recovery of operator DNA binding activity from denatured lactose repressor. *Biochemistry* **15**:4353.

Scaife, J. G. and J. R. Beckwith. 1967. Mutational alteration of the maximal level of *lac* operon expression. *Cold Spring Harbor Symp. Quant. Biol.* **31**:403.

Schmeissner, U., D. Ganem, and J. H. Miller. 1977a. Genetic studies of the *lac* repressor. II. Fine structure deletion map of the *lacI* gene, and its correlation with the physical map. *J. Mol. Biol.* **109**:303.

———. 1977b. Revised gene-protein map for the *lacI* gene-*lac* repressor system. *J. Mol. Biol.* **117**:572.

Schmitz, A., C. Coulondre, and J. H. Miller. 1978. Genetic studies of the *lac* repressor. V. Repressors which bind operator more tightly generated by suppression and reversion of nonsense mutations. *J. Mol. Biol.* (in press).

Schmitz, A., U. Schmeissner, J. H. Miller, and P. Lu. 1976. Mutations affecting the quaternary structure of the *lac* repressor. *J. Biol. Chem.* **251**:3359.

Shine, J. and L. Dalgarno. 1974. The 3′-terminal sequences of *Escherichia coli* 16S ribosomal RNA: Complementarity to nonsense triplets and ribosome binding sites. *Proc. Natl. Acad. Sci.* **71**:1342.

Smith, T. F. and J. R. Sadler. 1971. The nature of lactose operator constitutive mutations. *J. Mol. Biol.* **92**:93.

Sommer, H. 1977. Biochemical characterization of *lac* repressor proteins produced by suppression of two amber mutations. *J. Mol. Biol.* **109**:275.

Sommer, H., P. Lu, and J. H. Miller. 1976. *Lac* repressor: Fluorescence of the two tryptophans. *J. Biol. Chem.* **251**:3774.

Sommer, H., A. Schmitz, U. Schmeissner, J. H. Miller, and H. G. Wittman. 1978. Genetic studies of the *lac* repressor. VI. The B116 repressor: An altered *lac* repressor containing amino acids specified by both the *trp* and *lacI* leader regions. *J. Mol. Biol.* (in press).

Steege, D. A. 1977. 5′-Terminal nucleotide sequence of *Escherichia coli* lactose repressor mRNA: Features of translational initiation and reinitiation sites. *Proc. Natl. Acad. Sci.* **74**:4163.

Steitz, J. A., K. U. Sprague, D. A. Steege, R. C. Yuan, M. Laughrea, P. B. Moore, and A. J. Wahba. 1977. In *Nucleic acid-protein recognition* (ed. H. J. Vogel), p. 491. Academic Press, New York.

Streisinger, G., Y. Okada, J. Emrich, J. Newton, A. Tsuguta, E. Terzaghi, and M. Inouye. 1966. Frameshift mutations and the genetic code. *Cold Spring Harbor Symp. Quant. Biol.* **31**:77.

von Hippel, P. H., A. Revzin, C. A. Gross, and A. C. Wang. 1974. Non-specific DNA binding of genome regulating proteins as a biological control mechanism. I. The *lac* operon: Equilibrium aspects. *Proc. Natl. Acad. Sci.* **71**:4808.

Weber, K., T. Platt, D. Ganem, and J. H. Miller. 1972. Altered sequences changing the operator-binding properties of the *lac* repressor: Colinearity of the repressor protein with the *i*-gene map. *Proc. Natl. Acad. Sci.* **69**:3624.

Weber, K., J. G. Files, T. Platt, D. Ganem, and J. H. Miller. 1975. *Lac* repressor. In *Protein-ligand interactions* (ed. H. Sund and G. Blauer), p. 228. Walter de Gruyter, Berlin.

Went, F. C. 1901. *J. Wiss. Bot.* **36:**611.

Willson, C., D. Perrin, M. Cohn, F. Jacob, and J. Monod. 1964. Non-inducible mutants of the regulator gene in the "lactose" system of *Escherichia coli. J. Mol. Biol.* **8:**582.

Wollman, E. and F. Jacob. 1955. Sur le mécanisme du transfert de materiel génitique au cours de la recombinaison chez *Escherichia coli* K12. *C. R. Acad. Sci.* **240:**2449.

————. 1959. *La sexualité des bactéries.* Masson et Cie, Paris.

Yanofsky, C., J. Ito, and V. Horn. 1967. Amino acid replacements and the genetic code. *Cold Spring Harbor Symp. Quant. Biol.* **31:**151.

Zabin, I., A. Kepes, and J. Monod. 1959. On the enzymic acetylation of isopropyl-β-D-thiogalactoside and its association with galactoside permease. *Biochem. Biophys. Res. Commun.* **1:**289.

β-Galactosidase, the Lactose Permease Protein, and Thiogalactoside Transacetylase

Irving Zabin and Audrée V. Fowler
Department of Biological Chemistry, School of Medicine
and Molecular Biology Institute
University of California, Los Angeles 90024

INTRODUCTION

The three structural genes of the *lac* operon, *Z*, *Y*, and *A*, code for β-galactosidase, the lactose permease protein, and thiogalactoside transacetylase, respectively. Since the discussion of these gene products in *The Lactose Operon* (Zabin and Fowler 1970; Kennedy 1970), a considerable amount of work has been carried out, particularly on β-galactosidase. In 1970 the subunit structure of this enzyme was known with reasonable certainty, but some controversy remained. Now the primary structure has been completed. Much new information is available on β-galactosidase from strains with mutations in the *lacZ* gene, on complementation, and on immunological properties. Interesting fusion proteins have been described. Considerably less information has been accumulated on the *lacY* gene product, and in fact, the lactose permease protein has not yet been obtained in chemically pure form. The function of thiogalactoside transacetylase has been a mystery for a long time. Recently evidence has been presented for a possible physiological role in the cell. A detailed study of its enzymatic characteristics has been carried out, and a beginning has been made toward determining the amino acid sequence of this protein.

Such information on the three proteins is presented here and is discussed primarily from a biochemical point of view.

β-GALACTOSIDASE

Production and Isolation

β-Galactosidase (β-D-galactoside galactohydrolase E. C. 3.2.1.23) accounts for up to 5% of the total protein in haploid strains of *Escherichia coli*. Considerably higher levels can be obtained from certain partial diploids

(Fowler 1972a). When the strain A324-5 was grown on minimal medium containing succinate as carbon source, the amount of β-galactosidase produced was more than 20% of the soluble protein. Growth of the cells and isolation of the lactose proteins were found to be considerably more convenient and efficient with this strain than with other hyperproducing strains. The conditions for growth of the wild-type merodiploid were also used for merodiploid strains of *E. coli* containing mutations in the *lacZ* gene (Villarejo and Zabin 1974; Langley et al. 1975b).

The standard procedure for obtaining a large amount of enzyme has been ammonium sulfate fractionation and DEAE-cellulose chromatography. In some cases the protein was purified further by gel filtration on Sephadex. β-Galactosidase has also been purified on a free-flow electrophoresis apparatus (Fowler 1972a). Recently DEAE-Bio-Gel columns have been used in this laboratory with excellent results. Losses which occur on DEAE-cellulose due to irreversible absorption did not occur on DEAE-Bio-Gel, and yields were high.

Affinity chromatography has also been used for the isolation of β-galactosidase. Tomino and Paigen (1970) coupled β-aminophenyl β-D-thiogalactoside (a competitive inhibitor of β-galactosidase) to crosslinked γ globulin. The same substrate analog was used in an extensive study of affinity chromatography of β-galactosidase in which it was found that agarose was a good support for the analog whereas polyacrylamide was ineffective. The length of the "linker arm" was critical; 21 Å was the best length (Steers et al. 1971; Steers and Cuatrecasas 1974).

It has been pointed out that the purification of β-galactosidase by such columns is not true affinity chromatography but that hydrophobic and ionic interactions play a very large role in the binding of the protein to the adsorbent (Nishikawa and Bailon 1975). β-Galactosidase was bound so tenaciously to 1,6-diaminohexane linked to agarose that it could be eluted only with 4 M guanidine. Several ionic and neutral linker arms were also tested with similar results. Hydrophobic chromatography on agarose-L-valine has been used to purify β-galactosidase (Rimerman and Hatfield 1973). In this case proteins were applied to the column in 1 M potassium phosphate and eluted with a decreasing concentration gradient of the same salt. Although it was concluded by Nishikawa and Bailon (1975) that the binding of β-galactosidase to the substrate analog is somewhat fortuitous, it seems probable that affinity plays some role in the binding. Buffers containing lactose or substrate analogs *can* elute β-galactosidase from affinity columns, but rather inefficiently (Steers and Cuatrecasas 1974). No matter what the mechanism, these columns have been used not only for β-galactosidase but for the purification of β-galactosidase-specific polysomes (Melcher 1975) and for polypeptides from strains with mutations in the Z gene (Villarejo and Zabin 1974; Langley et al. 1975b).

Subunit and Quaternary Structure

The evidence that β-galactosidase is a tetramer of four identical subunits has been reviewed and is well documented (Zabin and Fowler 1970; Wallenfels and Weil 1972). Molecular-weight measurements of the native protein in the ultracentrifuge have ranged from about 490,000 to 540,000. It has been pointed out that the correct value is probably closer to the lower number, since enzyme preparations contained small amounts of heavier material (Wallenfels and Weil 1972). The original report on higher forms indicated that there were at least seven enzymatically active electrophoretic forms in extracts of wild-type strains (Appel et al. 1965). At least 30% of the enzyme isolated from the hyperproducing strain was found to be in higher aggregates (Fowler 1972a). Estimates of the subunit size in 8 M urea or 6 M guanidine vary similarly, from 118,000 to 147,000 daltons. From the sequence analysis (see below) the monomer molecular weight is about 116,350 and the tetramer about 465,400.

The effects of pH, ionic strength, D_2O, and protein concentration on the association-dissociation behavior of β-galactosidase have been studied in detail (Contaxis et al. 1973). At low ionic strength and/or low protein concentrations, the protein dissociated into monomers, and at high ionic strength and protein concentrations, the protein hyperassociated, i.e., formed aggregates higher than the tetramer. In 90% glycerol, β-galactosidase dissociated to inactive monomers. Active tetramer reformed upon removal of the glycerol (Contaxis and Reithel 1971).

The tetramer and the higher aggregates are probably the only active forms of the enzyme. This is suggested by several lines of evidence. Many proteins which are enzymatically inactive are found to be dimers. For example, proteins from the missense mutant 3310 and the deletion mutant M15 are dimers (Steers and Shifrin 1967; Langley et al. 1975b). The protein from the antibody-activatable mutant S30 is a dimer (B. Rotman and E. Macario, pers. comm.), and addition of antibody results in tetramer formation. Certain inactivating antibodies dissociate the native tetrameric enzyme (Roth and Rotman 1975a). Activation of M15 protein by anti-β-galactosidase can occur, and the active material is a tetramer (Accolla and Celada 1976; F. Celada and I. Zabin, unpubl.). Finally, when an active enzyme is formed by either ω or α complementation, it always exists as a tetramer (Ullmann and Perrin 1970; Langley and Zabin 1976). There was one report of an active dimer formed in the presence of Ag^+ (Kaneshiro et al. 1975), but the level of activity was not given. It seems possible that this is an equilibrium form and that during enzyme assay the isolated dimer might tetramerize. A "260-nm absorbing compound" bound to β-galactosidase has been described, with the suggestion that this may act as a stabilizer for the tetrameric form (Contaxis and Reithel 1974). However, this compound has not been characterized further.

Primary Structure

The proposed amino acid sequence of β-galactosidase is shown in Figure 1, and the composition in Table 1. The monomer contains 1021 residues in a single polypeptide chain—fewer than the 1170 assumed previously on the basis of physical measurements of molecular weight. The sequence determination was done by conventional biochemical procedures but was aided by complementation studies, by the use of termination mutants, by a new immunochemical method, and by a correlative study on the DNA sequence of part of the *lacZ* gene. The analysis was initiated by tryptic cleavage of carboxymethyl-β-galactosidase. From this digest, 60 peptides were isolated in pure form (Fowler and Zabin 1970). A second tryptic digest was prepared from protein which was first treated with maleic anhydride to react with lysine residues so that cleavage would occur only at arginine residues (Fowler 1972b). Eighteen additional peptides were obtained in pure form. Peptides from the two digests accounted for 968 amino acid residues of the subunit, and most of the smaller peptides (up to 20 residues) were sequenced by the manual Edman plus dansylation procedure. In addition, the amino- and carboxyl-terminal tryptic peptides were identified (Zabin and Fowler 1972). There are 75 unique tryptic

Table 1 Amino acid composition of β-galactosidase

	Analysis	Sequence[a]
Trytophan	27	39
Lysine	23	20
Histidine	31	34
Arginine	64	66
Aspartic acid	105	111
Threonine	59	56
Serine	60	60
Glutamic acid	124	119
Proline	62	64
Glycine	72	70
Alanine	81	76
Half-cystine	15	16
Valine	64	63
Methionine	23	23
Isoleucine	38	39
Leucine	96	96
Tyrosine	29	31
Phenylalanine	38	38
Total	1011	1021

[a]Calculated molecular weight is 116,349.

peptides, 3 residues of free lysine, and 2 residues of free arginine from Arg-Lys, Lys-Lys, and Lys-Arg bonds. Three peptides have Lys-Pro bonds and 3 peptides have Arg-Pro bonds, none of which are cleaved by trypsin.

To place the tryptic peptides in order, the carboxymethylated protein was treated with chymotrypsin (A. V. Fowler, unpubl.). The 71 chymotryptic peptides isolated ranged in size from 2 to 26 residues and, after sequencing, gave a number of overlaps with tryptic peptides.

Cleavage of β-galactosidase with cyanogen bromide (CNBr) should yield 24 peptides, since there are 23 methionine residues per subunit. In an earlier study, the gel-electrophoresis banding pattern after a preliminary gel-filtration step indicated 20 to 25 peptides (Steers et al. 1965). However, that value was probably high because bands were formed on the gel by both the homoserine and homoserine lactone forms of each peptide. Amino-terminal analysis of the cyanogen bromide cleavage products indicated 23 peptides with 11 different amino acids (Katze et al. 1966). Because of its small size and ether solubility, the amino-terminal cyanogen bromide peptide (CB1, Thr-Met) was easily isolated and identified. Twenty-three additional peptides, ranging up to 119 residues in size, have been isolated in pure form. Special techniques were developed for their purification (Fowler 1975). Chromatography on cellulose and Sephadex ion exchangers was used extensively, particularly in the presence of 8 M urea. Before ion-exchange chromatography, eight small peptides were separated by Sephadex G-25 filtration. The larger peptides, excluded by the gel, were chromatographed at pH 5.0 on a carboxymethylcellulose column in ammonium acetate buffer containing 8 M urea and were eluted with a salt gradient. The elution pattern of the 16 large CNBr peptides can be seen in Figure 2. Some of the peaks in the profile represented fragments not cleaved completely at certain methionine residues or peptides derived by cleavage at Asp-Pro bonds, which are very susceptible to low pH. Some peptides were pure at this stage, but most were obtained in pure form after gel filtration on Sephadex G-50. In some cases an additional ion-exchange step was necessary, and this was carried out on sulphopropyl (SP) Sephadex at pH 2.5 in ammonium formate buffer containing 8 M urea or on diethyl-(2-hydroxypropyl) aminoethyl (QAE) Sephadex at pH 8.4 in ammonium chloride. The criteria of purity for the peptides included amino-terminal analysis, electrophoresis on 7.5% cross-linked gels containing urea, and automatic-sequencer analysis. All of the CNBr peptides were sequenced by automatic-sequencer methods supplemented as necessary by further cleavages with trypsin, chymotrypsin, thermolysin, and a glutamic-acid-specific staphylococcal protease.

The CNBr peptides were placed in order mainly by comparison with the sequences in tryptic and chymotryptic peptides. The ordering was aided by other techniques. One of these was the use of α complementation and was based on the finding that a CNBr digest contained α-donor

```
          10                    20                    30
Thr-Met-Ile-Thr-Asp-Ser-Leu-Ala-Val-Val-Leu-Gln-Arg-Arg-Asp-Trp-Glu-Asn-Pro-Gly-Val-Thr-Gln-Leu-Asn-Arg-Leu-Ala-Ala-His-
CNBr1
MTS4

          40                    50                    60
Pro-Pro-Phe-Ala-Ser-Trp-Arg-Asn-Ser-Glu-Glu-Ala-Arg-Thr-Asp-Arg-Pro-Ser-Gln-Gln-Leu-Arg-Ser-Leu-Asn-Gly-Glu-Trp-Arg-Phe-
                                    CNBr2

          70                    80                    90
Ala-Trp-Phe-Pro-Ala-Pro-Glu-Ala-Val-Pro-Glu-Ser-Trp-Leu-Glu-Cys-Asp-Leu-Pro-Glu-Ala-Asp-Thr-Val-Val-Val-Pro-Ser-Asn-Trp-
                              MTIn8

          100                   110                   120
Gln-Met-His-Gly-Tyr-Asp-Ala-Pro-Ile-Tyr-Thr-Asn-Val-Thr-Tyr-Pro-Ile-Thr-Val-Asn-Pro-Pro-Phe-Val-Pro-Thr-Glu-Asn-Pro-Thr-

          130                   140                   150
Gly-Cys-Tyr-Ser-Leu-Thr-Phe-Asn-Val-Asp-Glu-Ser-Trp-Leu-Gln-Glu-Gly-Gln-Thr-Arg-Ile-Ile-Phe-Asp-Gly-Val-Asn-Ser-Ala-Phe-
                                    CNBr3

          160                   170                   180
His-Leu-Trp-Cys-Asn-Gly-Arg-Trp-Val-Gly-Tyr-Gly-Gln-Asp-Ser-Arg-Leu-Pro-Ser-Glu-Phe-Asp-Leu-Ser-Ala-Phe-Leu-Arg-Ala-Gly-

          190                   200                   210
Glu-Asn-Arg-Leu-Ala-Val-Met-Val-Leu-Arg-Trp-Ser-Asp-Gly-Ser-Tyr-Leu-Glu-Asp-Gln-Asp-Met-Trp-Arg-Met-Ser-Gly-Ile-Phe-Arg-
           TB14        CNBr4          TA12          CNBr5        TN3

          220                   230                   240
Asp-Val-Ser-Leu-Leu-His-Lys-Pro-Thr-Thr-Gln-Ile-Ser-Asp-Phe-His-Val-Ala-Thr-Arg-Phe-Asn-Asp-Asp-Phe-Ser-Arg-Ala-Val-Leu-
                              CNBr6

          250                   260                   270
Glu-Ala-Glu-Val-Gln-Met-Cys-Gly-Glu-Leu-Arg-Asp-Tyr-Leu-Arg-Val-Thr-Val-Ser-Leu-Trp-Gln-Gly-Glu-Thr-Gln-Val-Ala-Ser-Gly-
MTS2
```

Figure 1 (Continued on pages following.)

94

```
                              280                        290                        300
Thr-Ala-Pro-Phe-Gly-Gly-Glu-Ile-Ile-Asp-Glu-Arg-Gly-Gly-Tyr-Ala-Asp-Arg-Val-Thr-Leu-Arg-Leu-Asn-Val-Glu-Asn-Pro-Lys-Leu-

                              310                        320                        330
Trp-Ser-Ala-Glu-Ile-Pro-Asn-Leu-Tyr-Arg-Ala-Val-Val-Glu-Leu-His-Thr-Ala-Asp-Gly-Gln-Leu-Ile-Glu-Ala-Gly-Thr-Cys-Asp-Phe-
                                                                       CNBr7

                              340                        350                        360
Arg-Glu-Val-Arg-Ile-Glu-Asn-Gly-Leu-Leu-Leu-Leu-Asn-Gly-Lys-Pro-Leu-Leu-Ile-Arg-Gly-Val-Asn-Arg-His-Gln-His-His-Pro-Leu-

                              370                        380                        390
His-Gly-Gln-Val-Met-Asp-Glu-Gln-Thr-Met-Val-Gln-Asp-Ile-Leu-Leu-Met-Lys-Gln-Asn-Asn-Phe-Asn-Ala-Val-Arg-Cys-Ser-His-Tyr-
                  CNBr8          CT16A              CNBr9

                              400                        410                        420
Pro-Asn-His-Pro-Leu-Trp-Tyr-Thr-Leu-Cys-Asp-Arg-Tyr-Gly-Leu-Tyr-Val-Val-Asp-Glu-Ala-Asp-Ile-Glu-Thr-His-Gly-Met-Val-Pro-
                  CNBr10                              MTS6                           CNBr11

                              430                        440                        450
Met-Asn-Arg-Leu-Thr-Asp-Asp-Pro-Arg-Trp-Leu-Pro-Ala-Met-Ser-Glu-Arg-Val-Thr-Arg-Met-Val-Gln-Arg-Asp-Arg-Asn-His-Pro-Ser-
          CNBr12              TN23              CNBr13              TB16

                              460                        470                        480
Val-Ile-Ile-Trp-Ser-Leu-Gly-Asn-Glu-Ser-Gly-His-Gly-Ala-Asn-His-Asp-Ala-Leu-Tyr-Arg-Trp-Ile-Lys-Ser-Val-Asp-Pro-Ser-Arg-
                                                  CNBr14

                              490                        500                        510
Pro-Val-Gln-Tyr-Glu-Gly-Gly-Gly-Ala-Asp-Thr-Thr-Ala-Thr-Asp-Ile-Ile-Cys-Pro-Met-Tyr-Ala-Arg-Val-Asp-Glu-Asp-Gln-Pro-Phe-
                  MTS1
```

520   530   540
Pro-Ala-Val-Pro-Lys-Trp-Ser-Ile-Lys-Lys-Trp-Leu-Ser-Leu-Pro-Gly-Glu-Thr-Arg-Pro-Leu-Ile-Leu-Cys-Glu-Tyr-Ala-His-Ala-Met-
CNBr15   TN8

550   560   570
Gly-Asn-Ser-Leu-Gly-Gly-Phe-Ala-Lys-Tyr-Trp-Gln-Ala-Phe-Arg-Gln-Pro-Arg-Leu-Gln-Pro-Gly-Phe-Val-Trp-Asp-Trp-Val-Asp-
CNBr16

580   590   600
Gln-Ser-Leu-Ile-Lys-Tyr-Asp-Glu-Asn-Gly-Asn-Pro-Trp-Ser-Ala-Tyr-Gly-Gly-Asp-Phe-Gly-Asp-Thr-Pro-Asp-Asp-Arg-Gln-Phe-Cys-
C8

610   620   630
Met-Asn-Gly-Leu-Val-Phe-Ala-Asp-Arg-Thr-Pro-His-Pro-Ala-Leu-Thr-Glu-Ala-Lys-His-Gln-Gln-Gln-Phe-Phe-Gln-Phe-Arg-Leu-Ser-
CNBr17

640   650   660
Gly-Gln-Thr-Ile-Glu-Val-Thr-Ser-Glu-Tyr-Leu-Phe-Arg-His-Ser-Asp-Asn-Glu-Leu-Leu-His-Trp-Met-Val-Ala-Leu-Asp-Gly-Lys-Pro-
CT3A

670   680   690
Leu-Ala-Ser-Gly-Glu-Val-Pro-Leu-Asp-Val-Ala-Pro-Gln-Gly-Lys-Gln-Leu-Ile-Glu-Leu-Gln-Leu-Pro-Gln-Pro-Glu-Ser-Ala-Gly-
CNBr18

700   710   720
Pro-Leu-Trp-Leu-Thr-Val-Arg-Val-Val-Gln-Pro-Asn-Ala-Thr-Ala-Trp-Ser-Glu-Ala-Gly-His-Ile-Ser-Ala-Trp-Gln-Gln-Trp-Arg-Leu-

730   740   750
Ala-Glu-Asn-Leu-Ser-Val-Thr-Leu-Pro-Ala-Ala-Ser-His-Ala-Ile-Pro-His-Leu-Thr-Thr-Ser-Glu-Met-Asp-Phe-Cys-Ile-Glu-Leu-Gly-
TN1

760   770   780
Asn-Lys-Arg-Trp-Gln-Phe-Asn-Arg-Gln-Ser-Gly-Phe-Leu-Ser-Gln-Met-Trp-Ile-Gly-Asp-Lys-Lys-Gln-Leu-Leu-Thr-Pro-Leu-Arg-Asp-
CNBr19   TB6

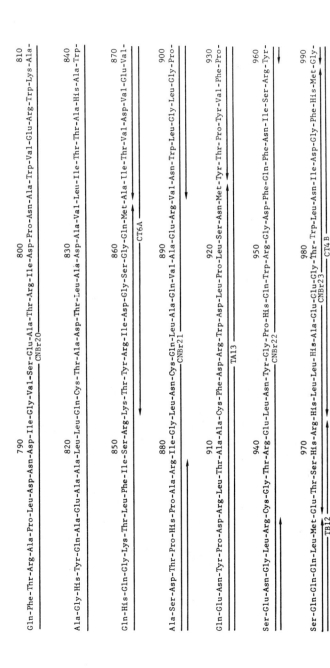

Figure 1 Amino acid sequence of β-galactosidase.

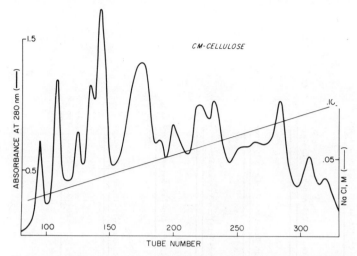

Figure 2   Carboxymethyl-cellulose chromatography of CNBr peptides of β-galactosidase. Peptides excluded from Sephadex G-25 were applied to a column (1.5 × 20 cm) in 0.02 M ammonium acetate (pH 5.0), 8 M urea and were eluted with a linear gradient of 0–0.15 M NaCl in the same buffer. Total volume 600 ml.

activity for an extract of the deletion mutant M15 (Lin et al. 1970). The purification of the complementing peptide could therefore be monitored by its biological activity. The isolation and sequence analysis of this peptide, CB2, which is derived from residues 3–92, have been reported (Langley et al. 1975a).

A second procedure involved the use of termination mutations such as *NG125*, which maps near the center of the *lacZ* gene. The resulting polypeptide of molecular weight about 60,000 corresponding to the amino-terminal half of β-galactosidase was isolated (Fowler and Zabin 1966; Villarejo and Zabin 1974). After treatment with CNBr, the products were chromatographed on carboxymethylcellulose under conditions identical to those used for the whole protein. The elution profile was used as a kind of fingerprint. The peptides which were identified could therefore be assigned to the amino-terminal half of the polypeptide chain (A. V. Fowler et al. unpubl.).

A third aid to the sequence determination was a new immunochemical method devised for this purpose (A. Brake et al., unpubl.). Antibodies have been prepared against many CNBr peptides, as described under Immunological Properties. Some of these have been used to find overlapping peptides. For example, a tryptic peptide which overlaps CB21 and CB22 was detected in the following way: Anti-CB21 was prepared and was tested by a binding assay with ^{125}I-labeled CB21. This binding was found to be inhibited by a tryptic digest. Fractionation of the digest yielded a specific inhibiting tryptic peptide. Sequence analysis of this peptide showed that it contained the carboxyl-terminal 31 residues of CB21 and the amino-terminal 13 residues of CB22 and was therefore the necessary overlap. Thus a considerable amount of time was saved by avoiding the necessity of examining many fractions in order to locate the desired peptide.

Finally, the sequence determination was helped by a correlative study on the DNA sequence of part of the *lacZ* gene by A. Maxam and W. Gilbert (at the meeting on Molecular Aspects of *lac* Operon Control, July 1976, Cold Spring Harbor). Amino acid residues 1–145 were found to agree with the assignments predicted from the DNA sequence. Several minor uncertainties could be resolved, for example, an amide assignment at residue 135. The region around amino acids 120–130 was particularly interesting since this corresponds to the DNA region of the second operator binding site (Reznikoff et al. 1974; Gilbert et al. 1975).

Completion of the sequence determination proves, of course, that there are no smaller subunits making up the monomer of β-galactosidase. The polypeptide chain of 1021 amino acid residues is the largest that has been sequenced up to this time. There are several unique features besides its large size. One is an extremely high content of 39 tryptophan residues. These are spread throughout the molecule, with the notable exception that only three occur between residues 204 and 430. The 16 cysteine and the 23 methionine residues are located randomly except that all the small CNBr peptides are within the first half of the molecule. Interestingly, there is only one lysine residue before residue 300, a Lys-Pro bond in CB6 (residues 217–218). Except for the carboxyl-terminal residue, the remaining lysines are clustered between residues 299 and 852. Since it is generally believed that all lysine residues are on the exterior of protein molecules, this suggests that the amino- and carboxyl-terminal regions of the polypeptide chain of β-galactosidase are buried within the molecule.

The most obvious homologous feature within the protein is a five-residue sequence, Thr-Pro-His-Pro-Ala, which appears beginning at residue 610 and again at residue 874. No other striking duplication is present, but a more extensive search for internal homology and homology to the *lac* repressor is being undertaken.

Reaction Mechanism

The bond cleaved by β-galactosidase is between the anomeric carbon (C1) and the glycosyl oxygen (Wallenfels and Malhotra 1961; Wallenfels and Weil 1972). The enzyme is specific for the β-D-galactopyranoside configuration, but the aglycone can vary quite widely; it can be another sugar, an aryl, or an alkyl group. In addition to C—O bonds, the enzyme also cleaves C—F and C—N bonds. It can also cleave C—S bonds if electron-withdrawing substituents are present on the aromatic ring. The enzyme acts as a transferase as well as a hydrolase. The galactosyl moiety can be transferred to monosaccharides, oligosaccharides, alkyl alcohols, and phenols. Mercaptoethanol is a very good acceptor, whereas Tris is a very poor acceptor. β-Galactosidase can also transfer the galactosyl moiety from the 4 position to the 6 position of glucose to form allolactose, the natural inducer of the *lac* operon. It has recently been shown that at low concentrations of lactose the rearrangement is achieved without release of glucose (Huber et al. 1976). These authors also found that at higher concentrations trisaccharides and tetrasaccharides of lactose and allolactose were produced. It was also shown that allolactose is a better substrate for β-galactosidase than lactose (Huber et al. 1975). The K_m's of lactose and allolactose are 5.5×10^{-3} M and 6.3×10^{-4} M, respectively. The V_{max} for o-nitrophenyl-β-D-galactosidase (ONPG) hydrolysis is 15 times higher than for lactose and about 12 times higher than for allolactose.

The effects of Na^+ and Mg^{++} on β-galactosidase have been well studied, but the necessity for these cations is still unclear. A monovalent cation is required for activity. Sodium ion enhances the affinity of the enzyme for the substrate as well as the maximum rate of hydrolysis (Neville and Ling 1967). Recently it has been shown that Na^+ does not bind to the free enzyme but requires substrate for binding (Hill and Huber 1974). The enzyme is activated by Mg^{++} but can function without any divalent metal ion. In a system containing Na^+ at optimal concentrations, divalent metal ions activate when assayed at low concentrations (Ca^{++}, Zn^{++}, Fe^{++}, Mn^{++}, and Co^{++} but not Cu^{++}, Pb^{++}, and Hg^{++}). One Mg^{++} is bound per monomer (Case et al. 1973).

The pH optimum of the enzyme is about 7.2. From the pH profile, it was concluded that two groups are important in the catalysis: one protonated group which ionizes in the alkaline range and one unprotonated group which ionizes in the acidic range (Tenu et al. 1971). A carboxylate has been suggested for the low-pK group. The pK of the alkaline group shifts from 8.4 in the presence of Mg^{++} to 6.5 in the absence of Mg^{++}. The nature of this group is unknown.

Hydrolysis by all glycosidases resembles acid-catalyzed hydrolysis in that cleavage of the glycosyl C—1 oxygen occurs. The mechanism of the reaction of β-galactosidase therefore has been looked upon as quite analogous to that of lysozyme. However, evidence has been accumulating suggesting that a galactosyl-enzyme intermediate is formed with β-galactosidase, whereas lysozyme forms a stabilized carbonium ion. A common intermediate appeared to be formed in the hydrolysis of various aryl-β-galactosides (Stokes and Wilson 1972). However, these studies could not differentiate between a galactosyl enzyme and a stabilized carbonium ion. The inhibitor D-galactal was shown to combine very slowly with β-galactosidase and then release 2-deoxygalactose, which suggested a galactosyl-enzyme-like intermediate (Wentworth and Wolferden 1974). A D_2O effect was also observed, which suggested a process involving formation of a bond from C to H or D, but the intermediate could not be trapped. A burst of ONPG hydrolysis stoichiometric with enzyme concentration was demonstrated when the reaction was carried out below 10°C in 50% dimethylsulfoxide (Fink and Angelides 1975). Such a burst indicates the existence of a galactosyl-enzyme intermediate. The Arrhenius plot for turnover gave an E_a of 26 ± 3 kcal/mole. Recently a burst of ONPG hydrolysis was also seen with β-galactosidase resulting from a *lacZ* missense mutation (J. M. Yon, pers. comm.). The mechanism can be written as follows:

$$E + S \underset{k_{-1}}{\overset{k_1}{\rightleftharpoons}} ES \xrightarrow{k_2} E - G + P_1 \xrightarrow{k_3} E + P_2.$$

Thus far, no residues in the active site of β-galactosidase have been identified. An early photooxidation study indicated that a histidine residue might be involved (Proctor 1962). However, as pointed out by Wallenfels and Weil (1972), destruction of residues other than histidine might have occurred. β-Galactosidase can be inactivated by the site-specific reagent N-bromoacetyl-β-D-galactopyranosylamine (Naider et al. 1972). This reagent was shown to react reversibly with a single methionine near the active site, but methionine is not part of the active site since norleucine can replace methionine without loss of activity. Studies with β-galactosidase fragments from termination mutants indicate that the reactive methionine is within the amino-terminal two-thirds of the molecule (Villarejo and Zabin 1973). The enzyme is inactivated by reaction with β-D-galactopyranosylmethyl-p-nitrophenyltriazene (Sinnott and Smith 1976) and is protected from inactivation by methyl-1-thio-β-D-galactoside. The reagent 2,6-anhydro-1-diazo-1-deoxy-D-glycero-L-manno-heptitol also inactivates β-galactoside, and the enzyme can similarly be protected by isopropyl-thio-β-D-galactoside (IPTG) (Brockhaus and Lehmann 1976). Both these reagents produce very active compounds which might react with almost any functional group in the area of the active site.

Proteins from Mutant Strains

Mutationally altered proteins have been especially useful in studying gene-protein and structure-function relationships involving β-galactosidase. By examination of termination mutant strains, it was shown that the gene and the protein are oriented so that operator-proximal and operator-distal ends of the *lacZ* gene specify amino and carboxyl termini of β-galactosidase (Fowler and Zabin 1966; Brown et al. 1967a). Fragments have been isolated and purified from a number of termination and deletion mutant strains (Berg et al. 1970; Villarejo and Zabin 1974). These polypeptide chains were found to have molecular weights and properties which could be predicted from the nature and position of the mutation. For example, from a strain carrying the amber mutation *NG200*, which maps about two-thirds of the distance to the *lacY* gene, a fragment was isolated with a molecular weight of 89,000 determined by sedimentation equilibrium in guanidine hydrochloride. This fragment reacts strongly against anti-β-galactosidase. Antibodies were prepared with the fragment as antigen and were found to be very similar to anti-β-galactosidase (Berg et al. 1970). Such results have indicated that many mutationally altered proteins, though they do not contain the complete sequence, nevertheless fold in a manner similar to that of the native molecule.

Many fragments bind to affinity columns with a galactoside ligand (Villarejo and Zabin 1973). Those chains (M15, NG200, X90; see Fig. 3) which contain all of the central (or β) region of the β-galactosidase molecule are retained on the column. Some polypeptides (NG125, X82, U163) which contain the sequence corresponding to the operator-proximal portion of the β region are retarded by the column, and some fragments (W4680, B9) containing none of this sequence are excluded. Although the behavior of these chains on the column might not represent "true" affinity as discussed above, it seems reasonable to believe that retention of a fragment on the column is due, at least in part, to the presence of a substrate binding site. If this is so, then it is evident that folding of the β region of the molecule is crucial to the formation of a binding site.

It is now well recognized that mutationally altered proteins may be rapidly degraded in bacteria (cf. Goldberg and Dice 1974; Goldberg and St. John 1976). Goldschmidt (1970), in pulse-chase experiments, followed the disappearance of the β-galactosidase chain from ochre mutant X90 using SDS gel electrophoresis to measure the amount of the incomplete chain. The rates of degradation of fragments from many termination and deletion mutants were determined by Lin and Zabin (1972) using as assay α complementation after CNBr treatment of cells. In this case it was assumed that the amount of amino-terminal segment of the chain was equivalent to the amount of the whole fragment. Though fragments in

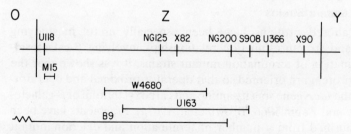

Figure 3 Map positions of β-galactosidase mutants.

general were found to be rapidly degraded, there were large differences in rates. For example, large termination fragments were relatively stable, but small ones had very short half-lives. In some cases the smaller fragments were not at all detectable in cell extracts. It was also of interest that fragments resulting from certain chain-termination mutations which map in the β region were degraded more rapidly than a fragment resulting from a neighboring mutation specifying a smaller chain. These results indicate that the fragments could not have random shapes; if they did, the rates of degradation would have been identical or quite similar. Proteolysis is apparently very sensitive to small differences in conformation. In partial diploids, complementing fragments may be partially protected from degration (Villarejo et al. 1972).

The mechanism of degradation is not known. Mutant strains (*deg⁻* or *degʳ⁻*) which have a reduced ability to degrade fragments have been isolated by Bukhari and Zipser (1973) by selecting Lac⁺ revertants from partial diploids containing complementing pairs of fragments. This mutation was subsequently found to be the same as *lon⁻* (Shineberg and Zipser 1973). It was also shown that the rate of disappearance of X90 fragment or of α-complementing donor peptide was less in strains carrying this mutation. Higher yields of isolated fragments were obtained from extracts of a termination mutant and a deletion mutant carrying the *deg⁻* mutation (Villarejo and Zabin 1974).

Mutations which create new sites in the *lacZ* gene for the reinitiation of polypeptide synthesis have been discovered and mapped (Grodzicker and Zipser 1968; Michels and Zipser 1969; Newton 1969). These "restart" fragments have been detected by their ability to act as donors in ω complementation but have not been characterized further. A mutation (*degʳ⁻*) in which these reinitiation fragments are more stable has also been detected (Apte et al. 1975), but the two *deg* mutations may very well be identical. It would be difficult to see on what basis termination and restart chains could be distinguished by proteolytic enzymes.

Since the rate of proteolysis depends partly on the conformation and/or degree of denaturation of the substrate, it is evident that not only protein derived from termination and deletion mutant strains but also protein from missense mutant strains may be subject to degradation. One of the criteria sometimes used to distinguish between termination and missense mutant strains is the cross-reactivity with antibody; the assumptions are that extracts of the former contain no cross-reacting material (CRM), while extracts of the latter do contain CRM. Both assumptions may be wrong. Clearly, if the missense mutation affects conformation drastically, the protein may become subject to degradation and extracts may be CRM⁻. In such cases, the amount of defective β-galactosidase remaining in extracts will be inversely proportional to the half-life of the rate of degradation.

A number of termination and missense mutants were examined by Truman and Bergquist (1976). Several of the latter were found to be CRM⁻. In other cases bands identical to β-galactosidase in molecular weight and absent in uninduced strains were detected on sodium dodecyl sulfate (SDS) gels. Such materials were also able to serve as α or ω donors in complementation. Reaction with antibody is thus not an adequate test by itself to distinguish between different classes of mutants.

Because β-galactosidase is such a large protein, it seems likely that many amino acid substitutions would perturb the structure to a small extent or not at all. According to Langridge (1974a), most missense mutations in β-galactosidase have little effect on activity unless the amino acid substituted is involved in substrate binding. Many amber and ochre mutations mapping throughout the gene can be suppressed by serine and glutamine suppressors with restoration of activity. Certain of the mutationally altered proteins have altered substrate binding, tertiary structure, and quaternary structure (Langridge 1968a,b, 1974b). Even the incorporation of selenomethionine in place of methionine into β-galactosidase results in normal activity and normal reaction with antibody, although the enzyme is more susceptible to denaturation by heat or urea and to attack by trypsin (Spizek et al. 1972). Norleucine also can replace methionine in β-galactosidase without loss of catalytic activity (Naider et al. 1972).

Complementation

Several reviews of β-galactosidase complementation have appeared (Ullmann and Perrin 1970; Zabin and Villarejo 1975). On the basis of early complementation experiments, the lacZ gene was divided into three regions, α, β, and ω. The α corresponds to the operator-proximal fourth, the ω corresponds to the terminal third, and the β region is the center of the gene. These are still useful designations even though the original basis for this definition has undergone some modification. Of cardinal importance to the proper interpretation of complementation data is the recognition that degradation of protein fragments may occur, sometimes very rapidly. Therefore a negative result must be interpreted with caution.

α Complementation has become much better understood in recent years. The usual acceptor for in vivo or in vitro α-complementation experiments is the defective β-galactosidase from strain M15 which has a deletion in the operator-proximal portion of the lacZ gene (Fig. 3). Donors are peptides containing the missing sequence. In the original experiments describing α complementation, only those termination mutations which mapped at least one-fourth of the distance into the lacZ gene resulted in sources of α donors (Ullmann et al. 1967). Later the surprising observation was made that autoclaved extracts of induced wild-type strains or of certain mutant strains contained a soluble peptide fraction which was an effective α donor. The molecular weight of the active material, determined in sucrose gradients, was about 7400 (Morrison and Zipser 1970). Following this observation, α-donor activity was found in cyanogen bromide digests of β-galactosidase (Lin et al. 1970). As discussed in the section on Primary Structure, the active peptide, CB2, is derived from residues 3–92 of the polypeptide chain (Langley et al. 1975a). An active peptide comprising residues 1–75 can also be obtained by treating β-galactosidase with 2-nitro-5-thiocyanobenzoic acid, which cleaves peptide chains at the amino-terminal side of cysteine residues (J. E. Snoke, unpubl.). Therefore, considerably less than the amino-terminal fourth of the polypeptide chain suffices for α complementation.

Both the autoclave procedure and the CNBr cleavage procedure have been used as assays for α-donor fragments. The autoclave method is probably simpler to use with large numbers of samples, but the cyanogen bromide method is much more sensitive. Extracts containing β-galactosidase treated with CNBr gave seven times more α-donor activity than an equal amount of extract treated in the autoclave (Lin and Zabin 1972).

The α-acceptor M15 protein was obtained in pure form by ammonium sulfate fractionation and affinity chromatography (Langley et al. 1975b). From this material a CNBr peptide was isolated which was identical to CB2 except that it lacked 31 amino acid residues, the β-galactosidase residues 11–41. Molecular-weight estimates by analytical ultracentrifugation were 134,000 in 6 M guanidine and 265,000 in 0.1 M phosphate (pH 7.2), 70 mM 2-mercaptoethanol. Therefore, under the latter conditions, M15 protein is a dimer.

Under optimum conditions, the combination of pure M15 protein and pure CB2 results in complemented enzyme with more than 50% of the specific activity of the native enzyme (Langley et al. 1975a). The mechanism of the interaction is of considerable interest. For several reasons it is unlikely that CB2 supplies amino acid residues for the catalytic site. Although M15 protein is essentially enzymatically inactive, it does have a trace of activity (Langley and Zabin 1976). This is increased by antibody to as much as 15% of that attained with CB2 (Accolla and Celada 1976). Also, fusion proteins such as the *lac* repressor–β-galactosidase protein (Müller-Hill and Kania 1974) lack part or all of the 11–41 portion of the sequence and still have β-galactosidase activity.

Studies of the properties and kinetics of α complementation suggest that CB2 causes a conformational change (Langley and Zabin 1976). Initial velocity studies indicate saturation kinetics when either component, CB2 or M15 protein, is fixed and limiting. The kinetics favor a model of rapid complex formation, followed by slow conformational change, as the mechanism of activation. The complemented enzyme has a stoichiometry of 1 CB2 : 1 M15 and a molecular weight in the ultracen-trifuge of 533,000. Therefore the interaction results in conversion of dimeric M15 protein to tetrameric enzyme. The complemented enzyme has the same K_m for substrate as wild-type enzyme but is less stable to heat or urea treatment. Formation of active enzyme is slow, requiring 3 hours at 28°C for completion. Once formed, the complemented enzyme is not readily dissociated.

α-Complemented enzyme is also stable in growing cells (Villarejo et al. 1972). An episome carrying the gene for the M15 protein was introduced into 14 recipient hosts, each carrying a termination mutation at a different site in the Z gene (Zamenhof and Villarejo 1972). All of the merodiploids had enzyme activity except for one in which the termination mutation maps very close to the operator locus. The amount of complemented enzyme formed varied from strain to strain and was apparently dependent in part on the tertiary structure of the termination fragment. It is interesting that the complemented enzymes were not homogeneous. On dissociation in urea and sedimentation in urea-sucrose gradients, two peaks of α-donor activity were seen. This suggests that exposed overlapping segments had been subjected to some proteolysis in the cell.

ω-Complementing acceptor proteins are those which contain the amino-terminal two-thirds (α plus β) of the β-galactosidase polypeptide chain but lack completely or partially the terminal third of the protein. ω Donors supply this missing carboxyl segment. In one case it was claimed that a peptide fragment of molecular weight 18,000, obtained by gel filtration of a crude extract of M15, can serve as ω donor for an extract containing the missense mutant protein S908 (Marinkovic and Tang 1971). However, none of these fragments were characterized further. It seems more likely that an intact ω fragment is required, and that this forms a globule which binds to the remainder of the molecule to form active enzyme as suggested by Goldberg (1970). When ω-complemented enzyme was isolated in pure form from the partial diploid 366/B9 (Fig. 3), its molecular weight by sedimentation equilibrium was found to be 595,000. Brief treatment of this material with papain eliminated overlapping sequences, and the molecular weight was reduced to that of the wild-type enzyme, 540,000 (Goldberg and Edelstein 1969; Goldberg 1969).

Complementation between wild-type subunits and polypeptides from missense mutants has also been examined. Positive complementation of an antibody-activatable mutant by normal β-galactosidase has been reported in heterogenotes (Hall 1973). The protein formed in vivo contained 60% more enzyme activity than could be accounted for on the basis of the wild-type subunits alone. In contrast, no activation of mutationally altered protein was observed in in vitro reconstitution experiments (Melchers and Messer 1971). With the assay of Rotman (1961), which measures the activity of single β-galactosidase molecules, it was shown that each wild-type subunit was independently active and that the mutant subunit was inactive (Melchers and Messer 1973). The lack of agreement between the in vivo and in vitro results may be related to the mode or conditions of assembly or simply to a difference in the protein studied.

Fusion Proteins

A number of hybrid or chimeric proteins with β-galactosidase activity have been produced by the fusion of a portion of the *lacZ* gene to another gene. The first and so far best-characterized molecule was isolated by Müller-Hill and Kania (1974) from Lac$^+$ revertants of an *E. coli* strain carrying the *lac* repressor mutation I^q and the *lacZ* gene termination mutation *U118*. These strains had fully active *lac* repressor and active β-galactosidase. From one such strain, a protein with both activities was obtained in almost pure form. Its mobility on SDS gels was less than that of β-galactosidase. The site of the fusion is not known, but the difference in relative molecular weights suggests that perhaps 30 amino acids are missing from the carboxyl-terminal area of the *lac* repressor protein and the amino-terminal portion of β-galactosidase. The site of the mutation in *U118* is similarly not yet known, but since *U118* and M15 do not give active β-galactosidase on recombination, the termination mutation must be within the area of the gene coding for the first 41 amino acid residues.

More than 100 *I-Z* fusions have now been detected by selecting for β-galactosidase activity (Müller-Hill et al. 1976). The chimeric proteins produced by these strains range in size from those containing only a small number of residues derived from *lac* repressor to others with almost the complete *lac* repressor chain. There is no reason to believe that the cut into *lacZ* occurs at the same site, but clearly it cannot extend far into the gene.

β-Galactosidase activity is more heat-unstable in these chimeric proteins than in the wild-type protein, as expected. The hybrids are precipitated by anti-β-galactosidase. They are tetramers, and this is a paradox. M15 protein is a dimer and lacks at least some of the same portion of the polypeptide chain. It requires an α-donor peptide such as CB2 or anti-β-galactosidase to tetramerize. It seems likely from studies with antibody (see below) that the CB2 segment is buried within the tetramer. Yet folding of the β-galactosidase part of the chimeras to tetramers occur even though this segment is deleted. It may be that only a relatively small number of amino acids are deleted from the β-galactosidase chain and that those required to allow the formation of tetramers are still in the molecule. Determination of the site of fusion is therefore of considerable interest. It is also of interest that the link between repressor and β-galactosidase is particularly sensitive to trypsin and that the β-galactosidase moiety retains activity after cleavage.

With the aid of bacteriophage Mu (Casadaban 1975, 1976), β-galactosidase has been converted to a membrane-bound state by fusion to a maltose transport protein (Silhavy et al. 1976). The hybrid protein is found in the cytoplasmic membrane and, because ONPG is not hydrolyzed by intact cells, it is probably on the inner surface. Gene fusions have also been produced between the *lac* and *ara* operons (Casadaban 1976), but the hybrid proteins have not yet been investigated.

Immunological Properties

Antibodies against wild-type β-galactosidase precipitate but do not inactivate the enzyme (Cohn and Torriani 1952), and they also enhance its heat stability (Melchers and Messer 1970a). The increased stability cannot be due simply to a change in physical state because the response depends on antibody dose (Celada and Strom 1972) and also occurs with Fab fragments, which do not precipitate (F. Celada and R. Strom, unpubl.). Apparently, then, the conformation of the protein is stabilized by the antibodies.

Recently it has been discovered that certain kinds of β-galactosidase antibodies cause the loss of enzyme activity (Roth and Rotman 1975a). These antibodies were prepared against enzyme from Lac⁺ revertants of strain S30, the producer of the antibody-activatable β-galactosidase (AMEF). The mechanism of the inactivation involves a dissociation of the native β-galactosidase, probably to a dimer, as demonstrated by sucrose density-gradient centrifugation of the protein-Fab complex (Roth and Rotman 1975b). It seems possible that such antibodies are directed against determinants concerned with quaternary associations in the molecule. By binding to these determinants, the antibodies, in effect, pry apart the molecule.

Although some inactivation occurs at low temperature, most of the effect requires temperatures above 25°C. Higher temperatures presumably would make intersubunit binding sites more available to complex formation with antibody. Also of interest is the observation that the mutationally altered enzymes from which these antibodies are prepared are generally much more heat-unstable than wild-type enzyme, which indicates that their structures are more open.

The availability of fragments from tryptic and cyanogen bromide digests has allowed another approach to the study of the conformation of β-galactosidase. Antibodies against peptides ranging in size from 15 to 96 residues have been prepared. Some of these react with the complete molecule and others do not (F. Celada et al., unpubl.). As a first approximation, it seems likely that such results can help to position specific portions of the polypeptide chain either on the surface or buried within the folded molecule. Antipeptide antibodies have also been useful in the sequence determination as discussed above.

The enzyme activity of AMEF is enhanced 500–1000-fold by anti-β-galactosidase (Rotman and Celada 1968). Since that original observation, a considerable amount of work has been carried out on the mechanism of activation. It has been shown that proteins from many missense strains can be activated (Messer and Melchers 1970a; Melchers and Messer 1970b). Eleven of these mutations have been mapped; seven fall into one group, two into another, and the remaining two elsewhere. The mutational sites farthest apart correspond to a distance of about three-fourths of the Z gene (Messer and Melchers 1970b). Measurement of the rates of activation of some of these enzymes suggests that the rate-limiting step of the activation process is a monomolecular reaction (Melchers et al. 1972). The simplest explanation for these observations is that the mutationally altered enzyme changes between two conformations and that the activating antibody binds and stabilizes the wild-type conformation. Antibodies made against proteins obtained from mutants do not activate the homologous protein, but several cases are known where activation does occur in heterologous combinations (Celada et al. 1974a).

A new and particularly interesting finding is that AMEF is a dimer which is converted to a tetramer on activation with anti-β-galactosidase (B. Rotman and E. Macario, pers. comm.). This is the converse of the inactivation of normal β-galactosidase by inactivating antibodies. The protein produced by deletion mutant strain M15 can itself be activated to some extent by anti-β-galactosidase (Accolla and Celada 1976). The activation is also accompanied by conversion of the dimeric M15 protein to the tetrameric form (F. Celada and I. Zabin, unpubl.).

Antibodies have effects on complementation. The yield of in vitro ω complementation can be increased more than fivefold by addition of anti-β-galactosidase or of the corresponding Fab fragments (Celada et al. 1974b). The yield of α complementation is not increased by antibodies, although there are effects on the kinetics of the reaction. Anti-ω fragment has been prepared; this reacts strongly with the whole enzyme, which indicates similarity between the tertiary structures of the ω peptide and the whole protein (Celada et al. 1974b). Antibodies prepared against the α-complementing peptide CB2 inhibit complementation and do not react with the enzyme, which suggests that the CB2 segment of the polypeptide chain is buried within the native protein (F. Celada et al., unpubl.).

An antigen cross-reacting to anti-β-galactosidase has been isolated from *E. coli* (Erickson and Steers 1972). This substance is a ribonucleoprotein with an amino acid composition and a molecular weight distinct from those of β-galactosidase. Its relationship to the latter is unknown.

THE LACTOSE PERMEASE PROTEIN

Several permease systems are responsible for the transport of α- and β-galactosides from outside to inside bacterial cells. By definition, the lactose permease is that system for which the *lacY* gene product is an integral part. The properties of the lactose permease system have been reviewed by Kepes (1971) and by Kennedy (1970). Despite intense investigation of the mechanism of transport and the structure and function of membranes in recent years, not very much is known of the *lacY* gene product as a protein.

The first direct demonstration of the *lacY* product as a membrane-bound protein, named the M protein (Fox and Kennedy 1965; Fox et al. 1967), was based on the facts that lactose transport is sensitive to sulfhydryl poisons and certain galactosides could protect against such reagents. The M protein was specifically labeled with N-ethyl-[^{14}C]maleimide after first treating thiodigalactoside-containing membrane fragments with unlabeled reagent. The fragments were then washed to remove the galactoside and thus expose the lactose permease sites. Partial purification of the labeled material was achieved by SDS extraction followed by gel filtration on Sephadex G-150. A single radioactive peak was obtained with a chemical purity of about 20–30% and an estimated molecular weight of about 30,000 (Jones and Kennedy 1969). The amount of M protein in whole cells of the ML strain was about 0.35% of the protein, or about 2–4% of the membrane protein.

A direct binding assay has also been developed (Kennedy et al. 1974) in which membrane fragments are equilibrated with [^{3}H]thio-digalactoside in phosphate buffer containing ^{32}P. The increment in ^{3}H to ^{32}P compared to control levels corresponds to the amount of M protein. From such assays it was calculated that the bacterial membrane contains approximately 9000 lactose permease binding sites per cell. This value was also obtained with the reagent N-bromoacetyl-β-D-[^{3}H]galactosylamide added to membrane fragments in experiments similar to those carried out with N-ethyl-maleimide (Yariv et al. 1972).

Several particularly interesting classes of compounds have been prepared by Kaback and coworkers to study the lactose permease system. One class consists of dansyl galactosides, which are fluorescent compounds. They bind to membrane vesicles; the binding is energy-dependent and inhibited by lactose (Kaback 1974; Schuldiner et al. 1975). The amount bound to membrane vesicles suggests that the binding protein may consist of 3–6% of the membrane protein, in agreement with the values reported by Kennedy and coworkers.

A second class of compounds are photoreactive azidophenylgalactosides. β-Nitro-4-azidophenyl-1-thio-β-D-galactopyranoside, for example, is a competitive inhibitor of lactose transport. Its uptake by membrane vesicles is markedly stimulated by D-lactate as energy source. When exposed to visible light in the presence of D-lactate, the transport system is irreversibly inactivated and the azido-containing ligand becomes covalently linked to the vesicles (Rudnick et al. 1975).

Is the carrier macromolecule which binds these galactosides in membrane vesicles the same as the M protein assayed in membrane fragments? One paradox is that lactose and thiomethylgalactoside are good substrates for the lactose permease, yet they do not protect against N-ethyl-maleimide inactivation. Because thiodigalactoside and melibiose do protect, it has been suggested that the protein contains two binding sites (Carter et al. 1968). Alternatively, the reactive sulfhydryl may not be directly in the substrate binding site, and thus not all sugars might protect (Yariv and Zipori 1972). A second paradox is that the initial binding of galactoside substrates to membrane vesicles required an energized state, but thiodigalactoside binding to M protein occurred in the absence of energy sources. It has been pointed out that the amount of thiodigalac-toside bound by the direct assay is considerably less than that expected from the amount of M protein measured by protection against N-ethyl-maleimide inactivation. Furthermore, an energized state might change the specificity of substrate binding. It should also be noted that genetic data of Langridge (1974c) agree with a single-site model.

There appears to be a growing realization that active transport by the lactose permease system is powered by an electrical potential (the "proton-motive force") across the cell membrane (Mitchell 1966; Harold 1972; Kaback 1974; Andrews and Lin 1976). This system must have many components. The place of the *lacY* gene product is apparently in the initial binding of the galactoside substrate.

The amount of M protein in membranes from F'*lac* strains appears to be about double that found in the wild type (Kennedy 1970). This suggests that lactose-protein-hyperproducing strains might contain additional lactose permease protein in the cytoplasm of these cells. No information is available concerning possible processing of protein before it is incorporated into the membrane. Certainly, isolation in pure form and chemical characterization of this elusive protein are badly needed. Some encouraging preliminary results on the purification have been obtained recently (M. Villarejo, pers. comm.).

THIOGALACTOSIDASE TRANSACETYLASE

Production and Isolation

This enzyme (acetyl-CoA:galactoside-6-O-acetyl-transferase [E. C. 2.3. 1.18]) is specified by the *lacA* gene, the third structural gene of the *lac* operon. Strain A324-5 produces large quantities of β-galactosidase, as discussed above (Fowler 1972a), and proportionately large amounts of transacetylase (Musso 1972), but a "natural polarity" exists. In either high- or low-producing strains, approximately 3–5 times more β-galactosidase subunits or monomers are synthesized than transacetylase subunits (Brown et al. 1967b). Since the β-galactosidase subunit is about 4 times the size of the transacetylase subunit, 12–20 times more by weight of the larger enzyme is formed. Transacetylase can be isolated in pure form rather easily by ammonium sulfate precipitation, ion-exchange Sephadex or cellulose chromatography, and gel filtration (Musso and Zabin 1973). Affinity columns containing thioester-linked coenzyme A (CoA) will bind the enzyme (I. Zabin, unpubl.).

To account for natural polarity in the lactose operon, transcription and translation initiation frequencies of β-galactosidase and transacetylase have been measured (D. Kennell and H. Riezman, pers. comm.). Ribosomes initiate more frequently to Z message than to A message, and A message decays faster than Z message. These two related processes explain the difference in rates of synthesis of the two enzymes.

Structure and Sequence

The enzyme is a dimer composed of two identical 30,000-dalton subunits and has the amino acid composition shown in Table 2. With the availability of larger amounts of transacetylase from strain A324-5, some information on the amino acid sequence has been obtained. An amino-terminal tripeptide, Asx-Met-Pro, was isolated in good yield (Musso 1972). Earlier findings of both aspartic acid (or asparagine) and methionine at the amino terminus (Brown et al. 1967c) were apparently due to removal of some of the aspartic acid (asparagine) by proteolysis during cell growth or during isolation of the protein.

A number of tryptic and cyanogen bromide peptides have also been separated in pure form. The partial amino acid sequences of the amino-terminal 25 residues and the carboxyl-terminal 15 residues are shown in Figure 4 (Musso 1972; R. E. Musso and I. Zabin, unpubl.).

Substrate Specificity and Reaction Mechanism

Thiogalactoside transacetylase catalyzes the transfer of acetyl groups from acetyl coenzyme A to an acceptor such as isopropyl thiogalactoside to form the ester, 6-O-acetyl-IPTG. The enzyme reaction was studied in some detail (Musso and Zabin 1973). Various divalent metal ions and chelators have negligible effects on the reaction. The Michaelis constant for acetyl coenzyme A and for IPTG were 1.8×10^{-4} M and 0.77 M, respectively. This suggests that acetyl-CoA is a natural substrate for the enzyme, but IPTG is not a natural acceptor. However, when a number of possible acceptors were compared with IPTG, none were found to saturate the enzyme at low concentrations. It is of interest that the rate

Table 2 Amino acid composition of
thiogalactoside transacetylase

	Residues/32,000 m.w.
Tryptophan	3
Lysine	14
Histidine	11
Arginine	14
Aspartic Acid	34
Threonine	15
Serine	14
Glutamic Acid	21
Proline	15
Glycine	22
Alanine	13
Half-cystine	3
Valine	26
Methionine	8
Isoleucine	20
Leucine	14
Tyrosine	11
Phenylalanine	10
Total	268

Data from Zabin (1963).

of acetylation of *p*-nitrophenyl-β-D-galactoside was found to be twice as
great as that of IPTG (Table 3). Substrate kinetics and product inhibition
studies were consistent with a reaction mechanism of the ordered bi-bi
type with acetyl-CoA and CoA as the first substrate and final product,
respectively.

Physiological Role

In animal tissues, acetylation reactions may be convenient modes of
detoxification. For example, foreign amines are excreted as *N*-acetyl

NH₂Asx-Met-Pro-Met-Thr-Glu-Arg-Ile-Arg-Ala-
Gly-Lys-Leu-Phe-Thr-Asx-Met-Cys-Glx-Gly-
Leu-Pro-Glx-Lys-Arg

Figure 4 Sequences at amino and carboxyl termini of thiogalactoside transacetylase.

Asx-Lys-His-Tyr-Tyr-
Phe-Lys-Asx-(Tyr, Ser, Val, Glx, Lys)-Ser-ValCOOH

Table 3 Substrate specificity of acetyl acceptors

Substrate	Concentration (mM)	IPTG reaction (%)
Lactose	28	0
Thioallolactose	50	2
1-*O*-β-D-Galactosyl-D-glycerol	10	9
UDP-galactose	3	0
p-Nitrophenyl-β-D-galactoside	10	210
p-Nitrophenyl-β-D-glucoside	5	51
p-Nitrophenyl-β-D-mannoside	5	1
p-Nitrophenyl-α-D-galactoside	10	32
p-Nitrophenyl-β-D-thiogalactoside	5	27

Data from Musso and Zabin (1973).

derivatives. A similar role for thiogalactoside transacetylase was considered (Zabin et al. 1962). The product of the reaction with IPTG as acceptor, 6-*O*-acetyl-IPTG, is an inert substance in *E. coli*. It is neither an inducer nor a substrate of the *lac* permease, and it diffuses passively from cells (Herzenberg 1961). However, acetyl compounds are formed at very low rates, the substrate specificity is very limited, and (as suggested from Michaelis constants) galactosides might not be true acceptor substrates. For these reasons the notion that detoxification is the raison d'être of this enzyme was discarded.

Recently, however, the interesting suggestion has been made that thiogalactoside transacetylase may confer a selective advantage on cells of *E. coli* growing on β-galactosides in the presence of nonmetabolizable analogs (Andrews and Lin 1976). By being acetylated, such analogs would be detoxified and excreted. In support of this idea, it was shown that the addition of IPTG to a mixed culture of *lacA⁺* and *lacA⁻* strains growing on lactose resulted in a 15-fold enrichment of the *lacA⁺* strain after 40 generations. This is a reasonable suggestion that may very well account for the role of transacetylase. The enzyme does catalyze the acetylation of many phenyl, thiophenyl, and nitrophenyl sugars (Table 3), some of which might be even more harmful to the bacterial cell. It should be informative to test such substrates also and to test additional mutants as well.

It is possible that thiolgalactoside transacetylase may have another function, but despite considerable searching no other differences between A⁺ and A⁻ strains have been discovered.

ACKNOWLEDGMENTS

It is a pleasure to acknowledge the contributions of the following collaborators: Steve Barta, Anthony J. Brake, Paulette Osborne, Val H.

Schaeffer, and Drs. Franco Celada, Joyce Hamlin, Keith E. Langley, Shin Lin, Richard E. Musso, John E. Snoke, and Merna R. Villarejo.

Works performed in this laboratory was supported in part by U.S. Public Health Service grants AI-04181, GM-1531, GM-00364, and GM-07104.

REFERENCES

Accolla, R. S. and F. Celada. 1976. Antibody-mediated activation of a deletion-mutant β-galactosidase defective in the α region. *FEBS Lett.* **67:**299.

Andrews, K. J. and E. C. C. Lin. 1976. Thiogalactoside transacetylase of the lactose operon as an enzyme for detoxification. *J. Bacteriol.* **128:**510.

Appel, S. H., D. H. Alpers, and G. M. Tomkins. 1965. Multiple molecular forms of β-galactosidase. *J. Mol. Biol.* **11:**12.

Apte, B. N., H. Rhodes, and D. Zipser. 1975. Mutation blocking the specific degradation of reinitiation polypeptides in *Escherichia coli.* *Nature* **257:**329.

Berg, A. P., A. V. Fowler, and I. Zabin. 1970. β-Galactosidase: Isolation of and antibodies to incomplete chains. *J. Bacteriol.* **101:**438.

Brockhaus, M. and J. Lehmann. 1976. 2,6-Anhydro-1-diazo-1-deoxy-D-glycero-L-manno-heptitol: A specific blocking agent for the active site of β-galactosidase. *FEBS Lett.* **62:**154.

Brown, J. L., D. M. Brown, and I. Zabin. 1967a. β-Galactosidase: Orientation and the carboxyl-terminal coding site in the gene. *Proc. Natl. Acad. Sci.* **58:**1139.

———. 1967b. Thiogalactoside transacetylase: Physical and chemical studies of subunit structure. *J. Biol. Chem.* **242:**4254.

Brown, J. L., S. Koorajian, and I. Zabin. 1967c. Thiogalactoside transacetylase: Amino- and carboxyl-terminal studies. *J. Biol. Chem.* **242:**4259.

Bukhari, A. and D. Zipser. 1973. Mutants of *Escherichia coli* with a defect in the degradation of nonsense fragments. *Nat. New Biol.* **243:**238.

Carter, J. R., C. F. Fox, and E. P. Kennedy. 1968. Interaction of sugars with the membrane protein component of the lactose transport system of *Escherichia coli.* *Proc. Natl. Acad. Sci.* **60:**725.

Casadaban, M. J. 1975. Fusion of the *Escherichia coli lac* genes to the ara promoter. General technique using bacteriophage Mu-1 insertions. *Proc. Natl. Acad. Sci.* **72:**809.

———. 1976. Transposition and fusion of the *lac* genes to selected promoters in *Escherichia coli* using bacteriophage lambda and Mu. *J. Mol. Biol.* **104:**541.

Case, G. S., M. L. Sinnott, and J. P. Tenu. 1973. Role of magnesium ions in β-galactosidase-catalyzed hydrolyses. Charge and shape of the β-galacto-pyranosyl binding site. *Biochem. J.* **133:**99.

Celada, F. and R. Strom. 1972. Antibody-induced conformational changes in proteins. *Q. Rev. Biophys.* **5:**395.

Celada, F., J. Radojkovic, and R. Strom. 1974a. Antibody-mediated activation of β-galactosidase mutants and complementing fragments. *J. Chim. Phys. Phys.-Chim. Biol.* **71:**1007.

Celada, F., A. Ullmann, and J. Monod. 1974b. Immunological study of complementary fragments of β-galactosidase. *Biochemistry* **13:**5543.

Cohn, M. and A. M. Torriani. 1952. Immunochemical studies with the β-galactosidase and structurally related proteins of *Escherichia coli. J. Immunol.* **69**:471.

Contaxis, C. C. and F. J. Reithel. 1971. Studies on protein multimers. The association-dissociation behaviour of β-galactosidase in glycerol. *Biochem. J.* **124**:623.

————. 1974. Protein multimers. VII. Stabilization of *Escherichia coli* β-galactosidase by a 260-nm absorbing compound in crude preparations. *Arch. Biochem. Biophys.* **160**:588.

Contaxis, C. C., D. McAfee, R. Goodrich, and F. J. Reithel. 1973. Protein multimers. V. Characterization of β-galactosidase self-association behavior with observations on apparent specific volume. *Int. J. Pept. Protein Res.* **5**:207.

Erickson, R. P. and E. Steers, Jr. 1972. Purification and properties of an antigen cross-reacting with *Escherichia coli* β-galactosidase. *Immunochemistry* **9**:29.

Fink, A. L. and K. J. Angelides. 1975. The β-galactosidase-catalyzed hydrolysis of *o*-nitrophenol-β-D-galactosidase at subzero temperatures: Evidence for a galactosyl-enzyme intermediate. *Biochem. Biophys. Res. Commun.* **64**:701.

Fowler, A. V. 1972a. High-level production of β-galactosidase by *Escherichia coli* merodiploids. *J. Bacteriol.* **112**:856.

————. 1972b. The amino acid sequence of β-galactosidase. II. Tryptic peptides of the maleylated protein and sequences of some tryptic peptides. *J. Biol. Chem.* **247**:5425.

————. 1975. Structural studies on *Escherichia coli* β-galactosidase. Separation of large cyanogen bromide peptides. *In Solid-phase methods of protein sequence analysis* (ed. R. A. Laursen), p. 169. Pierce Chemical Co., Rockford, Illinois.

Fowler, A. V. and I. Zabin. 1966. Co-linearity of β-galactosidase with its gene by immunological detection of incomplete polypeptide chains. *Science* **154**:3752.

————. 1970. The amino acid sequence of β-galactosidase. I. Isolation and composition of tryptic peptides. *J. Biol. Chem.* **245**:5032.

Fox, C. F. and E. P. Kennedy. 1965. Specific labeling and partial purification of the M protein, a component of the β-galactoside transport system of *Escherichia coli. Proc. Natl. Acad. Sci.* **54**:891.

Fox, C. F., J. R. Carter, and E. P. Kennedy. 1967. Genetic control of the membrane protein component of the lactose transport system of *Escherichia coli. Proc. Natl. Acad. Sci.* **57**:698.

Gilbert, W., J. Gralla, J. Majors, and A. Maxam. 1975. Lactose operator sequences and the action of *lac* repressor. In *Protein-ligand interactions*, p. 193. Walter de Gruyter, Berlin.

Goldberg, A. L. and J. F. Dice. 1974. Intracellular protein degradation in mammalian and bacterial cells. *Annu. Rev. Biochem.* **43**:835.

Goldberg, A. L. and A. C. St. John. 1976. Intracellular protein degradation in mammalian and bacterial cells: Part 2. *Annu. Rev. Biochem.* **45**:747.

Goldberg, M. E. 1969. Tertiary structure of *Escherichia coli* β-D-galactosidase. *J. Mol. Biol.* **46**:441.

————. 1970. Structural studies of ω-complemented β-galactosidase of *E. coli*. In *The lactose operon* (ed. J. R. Beckwith and D. Zipser), p. 273. Cold Spring Harbor Laboratory, Cold Spring Harbor, New York.

Goldberg, M. E. and S. J. Edelstein. 1969. Sedimentation equilibrium of paucidisperse systems. Subunit structure of complemented β-galactosidase. *J. Mol. Biol.* **46:**431.

Goldschmidt, R. 1970. *In vivo* degradation of nonsense fragments in *E. coli. Nature* **228:**1151.

Grodzicker, T. and D. Zipser. 1968. A mutation which creates a new site for the re-initiation of polypeptide synthesis in the *Z* gene of the *lac* operon of *Escherichia coli. J. Mol. Biol.* **38:**305.

Hall, B. G. 1973. *In vivo* complementation between wild-type and mutant β-galactosidase in *Escherichia coli. J. Bacteriol.* **114:**448.

Harold, F. M. 1972. Conservation and transformation of energy by bacterial membranes. *Bacteriol. Rev.* **36:**172.

Herzenberg, L. A. 1961. Isolation and identification of derivatives formed in the course of intracellular accumulation of thiogalactosides by *Escherichia coli. Arch. Biochem. Biophys.* **93:**314.

Hill, J. A. and R. E. Huber. 1974. Mechanism of sodium activation of *Escherichia coli* β-galactosidase and the inhibitory effect of high concentrations of magnesium on this activation. *Int. J. Biochem.* **5:**773.

Huber, R. E., G. Kurz, and K. Wallenfels. 1976. A quantitation of the factors which affect the hydrolase and transgalactosylase activities of β-galactosidase on lactose. *Biochemistry* **15:**1994.

Huber, R. E., K. Wallenfels, and G. Kurz. 1975. Action of β-galactosidase on allolactose. *Can. J. Biochem.* **53:**1035.

Jones, T. H. D. and E. P. Kennedy. 1969. Characterization of the membrane protein of the lactose transport system of *Escherichia coli. J. Biol. Chem.* **244:**5981.

Kaback, H. R. 1974. Transport studies in bacterial membrane vesicles. *Science* **186:**882.

Kaneshiro, C. M., C. A. Enns, M. G. Hahn, J. S. Peterson, and F. J. Reithel. 1975. Evidence for an active dimer of *Escherichia coli* β-galactosidase. *Biochem. J.* **151:**433.

Katze, J. S., S. Sridhara, and I. Zabin. 1966. An amino-terminal peptide of β-galactosidase: Its detection in crude extracts of wild-type and nonsense mutants of *Escherichia coli. J. Biol. Chem.* **241:**5341.

Kennedy, E. P. 1970. The lactose permease system of *Escherichia coli.* In *The lactose operon* (ed., J. R. Beckwith and D. Zipser), p. 49. Cold Spring Harbor Laboratory, Cold Spring Harbor, New York.

Kennedy, E. P., M. K. Rumley, and J. B. Armstrong. 1974. Direct measurement of the binding of labeled sugars to the lactose permease M protein. *J. Biol. Chem.* **249:**33.

Kepes, A. 1971. The β-galactoside permease of *Escherichia coli. J. Membr. Biol.* **4:**87.

Langley, K. E. and I. Zabin. 1976. β-Galactosidase α-complementation: Properties of the complemented enzyme and mechanism of the complementation reaction. *Biochemistry* **15:**4866.

Langley, K. E., A. V. Fowler, and I. Zabin. 1975a. Amino acid sequence of β-galactosidase. IV. Sequence of an α-complementing cyanogen bromide peptide, residues 3 to 92. *J. Biol. Chem.* **250:**2587.

Langley, K. E., M. R. Villarejo, A. V. Fowler, P. J. Zamenhof, and I. Zabin. 1975b. Molecular basis of β-galactosidase α-complementation. *Proc. Natl. Acad. Sci.* **72**:1254.

Langridge, J. 1968a. Genetic evidence for the disposition of the substrate binding site of β-galactosidase. *Proc. Natl. Acad. Sci.* **60**:1260.

———. 1968b. Genetic and enzymatic experiments relating to the tertiary structure of β-galactosidase. *J. Bacteriol.* **96**:1711.

———. 1974a. Mutation spectra and the neutrality of mutations. *Aust. J. Biol. Sci.* **27**:309.

———. 1974b. Genetic and enzymatic experiments relating to the quaternary structure of β-galactosidase. *Aust. J. Biol. Sci.* **27**:321.

———. 1974c. Characterization and intragenic position of mutations in the gene for galactoside permease of *Escherichia coli*. *Aust. J. Biol. Sci.* **27**:331.

Lin, S. and I. Zabin. 1972. β-Galactosidase: Rates of synthesis and degradation of incomplete chains. *J. Biol. Chem.* **247**:2205.

Lin, S., M. Villarejo, and I. Zabin. 1970. β-Galactosidase: α-Complementation of a deletion mutant with cyanogen bromide peptides. *Biochem. Biophys. Res. Commun.* **40**:249.

Marinkovic, D. V. and J. Tang. 1971. Specificity of *in vitro* complementation of β-galactosidase from mutant M15 of *Escherichia coli*. *Biochem. Biophys. Res. Commun.* **45**:1288.

Melcher, U. 1975. The purification of β-galactosidase-specific polysomes by affinity chromatography. *Anal. Biochem.* **64**:461.

Melchers, F. and W. Messer. 1970a. Enhanced stability against heat denaturation of *E. coli* wild type and mutant β-galactosidase in the presence of specific antibodies. *Biochem. Biophys. Res. Commun.* **40**:570.

———. 1970b. The activation of mutant β-galactosidase by specific antibodies. *Eur. J. Biochem.* **17**:267.

———. 1971. Hybrid enzyme molecules reconstituted from mixtures of wild-type and mutant *Escherichia coli* β-galactosidase. *J. Mol. Biol.* **61**:401.

———. 1973. Activity of individual molecules of hybrid β-galactosidase reconstituted from the wild-type and an inactive-mutant enzyme. *Eur. J. Biochem.* **34**:228.

Melchers, F., G. Koehler, and W. Messer. 1972. Stabilization of conformations of *Escherichia coli* β-galactosidase by specific antibodies. Restrictions in antigenic determinants and antibodies. *Colloq. Ges. Biol. Chem. Mosbach* **23**:409.

Messer, W. and F. Melchers. 1970a. The activation of mutant β-galactosidase by specific antibodies. In *The lactose operon* (ed. J. R. Beckwith and D. Zipser), p. 305. Cold Spring Harbor Laboratory, Cold Spring Harbor, New York.

———. 1970b. Genetic analysis of mutants producing defective β-galactosidase which can be activated by specific antibodies. *Mol. Gen. Genet.* **109**:152.

Michels, C. A. and D. Zipser. 1969. Mapping of polypeptide reinitiation sites within the β-galactosidase structural gene. *J. Mol. Biol.* **41**:341

Mitchell, P. 1966. Chemiosmotic coupling in oxidative and photosynthetic phosphorylation. *Biol. Rev. (Camb.)* **41**:445.

Morrison, S. L. and D. Zipser. 1970. Polypeptide products of nonsense mutations. I. Termination fragments from nonsense mutations in the *Z* gene of the *lac* operon of *Escherichia coli*. *J. Mol. Biol.* **50**:359.

Müller-Hill, B. and J. Kania. 1974. *Lac* repressor can be fused to β-galactosidase. *Nature* **249**:561.

Müller-Hill, B., G. Heidecker, and J. Kania. 1976. Repressor-galactosidase chimaeras. In *Proceedings of the Third John Innes Symposium: Structure-function relationships of proteins* (ed. R. Markham and R. W. Horne), p. 167. Elsevier/North-Holland, Amsterdam.

Musso, R. E. 1972. "Physiological and chemical studies on thiogalactoside transacetylase from *Escherichia coli.*" Ph.D. thesis, University of California, Los Angeles.

Musso, R. E. and I. Zabin. 1973. Substrate specificity and kinetic studies on thiogalactoside transacetylase. *Biochemistry* **12**:553.

Naider, F., Z. Bohak, and J. Yariv. 1972. Reversible alkylation of a methionyl residue near the active site of β-galactosidase. *Biochemistry* **11**:3202.

Neville, M. C. and G. N. Ling. 1967. Synergistic activation of β-galactosidase by Na$^+$ and Cs$^+$. *Arch. Biochem. Biophys.* **118**:596.

Newton, A. 1969. Re-initiation of polypeptide synthesis and polarity in the *lac* operon of *Escherichia coli. J. Mol. Biol.* **41**:329.

Nishikawa, A. H. and P. Bailon. 1975. Affinity purification methods. Nonspecific adsorption of proteins due to ionic groups in cyanogen bromide treated agarose. *Arch. Biochem. Biophys.* **168**:576.

Proctor, M. H. 1962. Histidine and β-galactosidase activity. *Biochim. Biophys. Acta* **59**:713.

Reznikoff, W. S., R. B. Winter, and C. K. Hurley. 1974. Location of the repressor binding sites in the *lac* operon. *Proc. Natl. Acad. Sci.* **71**:2314.

Rimerman, R. A. and G. W. Hatfield. 1973. Phosphate-induced protein chromatography. *Science* **182**:1268.

Roth, R. A. and B. Rotman. 1975a. Inactivation of normal β-D-galactosidase by antibodies to defective forms of the enzyme. *J. Biol. Chem.* **250**:7759.

————. 1975b. Dissociation of the tetrameric form of β-D-galactosidase by inactivating antibodies. *Biochem. Biophys. Res. Commun.* **67**:1384.

Rotman, M. B. 1961. Measurement of activity of single molecules of β-galactosidase. *Proc. Natl. Acad. Sci.* **47**:1981.

Rotman, M. B. and F. Celada. 1968. Formation of β-D-galactosidase mediated by specific antibody in a soluble extract of *E. coli* containing a defective *Z* gene product. *Proc. Natl. Acad. Sci.* **60**:660.

Rudnick, G., H. R. Kaback, and R. Weil. 1975. Mechanisms of active transport in isolated bacterial membrane vesicles. 22. Photoinactivation of the β-galactoside transport system in *Escherichia coli* membrane vesicles with 2-nitro-4-azidophenyl-1-thio-β-D-galactopyranoside. *J. Biol. Chem.* **250**:1371.

Schuldiner, S., G. K. Kerwar, R. Weil, and H. R. Kaback. 1975. Energy-dependent binding of dansyl-galactosides to the β-galactoside carrier protein. *J. Biol. Chem.* **250**:1361.

Shineberg, B. and D. Zipser. 1973. The *lon* gene and degradation of β-galactosidase nonsense fragments. *J. Bacteriol.* **116**:1469.

Silhavy, T. J., M. J. Casadaban, H. A. Shuman, and J. R. Beckwith. 1976. Conversion of β-galactosidase to a membrane-bound state by gene fusion. *Proc. Natl. Acad. Sci.* **73**:3423.

Sinnott, M. L. and P. J. Smith. 1976. Active-site directed irreversible inhibition of *E. coli* β-galactosidase by the "hot" carbonium ion precursor, β-D-galactopyranosylmethyl-*p*-nitrophenyltriazene. *J. Chem. Soc. Chem. Commun.* p. 223.

Spizek, J., Z. Technikova, J. Benes, and J. Janacek. 1972. Synthesis of β-galactosidase in *Escherichia coli* in the presence of methionine analogs. *Folia Microbiol.* **17**:143.

Steers, E., Jr. and P. Cuatrecasas. 1974. β-Galactosidase. *Methods Enzymol.* **34**:350.

Steers, E., Jr. and S. Shifrin. 1967. Characterization of the β-galactosidase from a lactose-negative, complementing mutant of *Escherichia coli* K12. *Biochim. Biophys. Acta* **133**:454.

Steers, E., Jr., P. Cuatrecasas, and H. Pollard. 1971. The purification of β-galactosidase from *Escherichia coli* by affinity chromatography. *J. Biol. Chem.* **246**:196.

Steers, E., Jr., G. R. Craven, C. B. Anfinsen, and J. L. Bethune. 1965. Evidence for non-identical chains in the β-galactosidase of *Escherichia coli* K12. *J. Biol. Chem.* **240**:2478.

Stokes, T. M. and I. B. Wilson. 1972. Common intermediates in the hydrolysis of β-galactosides by β-galactosidase from *Escherichia coli*. *Biochemistry* **11**:1061.

Tenu, J. P., O. M. Viratelle, J. Garnier, and J. Yon. 1971. pH dependence of the activity of β-galactosidase from *Escherichia coli*. *Eur. J. Biochem.* **20**:363.

Tomino, S. and K. Paigen. 1970. Isolation of β-thiogalactoside binding proteins of *E. coli* by specific adsorbents. In *The lactose operon* (ed. J. R. Beckwith and D. Zipser), p. 233. Cold Spring Harbor Laboratory, Cold Spring Harbor, New York.

Truman, P. and P. L. Bergquist. 1976. Genetic and biochemical characterization of some missense mutations in the *lac Z* gene of *Escherichia coli* K-12. *J. Bacteriol.* **126**:1063.

Ullmann, A. and D. Perrin. 1970. Complementation in β-galactosidase. In *The lactose operon* (ed. J. R. Beckwith and D. Zipser), p. 143. Cold Spring Harbor Laboratory, Cold Spring Harbor, New York.

Ullmann, A., F. Jacob, and J. Monod. 1967. Characterization by *in vitro* complementation of a peptide corresponding to an operator-proximal segment of the β-galactosidase structural gene of *Escherichia coli*. *J. Mol. Biol.* **24**:339.

Villarejo, M. and I. Zabin. 1973. Affinity chromatography of β-galactosidase fragments. *Nat. New Biol.* **242**:50.

———. 1974. β-Galactosidase from termination and deletion mutant strains. *J. Bacteriol.* **120**:466.

Villarejo, M., P. J. Zamenhof, and I. Zabin. 1972. β-Galactosidase: *In vivo* α-complementation. *J. Biol. Chem.* **247**:2212.

Wallenfels, K. and O. P. Malhotra. 1961. Galactosidases. In *Advances in carbohydrate chemistry* (ed. M. W. Wolfrom), p. 239. Academic Press, New York.

Wallenfels, K. and R. Weil. 1972. β-Galactosidase. In *The enzymes*, 3rd Ed. (ed. P. D. Boyer), vol. VII, p. 617. Academic Press, New York.

Wentworth, D. F. and R. Wolfenden. 1974. Slow binding of D-galactal, a reversible inhibitor of bacterial β-galactosidase. *Biochemistry* **13**:4715.

Yariv, J. and P. Zipori. 1972. Essential methionyl residue in the *lac*-permease of *Escherichia coli. FEBS Lett.* **24**:296.

Yariv, J., A. J. Kalb, and M. Yariv. 1972. Labeling of *lac*-permease. *FEBS Lett.* **27**:27.

Zabin, I. 1963. Crystalline thiogalactoside transacetylase. *J. Biol. Chem.* **238**:3300.

Zabin, I. and A. V. Fowler. 1970. β-Galactosidase and thiogalactoside transacetylase. In *The lactose operon* (ed. J. R. Beckwith and D. Zipser), p. 27. Cold Spring Harbor Laboratory, Cold Spring Harbor, New York.

———. 1972. The amino acid sequence of β-galactosidase. III. Sequences of amino- and carboxyl-terminal tryptic peptides. *J. Biol. Chem.* **247**:5432.

Zabin, I. and M. R. Villarejo. 1975. Protein complementation. *Annu. Rev. Biochem.* **44**:295.

Zabin, I., A. Kepes, and J. Monod. 1962. Thiogalactoside transacetylase. *J. Biol. Chem.* **237**:253.

Zamenhof, P. J. and M. Villarejo. 1972. Construction and properties of *Escherichia coli* strains exhibiting alpha-complementation of β-galactosidase fragments *in vivo. J. Bacteriol.* **110**:171.

Chemical Structure and Functional Organization of *lac* Repressor from *Escherichia coli*

Konrad Beyreuther
Institut für Genetik
Universität zu Köln
Köln, Germany

INTRODUCTION

Jacob and Monod (1961) proposed in their operon model that control genes would make repressors which would turn off the structural genes. This was an act of turning away from the hitherto discussed instructive theories of control. The essential and also new idea put forward was that the repressor acts as an intermediate to make the connection between the signal provided by the inducer or corepressor molecules and the target for the control, the operator. The signal molecules bind to the repressor and alter its affinity for the operator. If we want to understand these interactions, we have to answer the question about the molecular nature and chemical structure of both elements.

The isolations of nonsense mutations in the λ repressor *C*I gene (Jacob et al. 1962; Thomas and Lambert 1962) and in the *lac* repressor *I* gene (Bourgeois et al. 1965; Müller-Hill 1966) provided the first convincing genetic evidence for the nature of repressors. Suppression restored repressor activity and showed that the repressor genes encode proteins. The final proof was brought forth by Gilbert and Müller-Hill (1966) with the isolation of the *lac* repressor. They demonstrated that the repressor is a protein which binds β-D-galactosides in vitro and cosediments with *lac* operator DNA only in the absence of the gratuitous inducer isopropyl-1-thio-β-D-galactopyranoside (IPTG) (Gilbert and Müller-Hill 1966, 1967).

The amount of repressor made by the haploid wild-type cell is very small. The intracellular concentration of *lac* repressor was estimated by Gilbert and Müller-Hill (1966) to be on the order of 10^{-8} M. A wild-type *Escherichia coli* cell carrying one repressor-producing *I* gene would thus contain 10–20 *lac* repressor molecules. This corresponds to 0.002% of the total bacterial cellular protein, and 1 kg of *E. coli* cells would allow the isolation of not more than 3 mg of *lac* repressor. Approximately 1000 kg of cells, corresponding to about 10^{18} bacteria, would have been needed to perform the chemical studies described in this paper. This calculation does not include the amount of repressor needed for the analysis of the 20 mutationally altered repressors described later. It would have been nearly impossible to grow and work-up such large quantities of cells for repressor isolation. Fortunately, Müller-Hill (Müller-Hill et al. 1968) found a way to increase the amount of repressor normally present in a cell. This was achieved by means of two genetic manipulations. A strain was mutated to a form which produced ten times more repressor. The mutation alters the promoter of the I gene (Calos 1978). Then the number of copies of the I gene carrying this I^q mutation (q for quantity) was increased by incorporating the I gene into a λh80 chromosome which multiplies upon heat induction. Such a strain can synthesize 0.5% of its protein as lac repressor. Miller (1970) isolated another repressor-overproducing strain that makes 30–50 times the basal level and thus up to fivefold more than the I^q parent. Cells carrying this I^{sq} mutation (s for super) and the I^q mutation, placed upon the phage, initially produced up to 2.5% of their protein lac repressor. Most of the 4 g of repressor isolated in Cologne for the sequence analysis of the wild type was obtained from this strain. However, this strain is unstable for reasons not known, and in practice, the repressor content corresponds to about 1% of the total protein. Recently Müller-Hill (1975) isolated a strain which makes twofold more repressor than does the original $I^{q,sq}$. This is 100 times the basal level. When this mutation (I^{q1}) is placed upon the phage, cells produce up to 5% of their protein lac repressor.

The repressor-overproducing strains make the isolation of gram amounts of lac repressor straightforward (Müller-Hill et al. 1971) and provide the basis of the chemical studies of lac repressor described here. These studies of repressor structure have as their principal goal an understanding of the mechanism of specific protein-DNA interaction. One objective of this paper is to suggest that what we have learned about the chemical structures of lac repressor and mutationally altered lac repressors provides important clues to the functional organization of the repressor molecule and its DNA-binding site. Most attempts to attribute specific functional contributions to parts of the repressor sequence and to individual amino acid residues have centered around the operator-DNA-binding site. However, I will try to discuss the repressor as a whole and also to focus on the aggregation sites, the inducer-binding site, and the hinge region of the allosteric repressor protein, to the extent revealed by chemical studies. The work on repressor fragments and the genetic analysis of the repressor gene is described elsewhere in this volume (see Weber and Geisler; Miller).

PROPERTIES OF *lac* REPRESSOR

Purification

As mentioned in the Introduction, lac repressor is now an easily obtainable protein which can be isolated in gram amounts from strains overproducing repressor 100–1000-fold. The ability of the repressor to bind noncovalently and specifically to the inducer IPTG or to *lac* operator DNA permits a straightforward determination during the purification procedure (Gilbert and Müller-Hill 1966, 1967; Riggs et al. 1968).

Lac repressor has been obtained in the pure state from repressor-overproducing phage I^q, phage $I^{q,sq}$, and Phage I^{ql} E. *coli* K12 strains by fairly conventional methods of protein purification which are valid for nearly all DNA-binding proteins purified so far. These methods employ ammonium sulfate precipitations of DNase-treated crude extracts and ion-exchange column chromatography (Müller-Hill et al. 1971; Beyreuther et al. 1975). Since nonspecific DNA binding is a prerequisite for specific protein-DNA interaction and an inherent property of probably all regulatory DNA-binding proteins, the most effective purification step employs chromatography on phosphocellulose or DNA-cellulose. The binding of *lac* repressor to DNA-cellulose is similar to its binding to phosphocellulose, and the repressor is eluted at about the same ionic strength from both (Riggs and Bourgeois 1968; Müller-Hill et al. 1971; Lin and Riggs 1972). This also holds true for mutationally altered *lac* repressors with altered nonspecific DNA binding (Schlotmann et al. 1975; Schlotmann and Beyreuther 1977).

Since only 1–2% of the total soluble protein from E. *coli* binds to double-stranded DNA-cellulose (Alberts et al. 1969; D. Bielig and K. Beyreuther, unpubl.), the chromatographic step of the repressor purification should result in at least a 50-fold enrichment of DNA-binding proteins. Thus it should be possible to isolate *lac* repressor in pure state by selecting the proper conditions for elution. This was done and a single chromatographic step on phosphocellulose, for instance, was sufficient for complete separation of *lac* repressor from other proteins.

No differences have been observed in the elution profiles for *lac* repressor from wild type and three different repressor-overproducing strains (I^q, $I^{q,sq}$, and I^{ql}), and it is assumed that they are identical. Sequence analysis of these repressors indicated that this might indeed be the case. The amino-terminal sequences of wild-type repressor, extended for seven amino acids, and of repressor from mutants containing q1 extended for 83 amino acids, are identical to the sequences of repressors from q and q,sq mutants (Platt et al 1972; Adler et al. 1972; Beyreuther et al. 1973, 1975; M. Schlotmann and K. Beyreuther, unpubl.). The extrapolation of the DNA sequence of the *I* gene elucidated by Farabaugh (1978) provided the final proof that the protein sequence, determined from both q and q,sq mutants, was identical to that from the wild-type i[+], since the DNA sequence was determined from a plasmid constructed from the i[+] derivative (Calos 1978).

Lac repressor also binds to DEAE-cellulose but elutes at 0.15–0.17 M NaCl, together with the bulk of the proteins from E. *coli*. The use of DEAE-cellulose chromatography prior to chromatography on DNA-cellulose is recommended in order to separate the cellular DNA from the repressor-containing fraction, which in this case cannot be removed by dialysis following DNase treatment. Remaining DNase activity would otherwise destroy the immobilized DNA of DNA-cellulose.

The strong binding of *lac* repressor to DEAE-cellulose suggests that there are clusters of negatively charged side chains on the repressor surface. These clusters do not interfere with those of positive charge responsible for the binding to phosphocellulose and DNA-cellulose. This indicates a charge polarity on the repressor surface and might suggest that nonspecific DNA binding through side chains of basic amino acids could be directed by clusters of acidic amino acids.

Properties of Purified *lac* Repressor

Pure *lac* repressor can bind two types of ligands: β-D-galactosides, such as the inducer IPTG, and DNA containing the *lac* operator. *Lac* repressor is a tetrameric protein and consists of four identical subunits. It has four binding sites per tetramer for the inducer IPTG (Riggs and Bourgeois 1968; Müller-Hill et al. 1971). Only the 7S tetramer binds to *lac* operator DNA (Riggs and Bourgeois 1968), but two of the four subunits of repressor might be sufficient to recognize *lac* operator (Geisler and Weber 1976; Kania and Brown 1976). *Lac* repressor dimer subunits (4.5S repressor) and monomers (3.5S repressor) are found after treatment with sodium dodecyl sulfate (SDS) (Hamada et al. 1973). Such dimers and monomers bind inducer but do not bind to *lac* operator.

The operator-binding capacity of purified *lac* repressor is unstable, whereas the inducer-binding capacity is very stable. The loss of operator binding might be due to irreversible aggregation of repressor tetramers (Müller-Hill et al. 1971) to extensive but specific deamidation (Beyreuther et al. 1973, 1975) and to partial proteolytic degradation (Files and Weber 1976; Schlotmann and Beyreuther 1977).

The average charge of *lac* repressor is neutral at pH 7.6, the isoelectric point of *lac* repressor (D. Bielig and K. Beyreuther, unpubl.). Since *lac* repressor has to be stored at neutral pH (pH 7.0–7.5) to avoid rapid deamidation and denaturation, precipitates of repressor aggregates are easily formed. This can be avoided by storing the ammonium sulfate precipitates of the repressor at −20°C or rapidly frozen repressor solution in liquid nitrogen at −70°C. The operator-binding activity of *lac* repressor might thus be kept at the expected 1:1 stoichiometric binding to *lac* operator DNA (Rosenberg et al. 1977).

Composition

The amino acid composition of *lac* repressor (Table 1) is not very distinct from that of an "average" protein, as determined by distribution of amino acids in 68 eukaryotic and prokaryotic proteins (Jukes et al. 1975). This is

Table 1 Amino acid composition of *lac* repressor

Amino acid	Moles/mole	Percent/mole
Aspartic acid	17	4.7
Asparagine	12	3.3
Threonine	19	5.3
Serine	32	8.9
Glutamic acid	15	4.2
Glutamine	28	7.8
Proline	14	3.9
Glycine	22	6.1
Alanine	44	12.2
Cysteine	3	0.8
Valine	34	9.4
Methionine	10	2.8
Isoleucine	18	5.0
Leucine	41	11.4
Tyrosine	8	2.2
Phenylalanine	4	1.1
Histidine	7	1.9
Lysine	11	3.1
Arginine	19	5.3
Tryptophan	2	0.6
Total	360	

not unexpected since all organisms have solved the problem of meeting adaptive challenge in much the same way. They kept the amino acid composition of individual proteins as near to the genetic code frequencies as possible within the limits set by function (Holmquist and Moise 1975). Thus the distribution of amino acids in proteins is nonrandom and also not dependent on length or species of origin.

What are the compositional deviations of *lac* repressor? Only the values for lysine, glutamine, glutamic acid, aspartic acid, and the aromatic amino acids deviate. The low lysine content of *lac* repressor leads to an imbalance of arginine to lysine residues (Table 1) but not of basic to acidic amino acids, since both the glutamic acid and the aspartic acid contents are lower than expected from the composition of the average. If these amino acids were in proportion to their average occurrence in proteins, there would be 11% for the basic amino acids and 11.3% for the acidic amino acids. These values are decreased in *lac* repressor to 8.4% and 8.6%, respectively. Thus, the overall number of charged residues in *lac* repressor is decreased, but the charge neutrality at physiological pH is maintained if compared to other proteins (Table 1). This might explain the solubility problems encountered at repressor concentrations exceeding 5–10 mg/ml and also the high aggregation tendency of pure *lac* repressor.

Amino Acid Sequence

One of the prerequisites for the interpretation of a high-resolution X-ray analysis of a protein is the knowledge of its amino acid sequence. The sequence of a protein also allows conclusions on the sequence of the encoding DNA and its transcript and is therefore of special interest for the geneticist working on the same system. Knowledge of the sequence of the *lac* repressor from *E. coli* has, for instance, facilitated the elucidation of the function of several mutagens (Müller-Hill et al. 1975; Miller et al. 1975, 1977; Coulondre and Miller 1977a); the identification of translational reinitiation products past a mutationally created nonsense codon (Platt et al. 1972; Files et al. 1974; Weber et al 1975); the characterization of repressor fragments obtained after limited proteolysis in vitro of *lac* repressor with trypsin (Platt et al. 1973; Files and Weber 1976) and other proteases (Beyreuther 1975); the localization of amino acid substitutions in mutationally altered repressors (Weber et al. 1972; Ganem et al. 1973; Files et al. 1974; Müller-Hill et al. 1975, 1977; Schlotmann et al. 1975) the localization of the sites after chemical modification of *lac* repressor (Fanning 1975; Yang et al. 1977; Alexander et al. 1977; O'Gorman and Matthews 1977); and also the DNA- and RNA-sequence analysis of the *I* gene and its mRNA (Steege 1977; Farabaugh 1978).

The amino acid sequence of *lac* repressor was determined with conventional methods including enzymatic digestions of denatured carboxymethylated *lac* repressor and specific chemical cleavage at methionine residues with cyanogen bromide and at tryptophan residues with N-bromosuccinimide or BNPS-skatole (2-[2-nitrophenyl-sulfenyl]-3-methyl-3'-bromo-indolenine skatole) (Beyreuther et al. 1973, 1975; Beyreuther 1978).

The peptide map (fingerprint) of the tryptic hydrolysate of carboxymethylated *lac* repressor, as shown schematically in Figure 1, reveals the presence of 29 soluble fragments. Only two fragments are not soluble under the conditions employed for fingerprinting (Beyreuther et al. 1975). Trypsin, which cleaves peptide bonds at the carboxy terminus of both arginine and lysine residues, is in fact expected to produce 31 peptides (see the amino acid composition of *lac* repressor in Table 1). However, among the 31 peptides are two ditryptic peptides: a unique fragment containing a Lys-Pro sequence which is resistant to tryptic hydrolysis and a partial cleavage product with the sequence Arg-Lys (spot 1, Fig. 1) which is cleaved, as represented by two spots (spots 2, 3, Fig. 1).

Thus the number of unique tryptic peptides is 30 and not 31. A

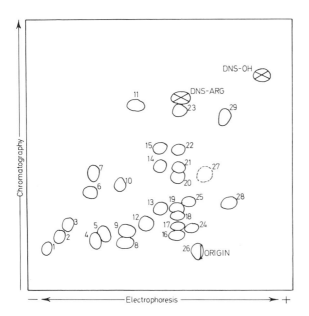

Figure 1 Fingerprint of the tryptic hydrolysate of *S*-[^{14}C]carboxyamido-methylated *lac* repressor. Thin-layer electrophoresis was performed at pH 6.5 and followed by ascending chromatography in butan-1-ol/pyridine/water (35/35/30, v/v/v). The numbers represent peptides which were isolated (Beyreuther et al. 1975). Peptides 1–15 are basic, 16–23 neutral, and 24–29 acidic at pH 6.5. Dansyl arginine (DNS-ARG) and dimethyl-aminonaphthalene-5-sulfonic acid (DNS-OH) were used as fluorescent markers. The electrophoretic mobilities of the peptides were calculated on the basis of the mobilities of these markers; the molecular weights of the peptides were then derived from these mobilities. (Reproduced, with permission, from Beyreuther et al. 1975.)

majority of these peptides (26 fragments) were soluble at pH 8.5 and pH 3.5 and were separated on Dowex 50X7 (Fig. 2). The remaining fraction (insoluble at pH 8.5 or pH 3.5) contained the large tryptic peptides (5 fragments) which were separated by gel filtration (Beyreuther et al. 1975). The sequences of the purified smaller tryptic fragments of up to 20 residues were determined by manual techniques that have been described in detail (Beyreuther et al. 1973). Some of the larger tryptic fragments had to be further fragmented with enzymes, and their sequences were deduced from that of the breakdown products. The order of the tryptic peptides was then determined with the help of cyanogen bromide cleavage products. We separated five large cyanogen bromide fragments including one partial cleavage product (CB 1, Table 2) on Sephadex G-75 (Fig. 3) and digested the four unique fragments (CB 2–CB 5, Table 2) with trypsin, chymotrypsin, and thermolysin. The chymotryptic and thermolytic peptides were those that gave decisive information for the order of the

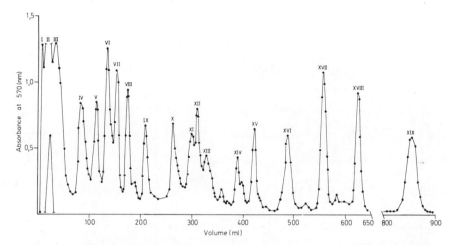

Figure 2 Chromatography of the soluble tryptic peptides on a column (10.5 × 0.9 cm) of Dowex 50X7 at 55°C. The solid line represents the curve obtained by alkaline hydrolysis followed by neutralization and reaction with ninhydrin; 2% was used for reaction with ninhydrin. The column was loaded with 55 mg of tryptic peptides from *S*-carboxyamidomethylated *lac* repressor protein. The numbers above the peaks represent peptides which were isolated. Four fractions containing more than one peptide (II, III, IV, XVII) were subjected to thin-layer electrophoresis or chromatography and yielded ten peptides (Beyreuther et al. 1975).

Table 2 Properties of the large cyanogen bromide fragments of *lac* repressor

Cyanogen bromide fragment	Residues	Position in the sequence	Sequence determined automatically	Percentage of antigenic determinants	Percentage of repressor sequence
CB 1 (FII)	183	43–225	1–54	N.D.[a]	50.8
CB 2 (FIII)	127	99–225	1–52	36	35.3
CB 3 (FIV)	93	255–346	1–42	23	25.8
CB 4 (FV)	56	43–98	1–25	10	15.5
CB 5 (FVI)	41	2–42	1–39	23	11.4

The percentage of antigenic determinants was determined as follows: The corresponding cyanogen bromide fragment was added to the precipitation reaction of *lac* repressor and purified rabbit antirepressor IgG, and the inhibition of repressor precipitation measured as a function of increasing fragment concentration. The values correspond to those reached at the plateau.

[a] N.D. = not determined.

130

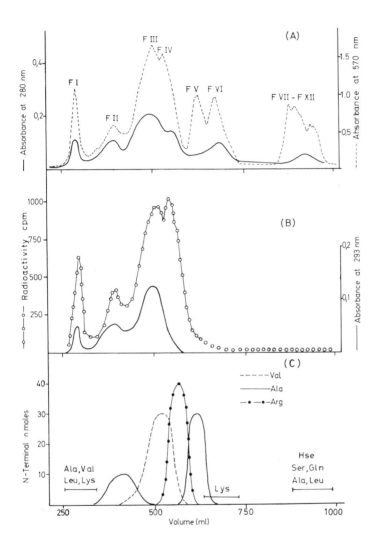

Figure 3 Separation of cyanogen bromide fragments. Cyanogen bromide fragments (60 mg) from S-[^{14}C]carboxyamidomethylated *lac* repressor were chromatographed on a column of Sephadex G-75 (2 × 200 cm). The effluent was recorded at 280 nm (*A*, ———), by ninhydrin analysis of 0.25% after alkaline hydrolysis (*A*, – – – –), at 293 nm (*B*, ———), by counting 1.25% in a liquid scintillation counter (*B*, ○), and by analysis of the N-terminal amino acid residues. The numbers above the peaks in *A* represent peptides which were isolated (Table 2). (Reprinted, with permission, from Beyreuther et al. 1975.)

tryptic peptides. Automated Edman degradation in a sequencer allowed the identification of up to 60 steps which corresponded to about 50% of the sequences of the cyanogen bromide fragments (Table 2). Thus the isolation of suitable peptides for automated sequence analysis allowed us to determine about 60% of the repressor sequence with this method (Beyreuther et al. 1975).

The sequence of *lac* repressor shown in Figure 5 differs from that reported earlier (Beyreuther et al. 1973; Beyreuther 1978). A reexamination of the peptide containing residues 208–216 (Fig. 5) showed that position 215 was a glutamic acid residue instead of glutamine (Beyreuther et al. 1975; J. G. Files, unpubl.). Moreover, the existence of an extra peptide with the sequence Gln-Met in the region directly following residue 230 was revealed by DNA sequence analysis of the *I* gene (Farabaugh 1978). Both of these modifications were suggested by genetic experiments (Miller et al. 1977; Coulondre and Miller 1977a). Furthermore, the DNA sequence of the *I* gene showed that we also missed an undecapeptide spanning residues 148–158 in the original sequence (Farabaugh 1978). I was recently able to confirm these results in the following way (Beyreuther 1978). The dipeptide in question (residues 231–232) should appear as an extra cyanogen bromide fragment with the sequence glutamine-homoserine. Homoserine originates from methionine after treatment with cyanogen bromide (Gross and Witkop 1962). But we did not find a peptide with the expected sequence. It is possible that the amino-terminal glutaminyl residue cyclized to pyrrolidone carboxylic acid, and thus the peptide was not detectable with conventional methods. The acidic reaction conditions for cyanogen bromide cleavage are known to favor the formation of pyrrolidone carboxylic acid from glutamine. So we decided to check the repressor sequence in question using fragments obtained after cleavage with BNPS-skatole. This reagent cleaves tryptophanyl bonds (Omenn et al. 1970). *Lac* repressor with two tryptophanyl residues yielded the expected three major fragments after treatment with BNPS-skatole. The fragments were separated on Bio-Gel P-150 as shown in Figure 4. Automated sequence analysis of fragment C (Fig. 4) containing the C-terminal third of the repressor sequence (residues 221–360) revealed the presence of the extra glutamine-methionine sequence (residues 231–232). Fraction B containing the fragment derived from sequence 1–201 was treated with trypsin. The largest tryptic peptide should include the sought-after undecapeptide. This tryptic peptide, spanning residues 119–168, was isolated by chromatography on Sephadex G-50 and cleaved with peptidyl-L-glutamate hydrolase, an endopeptidase cleaving specifically peptide bonds at glutamic acid residues at pH 4.0 (Houmard and Drapeau 1972). Three peptides were isolated and sequenced. The results confirm that of the DNA sequence analysis of the *I* gene by Farabaugh (1978). Thus the *lac* repressor subunit consists of 360

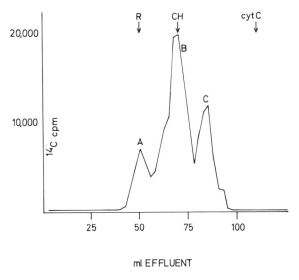

Figure 4 Separation of peptides obtained by cleavage of 20 mg S-[^{14}C]carboxy-amidomethylated *lac* repressor with BNPS-skatole (cleavage at the two trypto-phans). Chromatography on a column of Bio-Gel P-150 (2 × 81 cm) in 6 M guanidine hydrochloride; 0.2% were counted in a liquid scintillation counter. (*A*) Contains uncleaved *lac* repressor; (*B*) contains the fragment consising of residues 1–201 (the shoulder of peak *B* contained the partial cleavage product consisting of residues 1–220); (*C*) contains the fragment derived from the part of the sequence corresponding to residues 221–360. The elution of *lac* repressor (R), chymotrypsinogen (CH, m.w. 25,000), and cytochrome C (cyt C, m.w. 12,500) is indicated by arrows.

residues. They correspond to a subunit molecular weight of 38,600 daltons.

Characteristics of the Sequence

As mentioned above, the amino acid composition of *lac* repressor (Table 1) contains fewer charged residues than expected for an average protein. What is more astonishing is that the middle of the molecule, residues 100 to about 270, shows this diminution only for the basic residues (11.5% acidic residues, 6% basic residues), whereas the amino-terminal part (residues 1–60) and the carboxy-terminal region (residues 281–360) have exactly the opposite character (12% basic residues, 8% and 5% acidic residues, respectively). The region from residue 61 to residue 99 is highly hydrophobic and apolar (Fig. 5). This part of the sequence also contains none of the aromatic amino acids tyrosine, phenylalanine, and tryptophan. The amino-terminal part, in contrast, contains 50% of all tyrosine residues.

```
Met Lys Pro Val Thr Leu Tyr Asp Val Ala Glu Tyr Ala Gly Val
                                     10
Ser Tyr Gln Thr Val Ser Arg Val Val Asn Gln Ala Ser His Val
                20                                        30
Ser Ala Lys Thr Arg Glu Lys Val Glu Ala Ala Met Ala Glu Leu
                          40
Asn Tyr Ile Pro Asn Arg Val Ala Gln Gln Leu Ala Gly Lys Gln
                50                                        60
Ser Leu Leu Ile Gly Val Ala Thr Ser Ser Leu Ala Leu His Ala
                          70
Pro Ser Gln Ile Val Ala Ala Ile Lys Ser Arg Ala Asp Gln Leu
                80                                        90
Gly Ala Ser Val Val Val Ser Met Val Glu Arg Ser Gly Val Glu
                          100
Ala Cys Lys Ala Ala Val His Asn Leu Leu Ala Gln Arg Val Ser
          110                                       120
Gly Leu Ile Ile Asn Tyr Pro Leu Asp Asp Gln Asp Ala Ile Ala
                          130
Val Glu Ala Ala Cys Thr Asn Val Pro Ala Leu Phe Leu Asp Val
          140                                       150
Ser Asp Gln Thr Pro Ile Asn Ser Ile Ile Phe Ser His Glu Asp
                          160
Gly Thr Arg Leu Gly Val Glu His Leu Val Ala Leu Gly His Gln
              170                                   180
Gln Ile Ala Leu Leu Ala Gly Pro Leu Ser Ser Val Ser Ala Arg
                          190
Leu Arg Leu Ala Gly Trp His Lys Tyr Leu Thr Arg Asn Gln Ile
              200                                   210
Gln Pro Ile Ala Glu Arg Glu Gly Asp Trp Ser Ala Met Ser Gly
                          220
Phe Gln Gln Thr Met Gln Met Leu Asn Glu Gly Ile Val Pro Thr
              230                                   240
Ala Met Leu Val Ala Asn Asp Gln Met Ala Leu Gly Ala Met Arg
                          250
Ala Ile Thr Glu Ser Gly Leu Arg Val Gly Ala Asp Ile Ser Val
              260                                   270
Val Gly Tyr Asp Asp Thr Glu Asp Ser Ser Cys Tyr Ile Pro Pro
                          280
Leu Thr Thr Ile Lys Gln Asp Phe Arg Leu Leu Gly Gln Thr Ser
              290                                   300
Val Asp Arg Leu Leu Gln Leu Ser Gln Gly Gln Ala Val Lys Gly
                          310
Asn Gln Leu Leu Pro Val Ser Leu Val Lys Arg Lys Thr Thr Leu
              320                                   330
Ala Pro Asn Thr Gln Thr Ala Ser Pro Arg Ala Leu Ala Asp Ser
                          340
Leu Met Gln Leu Ala Arg Gln Val Ser Arg Leu Glu Ser Gly Gln
              350                                   360
```

Figure 5 Amino acid sequence of *lac* repressor.

Chou and coworkers (1975) have used the sequence to predict the secondary structure of *lac* repressor. They proposed a high content of β-structure for sequences 61–99 and 215–294 with an average length of 10 residues per β-sheet. Helical regions were predicted mainly for the amino-terminal part, residues 1–60, and the middle part, residues 105–206.

The sequence of *lac* repressor shows no significant similarity with that of any of the histones or other DNA-binding proteins. A significant similarity would include common sequences of more than four residues. There is no obvious indication that *lac* repressor has evolved out of a recently duplicated part of the *Z* gene, which produces β-galactosidase. The enzyme shows no significant sequence homology for *lac* repressor (Beyreuther et al. 1973; Fowler and Zabin 1977). This explains why there is no cross-reaction between β-galactosidase, *lac* repressor, and their respective antibodies (Müller-Hill 1971).

One might also compare the sequence of *lac* repressor with the sequence of lambda repressor (Beyreuther and Gronenborn 1976). The complete sequence of the lambda repressor protein was recently worked out by R. T. Sauer (Sauer and Anderegg 1978). The sequences of the two repressors show almost no similarities and there is thus no indication that both proteins have evolved out of a common ancestor. However, the functional organization, as revealed by genetic studies and biochemical analyses of both repressors, shows a striking similarity for both repressors (Eshima et al. 1972; Oppenheim and Noff 1975; Beyreuther and Gronenborn 1976; Müller-Hill et al. 1977).

FUNCTIONAL ANALYSIS OF *lac* REPRESSOR

The functional sites of *lac* repressor which are of special interest for the geneticist and the biochemist are the two ligand-binding sites: the operator- and inducer-binding sites, the transmitter region which links the two ligand-binding activities and the aggregation sites. The analysis of these sites requires their modification, which can be done with chemical and genetic methods.

Not much work has been done on the chemical modification of *lac* repressor, compared to the genetic analysis of the *I* gene and the analysis of mutationally altered *lac* repressors. Rando (1971) described a reagent for affinity labeling of the inducer-binding site, and Lin and Riggs (1974) described a method for affinity labeling of the operator-binding site with bromouracil-containing *lac* operator DNA. The amino acids involved in these reactions have not yet been identified.

Iodination of *lac* repressor leads to loss of operator binding if 1.5 moles of iodine is incorporated per mole of subunit (Fanning 1975). Only three of the eight tyrosine residues, tyrosine 7, 12, and 17, were modified.

The iodinated *lac* repressor does not bind to double-stranded DNA-cellulose, indicating that the bulky iodine atoms abolish binding to the DNA backbone (Beyreuther 1975). However, iodination of *lac* repressor also leads to side reactions, such as intersubunit cross-linking, as revealed by the appearance of stable, covalently linked dimer, trimer, and tetramer subunits and of higher aggregates on SDS-polyacrylamide gels (Kania and Brown 1976). The cross-links are presumably not intersubunit disulfide bridges, since reduction of the iodination products with β-mercapto-ethanol did not alter the pattern on the gel. The loss of operator-binding activity and the polymerization of repressor upon nitration of *lac* repressor with tetranitromethane have also been reported if tyrosines 7, 12, and 17, and presumably also tyrosine 47, are modified (Alexander et al. 1977). However, inducer binding remained essentially unaltered. Thus these results corroborate that tyrosine residues 7, 12, and 17 are exposed, as found by the iodination experiments. Both reactions, leading to modifications of tyrosine residues, result in loss of operator-binding activity and of intersubunit cross-linking, whereas inducer-binding activity remains. Recently, modification of the three cysteine residues for spectral studies has also been described (Yang et al. 1977; Sams et al. 1977). Inducer- and operator-binding activities remain intact, suggesting that the three cysteine residues (107, 140, 281) of the monomer are not constituents of the two ligand-binding sites. On the other hand, nitrophenol reporter groups, introduced at the sites of these cysteine residues, could be used in spectral studies as probes for conformational changes upon binding of inducer and anti-inducer (Sams et al. 1977). Selective modification of the cysteine residues is possible. Cysteine 281 reacts with 2-chloromercuri-4-nitrophenol using one equivalent of this reagent. When two or more equivalents of the alkylating agent are used, cysteines 107 (70%) and 140 (40%) are also modified. The converse was found with 2-bromoacetamide-4-nitrophenol: Cysteine 281 appears to be unreactive and cysteine 140 (85%) is primarily affected in the absence of inducer; but if the reaction is carried out in the presence of inducer, the reactivity of cysteine 107 is increased to near 80%. The different reactivities are a reflection of the environments of the three cysteines in the molecule. The two mercurinitrophenol-reactive cysteines, 107 and 281, are both found in the primary structure in regions containing polar and charged amino acid side chains, whereas the acetimidenitrophenol-reactive cysteine 140 occurs in a quite apolar region (Fig. 5). However, none of these residues reacts with iodoacetate, suggesting that they are not readily available to the solvent.

Treatment of *lac* repressor with N-bromosuccinimide resulted in the oxidation of one of the two tryptophan residues (tryptophan 220) in the monomer (O'Gorman and Matthews 1977). Addition of inducer IPTG but not of anti-inducer *o*-nitrophenyl-β-D-fucoside (ONPF) protected this tryptophan from oxidation. The oxidation of tryptophan 220 did not alter the affinity of repressor for inducer. This suggests that the reactivity of tryptophan 220 is altered not by direct steric hindrance but rather by a conformational change that results upon inducer binding. This conclusion agrees with spectral studies of mutationally altered repressors which indicated that tryptophan 220 is not part of the inducer-binding site (Sommer et al 1976). It has also been reported that low concentrations of *N*-bromosuccinimide destroy operator-binding activity without affecting the ability of the repressor to bind nonspecifically to DNA. However, this effect could not be attributed to a specific residue (O'Gorman and Matthews 1977).

Unfortunately, only a few amino acids can be modified with chemical methods and often several residues react at once. The genetic approach, on the other hand, is more specific and not restricted to a fraction of the 20 amino acids. The use of mutants offers the possibility to exchange nearly every amino acid, and proper selection techniques allow the isolation of mutants affected in specific functions. The elegance of the genetic analysis is described by Miller (this volume). I will focus here on the biochemical analysis of the two major classes of mutations affecting the two binding activities of the *lac* repressor.

Biochemical Analysis of Mutationally Altered *lac* Repressors

We have previously sequenced 20 i^{-d} and i^s repressors in order to localize the borders of the operator-binding site of the repressor monomer (Müller-Hill et al 1975, 1977). Weber and coworkers have sequenced an additional four i^{-d} repressors (Weber et al 1972; Files et al. 1974). Such an analysis makes sense only if the operator-binding site of the repressor may be at least partially uncoupled from the inducer-binding site, and if alterations in the operator-binding site do not affect aggregation sites. In the i^{-d} and i^s repressors, the two ligand-binding sites are in fact partially independent.

The nonrepressing and *trans*-dominant i^{-d} mutants show in vitro inducer-binding activity but no operator binding (Adler et al. 1972). The i^s repressors are, on the other hand, dominant *lac* negatives with weakened or undetectable affinity for inducer in vivo and in vitro (Willson et al. 1964; Gilbert and Müller-Hill 1966; Jobe et al. 1972). The i^s repressors bind to *lac* operator at least as well as the wild-type repressor (Jobe et al. 1972). They obviously have an intact operator-binding site but a damaged inducer-binding site, whereas the i^{-d} class of altered repressors has an intact inducer-binding site and a damaged operator-binding site. Both types of mutationally altered repressors have not lost the ability to form tetramers (Adler et al. 1972; Schmitz et al. 1976). If all mutations affecting operator binding but not inducer binding and aggregation belong to the class of I^{-d} mutations, then the amino acid exchanges leading to those defects should specify the operator-binding sites of the *lac* repressor. A similar argument can be made for the inducer-binding site and the i[s] class of mutants. Since there is evidence for at least partial uncoupling of both ligand-binding sites in mutationally altered *lac* repressors, an unambiguous assignment of residues to one of the two sites should be possible by sequencing all possible altered repressors of each of the two classes. Fortunately, this rather laborious way to analyze an active site is not necessary for the location of the operator-binding site of *lac* repressor.

The genetic analysis of I^{-d} mutations has revealed that they occur only in the part of the *I* gene coding for the amino-terminal region of the repressor, whereas I^s mutations map in a number of clusters throughout the gene (Pfahl 1972; Pfahl et al. 1974; Miller et al. 1975; Miller, this volume). In the regions where the last I^{-d} mutations map, the first I^s mutations are found. This indicates a possible overlapping of the two activities of the repressor. However, as discussed later, sequence analysis of mutationally altered repressors showed that this is not the case.

If in fact the majority of the I^{-d} mutations affect the amino-terminal region of the repressor sequence, then the borders of this site, and possibly the extension of it, should be specified simply by sequencing the i[−d] repressors mapping nearest the amino and carboxy termini. But this holds true only for mutations which abolish operator binding but not other properties of the repressor, since one could imagine that the structure of the operator-binding site might also be altered by damage to the aggregation sites or the inducer-binding site. The reverse situation might also be possible: amino acid substitutions in the operator-binding site could also damage the other sites. Slight alterations might be overlooked, particularly if a property, such as aggregation, is difficult to analyze. However, drastic effects are easy to detect. Therefore, the sought-after candidates are fully constitutive, strong I^{-d} mutations with drastically lowered (by a factor of 10^4) affinity for the operator and with aggregation and inducer-binding properties like wild type (Adler et al. 1972; Müller-Hill et al. 1975; Müller-Hill 1975). I^{-d} mutations leading to repressors which are still inducible (weak I^{-d} mutations) might occur elsewhere in the gene and also lie outside the binding site as mentioned before. They do not necessarily specify the operator-binding site of the repressor.

The genetic mapping by Pfahl (1972), which placed the operator-binding site of the repressor monomer in the amino-terminal region, was supported by protein-chemical mapping of I^{-d} mutations by Weber and coworkers in 1972. Their sequence analyses clearly showed for the first time that the amino acid substitutions in three strong i[−d] repressors are indeed found in the amino-terminal part of the repressor (Weber et al. 1972). The sequencing method used by these authors is based on limited proteolytic digestion of *lac* repressor by trypsin which produces five peptides comprising the amino-terminal 59 residues and those three peptides comprising the carboxy-terminal 20 residues (Platt et al. 1973; Beyreuther et al. 1973). Thus only 79 of the 360 residues of the repressor subunit had to be inspected in order to localize the substitutions. We also used this elegant technique to localize the amino acid exchanges in the strong i^{-d} mutationally altered repressors BG3, BG1, BG4, and JD24, listed in Table 3. The exchanges leading to the furthermost carboxy-terminal-mapping, strong I^{-d} mutations *BG78* and *BG135* could not be localized with this method. The tryptic fragment containing residues 52–59 (Fig. 5) was not found in the digest of native BG78 and BG135 repressor. Automated sequence analysis of the residual core fraction,

Table 3 Properties of mutationally altered *lac* repressor proteins lacking operator binding (strong i^{-d} repressors)

Mutant	Deletion group of mutation	Residue exchanged	Base pair exchanged	Stability in vivo	Nonspecific DNA binding
BG29	2	Thr-5/Met	C-2/U	degraded[a]	reduced
BG2	3	Val-9/Ile	G-1/A	degraded	reduced
BG15	3			degraded	reduced
BG19	3			degraded	reduced
BG24	3			degraded	absent
BG25	3			degraded	absent
BG5	4			degraded	reduced
BG14	4			degraded	reduced
BG13	5			degraded	reduced
BG20	5			stable	
BG11	6			degraded	absent
BG12	6	His-29/Tyr	C-1/U	degraded	reduced
op2	6			stable	absent
BG23	7			degraded	absent
BG1	7	Ala-53/Thr	G-1/A	stable	normal
BG3	7	Ala-53/Val	C-2/U	stable	normal
BG4	7	Ala-53/Thr	G-1/A	stable	normal
JD24	7	Gln-54, Gln-55, Leu-56 deleted		stable	normal
BG78	9	Gly-58/Asp	G-2/A	stable	normal
BG135	9	Gly-58/Ser	G-1/A	stable	normal

The mutants were isolated by Davies and Jacob (1968), Pfahl (1972), and Pfahl et al. (1974). Deletion-group mapping results are taken from Pfahl (1972) and Pfahl et al. (1974) (see also Müller-Hill et al. 1975, 1977; Schlotmann et al. 1975; Schlotmann 1977). All mutants except op2 and JD24 (spontaneous) were isolated after NG mutagenesis.

[a]Limited mutant-specific degradation leading to the removal of about 20, 40, and 60 amino-terminal residues from the mutationally altered repressor.

residues 52–340, revealed that both mutationally altered repressors carry exchanges of glycine 58. It is changed into serine in the BG135 repressor and into aspartic acid in the BG78 repressor (Table 3). An amino acid exchange, near the amino terminus, of threonine 5 to methionine has been reported by Files et al. (1974) in an ethylmethane-sulfonate-derived, mutationally altered repressor. The furthermost amino-terminal-mapping, strong I^{-d} mutation from the collection of Gronenborn and Pfahl (Pfahl et al. 1974) has also been shown to cause an exchange of threonine 5 to methionine (Schlotmann 1977). Do these exchanges define the amino- and carboxy-terminal borders of the operator-binding site of the repressor? BG78 and BG135 are the two rightmost-mapping strong I^{-d} mutations and are isolated from N-methyl-N'-nitro-N-nitrosoguanidine (NG)-derived mutants (Pfahl et al. 1974; Müller-Hill 1975). The vast majority of mutations observed after NG mutagenesis in E. coli, including all 16 substitutions sequenced in my laboratory, have been G/C-to-A/T base exchanges (Miller et al. 1975; Müller-Hill et al. 1975, 1977; Coulondre and Miller 1977b). We therefore would not expect missense mutations at triplets coding for Asn, Gln, Ile, Lys, Phe, Tyr, or Trp in NG-derived mutants (see also Smith et al. 1971). Thus the carboxy-terminal boundary of the operator-binding site might be either glycine 58, lysine 59, or glutamine 60, since at the triplets for lysine and glutamine no mutational changes are expected from the action of NG. The next residue, serine 61, is not in question (see below and Table 4). The amino-terminal border might well be threonine 5, as suggested by the sequence analyses of the mutants, since the codon of the preceding valine residue 4 is expected to be changed after mutagenesis with NG. The next valine residue in position 9 of the sequence is substituted by isoleucine in mutationally altered repressor BG2 (Table 3).

From the sequence analysis of repressors resulting from strong I^{-d} mutations, we may now conclude that the operator-binding site, or at least its major part, is located between residues 5 and 58–60. This fulfills nicely the earlier predictions of Adler et al. (1972) which placed the operator-binding site between residues 1 and 50. Similar results have been obtained by Miller and coworkers in a more extensive study on the suppression of nonsense mutations in the lacI gene (Miller et al. 1975, 1977) and by Weber and coworkers on the biochemical analysis of repressor fragments (Weber et al. 1975; Files and Weber 1976; Geisler and Weber 1977).

We may now ask whether in the strong i^{-d} mutants the specific or the nonspecific binding to lac operator DNA is destroyed. All the mutationally altered repressors listed in Table 3 were tested for binding to phosphocellulose because we found that, in all cases, when repressor binds to phosphocellulose it also binds to double-stranded DNA-cellulose, and when there is no phosphocellulose binding detectable there exists no detectable binding to double-stranded DNA-cellulose (Schlot-mann et al. 1975; Schlotmann and Beyreuther 1977). Using this assay we could determine the region of the protein responsible for nonspecific DNA binding. Among the repressors with exchanges (amino terminal to residue 53) are those which show altered binding to phosphocellulose, i.e., altered nonspecific DNA binding. We did not find any i^{-d} repressor with sequence alterations beyond residue 53 that did not bind to phosphocel-lulose (Table 3). This also holds true for the eight weak i^{-d} repressors sequenced in my laboratory (Table 4). There seem to exist only a few positions for mutations in the amino-terminal part (5–53) leading to repressors capable of normal nonspecific DNA binding. Two such strong i^{-d} mutants have been described by Weber et al. (1972) with exchanges of serine 16 by proline and threonine 19 by alanine. I suggest that these exchanges at positions 16 and 19 are in the specific operator-recognition site of the repressor. The two residues flank one of the three tyrosine residues which are accessible to both iodination and nitration (Fanning 1975; Alexander et al. 1977). Thus it is likely that serine 16 and threonine 19 are also on the surface of the DNA-binding site. Substitution of these

Table 4 Properties of mutationally altered *lac* repressor proteins with reduced operator binding (weak i^{-d} mutants) and of mutationally altered *lac* repressor proteins with altered inducer binding (i^s mutants)

Mutant	Deletion group of mutation	Geno-type	Inducer binding	Residue exchanged	Base pair exchanged	Mutagen
BG46	9	weak I^{-d}	normal	Ala-57/Thr	G-1/A	NG
BG109	9	weak I^{-d}	normal	Ala-57/Thr	G-1/A	NG
BG56	10	weak I^{-d}	reduced	Pro-76/Leu	C-1/U	spontaneous
BG26	9	weak I^{-d}	normal	Ser-77/Leu	C-2/U	NG
BG124	10	weak I^{-d}	normal	Ser-77/Leu	C-2/U	NG
BG200	10	weak I^{-d}	increased	Ala-81/Val	C-2/U	NG
BG185	11	weak I^{-d}	increased	Ala-81/Val	C-2/U	NG
BG52	13	weak I^{-d}	normal	Arg-118/His	G-2/A	spontaneous
X86[a]	9/10	I^s/I^r	normal	Ser-61/Leu	C-2/U	X-ray
MP77	10	I^s	none[b]	His-74/Tyr	C-1/U	NG
MP78	10	I^s	none	Ala-75/Val	C-2/U	NG

Map positions are from Pfahl et al. (1974) and from Bourgeois and Pfahl (1976). For other references, see Table 3. Nonspecific DNA binding of all mutants is similar to that of the wild type.

[a]Induction patterns of X86 repressor are described by Chamness and Willson (1970). The operator binding of this repressor is 40 times tighter than the binding of wild-type repressor (Jobe and Bourgeois 1972). The sequence of X86 repressor has been determined independently by Files and Weber (1976).

[b]Inducer binding is 7% of that of the wild type in the presence of rabbit antiserum against wild-type repressor (I. Triesch, pers. comm.).

residues abolishes operator recognition but not nonspecific DNA binding, since both mutationally altered repressors bind like wild type to phosphocellulose (Weber et al. 1972; K. Weber, pers. comm.). The replacement of "binding" residues by "nonbinding" residues might also change the secondary structure. However, a drastic change in secondary structure should have affected nonspecific binding as well as specific binding, which is not the case.

We may conclude that the operator-binding site (residues 5–60) of the repressor monomer is divided into subregions: a region responsible for nonspecific and specific DNA recognition between residues 5 and 53, and a region between residues 53 and 60 which may be involved only in specific recognition of the operator.

The positive proof that the nonspecific binding region of *lac* repressor indeed resides in the amino-terminal part was recently provided by Müller-Hill and coworkers (1976), using chimaeras which contain amino-terminal pieces of *lac* repressor fused to β-galactosidase, and by Geisler and Weber (1977), using isolated intact amino-terminal parts (headpieces) of *lac* repressor.

No I^s mutations have been found which lower IPTG binding significantly and which map in the first 20% of the gene. The earliest mutations of this type result from mutations I^s77 and I^s78 (Pfahl et al. 1974; Bourgeois and Pfahl 1976) and have amino acid exchanges in position 74 and 75 (Table 4). We also found several weak I^{-d} mutations in this region which lead to repressors with altered operator and inducer binding (Table 4). The failure to find strong I^d mutations in the same region as the earliest I^s mutations, coupled with the finding that repressor fragments missing the initial 59 or 61 residues still bind to IPTG with normal affinity (Weber et al. 1975; Weber and Geisler, this volume), strongly suggests that the residues belonging to the operator-binding site do not overlap and are not shared by those belonging to the inducer-binding site. (Weak I^{-d} mutations do not necessarily occur in the operator-binding site, as indicated by those mutationally altered repressors which have both active sites altered; BG56, BG200, BG185 in Table 4.)

In Vivo Degradation of Mutationally Altered *lac* Repressors

So far, stable i^{-d} repressors have been analyzed which could easily be purified by the conventional method described for wild type. However, we found that some i^{-d} repressors exhibited a broader elution profile from phosphocellulose than that of wild-type repressor, indicating that degradation might have occurred. Recently, Schlotmann (1977) has indeed shown that i^{-d} repressors exist which are degraded in vivo. Some of these unstable repressors are listed in Table 3. Interestingly, these repressors are degraded in a limited mutant-specific way, and the proteolytic degradation does not affect the whole polypeptide chain as shown, for instance, for L_1 repressor (Platt et al. 1970). The resulting tetrameric, inducer-binding fragments resemble those of the proteolytic core fragments of *lac* repressor obtained in vitro (Files and Weber 1976; Schlotmann and Beyreuther 1977).

The processing of i^{-d} mutationally altered *lac* repressors is presumably a cotranslational event, since we did not observe a time-dependent appearance of the fragments in a pulse-chase experiment. Sequence analyses of in-vivo-generated i^{-d} repressor fragments revealed that only parts of the amino-terminal segments were removed. Three major size classes of fragments were identified: fragments lacking approximately 20 residues (m.w. 37,000), 40 residues (m.w. 35,000), and 60 residues (m.w. 32,000).

It is worthwhile to stress that the majority of these repressors which are unstable in vivo map in the part of the *I* gene corresponding to residues 1–51 of the sequence (Table 3). This part is responsible for nonspecific binding to DNA. It therefore seems likely that this region forms a structure of its own, as suggested by Adler et al. (1972). The immunological properties of the amino-terminal-derived cyanogen bromide fragment, residues 2–42 (CB 5 in Table 2), would be in agreement with this assumption. The direct proof that the amino-terminal 51 residues of the repressor subunit have a defined secondary structure was provided by Geisler and Weber (1977) with the isolation and characterization of the headpiece. The amino-terminal DNA-binding domain of the labile i^{-d} repressors might not be folded with the same speed as that of wild type and therefore become susceptible to intracellular proteolysis until folding is complete.

Repressor restart fragments are also stable in vivo and have been isolated in three size classes lacking 23, 42, and 61 amino-terminal residues. They have the same properties as the in-vivo- and in-vitro-generated wild-type and mutationally altered repressor fragments (Platt et al. 1972; Files et al. 1974; Weber et al. 1975). The ease with which approximately 20, 40, and 60 amino-terminal residues are removed in vivo and in vitro and the isolation of stable repressor fragments lacking these residues suggest that structurally independent segments exist in *lac* repressor. This might also be a reflection of a stepwise folding process of the DNA-binding domain of *lac* repressor during translation in units of approximately this length.

Conformational Change of the Operator-binding Site as Revealed by Chemical Studies

Lac repressor is an allosteric protein which exists in at least two conformations: an operator-binding form (R^o) and an inducer-binding form (R^i). The R^o conformation is capable of binding to operator and the R^i conformation is capable of binding inducer. Physicochemical measurements have revealed that a conformational transition occurs between two states of *lac* repressor (Laiken et al. 1972; Oshima et al. 1972; Matthews et al. 1973; Wu et al. 1976). But these studies, depending on changes of fluorescence or ultraviolet (UV)-absorption of the two tryptophans of *lac* repressor (residues 201 and 220), do not allow conclusions as to which residues are involved in the interconversion.

We have used a chemical approach, limited proteolytic digestion of *lac* repressor by chymotrypsin, as a probe for the allosteric change. This assay is based on the finding of Platt et al. (1972) that limited digestion of native *lac* repressor with trypsin releases amino-terminal and carboxy-terminal peptides and produces tetrameric core fragments, devoid of operator binding, that bind inducer.

The chymotryptic proteolysis of native wild-type *lac* repressor at 37°C is different for inducer-liganded and anti-inducer-liganded repressors (Beyreuther 1975; Müller-Hill et al. 1975, 1977). We found that core fragments produced by treatment of unliganded *lac* repressor with chymotrypsin are similar to those obtained in the presence of the inducer IPTG (Table 5). Under these conditions, the repressor is more or less resistant to proteolytic attack. The same digestion but in the presence of the anti-inducer ONPF results in a complete, rapid release of the

Table 5 Chymotryptic cores of *lac* repressor

Ligand	Core fragment amino terminus	carboxy terminus	Percent
No ligand	Gln-18 --	Gln-360	26
	Asn-46 ----------------------------------	Gln-360	22
	Ala-57 -------------------------------	Gln-360	52
IPTG (0.1 M)	Gln-18 --	Gln-360	19
	Asn-46 ----------------------------------	Gln-360	23
	Ala-57 -------------------------------	Gln-360	58
ONPF (0.01 M)	Ala-57 -------------------------------	Leu-323	81
	Ala-57 ----------------------------	Leu-296	17

Lac repressor (4 mg/ml in 0.1 M ammonium bicarbonate buffer, pH 8.0) was digested with chymotrypsin (1% w/w) for 5 min at 37°C in the presence of the inducer IPTG and the anti-inducer ONPF, and in the absence of ligands. The reaction was stopped by lowering the pH to 3.0, and the digest was chromatographed on Sephadex G-50 (1 M acetic acid as eluant). The core fraction (eluting with the front) was subjected to automated sequence analysis (amino-terminal cleavage sites) and digested with carboxypeptidase C (carboxy-terminal cleavage sites). C-terminal cleavage sites were also deduced from the released (C-terminal derived) peptides which eluted after core on Sephadex G-50 (Müller-Hill et al. 1975; K. Beyreuther, unpubl.).

amino-terminal residues 1–56, as determined by automated sequence analysis of the resulting core (Table 5). In addition to the release of amino-terminal repressor parts under the conditions specified in Table 5, there is also a release of carboxy-terminal-derived peptides in the presence of ONPF. ONPF is known to bind to operator-bound repressor, stabilizing the complex (Müller-Hill et al. 1964), and was used instead of *lac* operator DNA, which was not available in sufficient quantities for these experiments. ONPF competes with IPTG for binding, suggesting that both effectors bind at the same site. The difference between the native proteolysis in the presence of ONPF and that of free and IPTG-bound repressor was used as a measure for the repressor conformation. We define the R^i conformation as one which allows not more than 50–60% cleavage at leucine 56, producing tetrameric, inducer-binding core fragments. Repressor in the R^o conformation stabilized, for instance, by ONPF leads to 100% release of 56 amino-terminal residues by chymotrypsin. Thus we were able to test some of the mutationally altered repressors and to ask whether the sequence alteration had any influence on repressor conformation. For instance, we expect that some of the i^s repressors might be permanently present in the R^o conformation and might show the typical proteolytic pattern of the R^o form. We also expect that some of the i^{-d} repressors might exhibit a pattern characteristic of the R^i form even in the presence of the anti-inducer ONPF if the hinge region is affected.

We have tested some of the sequenced mutationally altered repressors, and the results are listed in Table 6. There is a group of mutationally altered repressors which behave just like wild type. To this group belong all the tested weak i^{-d} repressors and the strong i^{-d} mutationally altered repressors with amino acid alterations before residue 53. Iodinated *lac* repressor behaves the same only if tyrosine residues 7, 12, and 17 are modified (Beyreuther 1975). Another group of mutationally altered repressors, including all tested strong i^{-d} repressors with amino acid exchanges between residues 53 and 58, does not show the characteristic rapid removal of the 56 amino-terminal residues in the presence of ONPF. The two i^s mutationally altered repressors analyzed thus far do not bind IPTG or ONPF and were found only in the R^o form. Mutationally altered X86 repressor differs only in the unliganded form from the wild type (Table 6).

How can we understand these results? We have seen (above) that the amino-terminal part of *lac* repressor is involved in specific and nonspecific DNA binding and that amino acid alterations in the region between residues 53 and 58 completely abolish specific binding with no concomitant loss of nonspecific binding. Some of the i^{-d} mutationally altered repressors which have amino acid substitutions before residue 53 are damaged, to some extent, in nonspecific DNA binding. Furthermore, in

Table 6 Chymotryptic cores of mutationally altered *lac* repressors

Repressor	Conformation			Allosteric properties
	no ligand	inducer	anti-inducer	
Wild type	R^i	R^i	R^o	normal
BG2 (strong i^{-d}) (Val-9/Ile)	R^i	R^i	R^o	normal
BG124 (weak i^{-d}) (Ser-77/Leu)	R^i	R^i	R^o	normal
Iodinated wild type	R^i	R^i	R^o	normal
BG1 (strong i^{-d}) (Ala-53/Thr)	R^i	R^i	R^i	altered
BG78 (strong i^{-d}) (Gly-58/Asp)	R^i	R^i	R^i	altered
BG135 (strong i^{-d}) (Gly-58/Ser)	R^i	R^i	R^i	altered
MP77 (i^s) (His-74/Tyr)	R^o	R^o	R^o	altered
X86 ($i^{s/r}$) (Ser-61/Leu)	R^o	R^i	R^o	altered

R^i refers to core fragments similar to those produced from wild-type repressor in the presence of the inducer IPTG or in the absence of ligands; it denotes the inducer-binding conformation. R^o indicates that the core fragments produced resemble those produced from wild-type repressor in the presence of the anti-inducer ONPF; it denotes the operator-binding conformation. For comparison and conditions, see Table 5.

the presence of IPTG, the binding constant of *lac* repressor for *lac* operator is reduced by several orders of magnitude, but the binding to other DNAs is not altered (Lin and Riggs 1972; von Hippel et al. 1975; Beyreuther 1975). Therefore we can conclude that the *lac* repressor–inducer complex is altered only in the specific recongition of operator, and not in the binding to the backbone of the DNA. The observation that chymotrypsin cuts preferentially after leucine residue 56 when the repressor is liganded with the anti-inducer ONPF, but not in the presence of the inducer IPTG, suggests that it is the region between residues 53 and 58 which changes its conformation upon induction. This hypothesis is strengthened by the result that two i^s repressors which have residues 74 or 75 exchanged behave toward chymotrypsin like ONPF-liganded wild-type repressor, and by the finding that strong i^{-d} mutationally altered repressors with exchanges of residues 53 and 58 behave in the presence of ONPF like unliganded wild-type repressor. These results seem to indicate that the two i^s repressors are frozen in the R^o form and the i^{-d} repressors are frozen in the R^i form.

The treatment of repressor resulting from i^s77 with several proteases, including chymotrypsin, trypsin, and thermolysin, produces core fragments which bind inducer weakly. The effect is increased if leucine 56 is removed (Table 7). Thus the removal of the DNA-binding site improves inducer binding in this case.

All analyzed strong i^{-d} repressors with alterations (carboxy terminal of residue 52) are frozen in the R^i form. These mutationally altered repressors bind ONPF, but do not respond. Mutationally altered i^{-d} repressors whose exchanges are between residues 1 and 52 and all weak i^{-d} repressors tested so far, including BG46 which has alanine 57 replaced by threonine, behave like wild-type repressor and have no drastically altered allosteric properties. We might therefore conclude that the part of the repressor formed by residues 53–58 forms the hinge region which is deformed during binding of inducer. This might be the molecular explanation of induction. Residues to the carboxy terminal of lysine 59, including serine 61, histidine 74, and alanine 75, might be part of the region which transmits the signals from the inducer-binding site to the flexible part of the operator-binding site (the hinge region) and vice versa.

Aggregation Sites

Proteolysis of *lac* repressor also leads to a release of carboxy-terminal-derived peptides (Beyreuther et al. 1973; Files and Weber 1976)

Table 7 Inducer-binding properties of i^s77 mutationally altered *lac* repressor

Repressor protein	Amino-terminal residues removed	IPTG-binding specific activity[a] (%/mg/ml)
Wild type	0	1300
Wild type T-C core	59	2000
i^s77	0	<0.5
i^s77 TL core	55	8
i^s77 T core	$\begin{cases} 51 \\ 59 \end{cases}$ (equimolar)	16
i^s77 C core	56	32
i^s77 T-C core	59	35

The i^s77 repressor has histidine 74 replaced by tyrosine and has the conformation R^o as defined in Table 6. IPTG-binding assays have been carried out as described by Gilbert and Müller-Hill (1966). The repressor core fragments were obtained under the conditions specified in Table 5 (no ligand). The proteases used were trypsin (T), chymotrypsin (C), and thermolysin (TL).
[a]As defined by Müller-Hill et al. (1968).

Prolonged digestion with trypsin or chymotrypsin leads to core fragments which are no longer tetramers. Both proteases produce dimeric core fragments after 60-minute digestion at 37°C and monomeric core fragments after 330-minute digestion (Table 8). The monomeric core produced with chymotrypsin lacks 65 residues from the carboxy-terminal end and does not bind inducer. The dimeric repressor core fragments have lost 35 residues (tryptic core) and 37 residues (chymotryptic core) from the carboxy terminus. ·

The results presented in Table 8 indicate that a transition of *lac* repressor from one conformation to the other influences not only the proteolytic susceptibility of the "inducible" part of the amino-terminal operator-binding site (the hinge region) but presumably also that of some residues participating in aggregation. I expect this to be important for the proper spacing of the subunits in *lac* repressor tetramers for operator binding. Such a change in the quaternary structure as a consequence of a "rolling" of subunits is known to occur in hemoglobin (Perutz 1970).

Mutations resulting in aggregation defects are described by Miller (Schmitz et al. 1976). They map in the part of the *I* gene which specifies a region of the repressor close to that removed in the monomeric core fragments. Thus it is possible to assume that the carboxy-terminal part of *lac*

Table 8 Quaternary structure of proteolytic cores

Protease	Ligand	Digestion time (min)	Core (%)	Residues released from C terminus[a]	Inducer binding
Trypsin	IPTG (0.1 M)	60	25 tetramer	no	wt[b]
	IPTG (0.1 M)	60	75 dimer	35	1.5x wt
	ONPF (0.01 M)	60	100 dimer	35	1.5x wt
Chymotrypsin	IPTG (0.1 M)	60	5 tetramer	no	wt
	IPTG (0.1 M)	60	90 dimer	37	1.5x wt
	IPTG (0.1 M)	60	5 monomer	64	absent
	IPTG (0.1 M)	330	100 dimer	37	1.5x wt
	ONPF (0.01 M)	60	40 dimer	37	1.5x wt
	ONPF (0.01 M)	60	60 monomer	64	absent
	ONPF (0.01 M)	330	8 dimer	37	1.5x wt
	ONPF (0.01 M)	330	92 monomer	64	absent

Core fragments were analyzed by sedimentation in glycerol gradients and by chromatography on Sephadex G-200. Inducer binding of wild-type repressor (wt) was assumed as 1350 (sp. act. according to Gilbert and Müller-Hill [1966]; Müller-Hill et al. [1971]).
[a]See also Table 5 for the sequence of the core fragments.
[b]wt = Wild type.

repressor is involved in the aggregation of the subunits and that the aggregation sites might be in "allosteric" contact with the ligand-binding sites.

CONCLUDING REMARKS

The protein-chemical analysis of wild-type and mutationally altered *lac* repressors has yielded the answers to questions such as, To which parts of the sequence do the two ligand-binding sites, the aggregation sites, the hinge region, and the transmitter region extend? However, at present, a precise answer can be provided only for the operator-DNA-binding site on which most of the experiments described were focused. The general conclusion is that the operator-binding site of the *lac* repressor monomer consists of two functionally distinct parts: (1) a structurally rigid, "noninducible" subregion which is presumably formed from the amino-terminal repressor sequence 1–51; (2) a structurally flexible, "inducible" part composed of residues 52–60 (Table 9).

The latter functional part of the DNA-binding site might be identical with the hinge region or at least a part of it. The inducible part exists in two conformations, one capable of interacting specifically with the bases of the operator DNA and the other preventing this upon binding of inducer. The noninducible part of the DNA-binding site also participates in base recognition and interacts with the phosphate groups of the DNA backbone by using some of the basic residues from sequence 22–51 of the subunits.

The transmitter region is presumably located adjacent to the inducible part of the DNA-binding site. Some of the residues of sequence 61–81 might belong to this region which transmits the signal between the two binding sites upon binding of ligands. In other words, the DNA-binding site is separated from the inducer-binding site by a region which triggers the conformation of the inducible part of the operator-binding site. The existence of an operator-binding, inducer-nonbinding i^s repressor which binds inducer if the DNA-binding site is removed provided biochemical evidence that both activities exclude each other. That means each of the

Table 9 Functional organization of the operator-binding site of the *lac* repressor subunit

Operator DNA-binding site	Sequence
Noninducible	1–51
Inducible	52–60

two conformations exhibits only one binding activity; therefore, repressor in the operator-binding conformation does not bind inducer, and vice versa.

A precise assignment of the aggregation sites to the sequence is not possible with the results discussed in this paper. However, genetic and biochemical evidence points to the carboxy-terminal sequence 280–360 as a region possibly contributing to aggregation. Inducer binding may affect aggregation, as indicated by the in vitro proteolysis experiments.

Up to now, little positive evidence has been obtained by chemical analysis for the localization of the inducer-binding site to specific parts of the sequence. However, a large amount of negative and positive evidence has accumulated which places the inducer-binding site outside of the DNA-binding site and also outside of the sequence 323–360.

Since 1972, increasing evidence has been obtained in favor of an independent tertiary structure for the part of the repressor monomer carrying the DNA-binding site and for the part carrying the inducer-binding site and the aggregational sites. They might exist as two globular domains. If that holds true, we might ask how the globule which carries the operator-binding site might appear. I suggest that the operator-DNA-binding site of the repressor looks rather like a plaster cast of the operator DNA. Such an active site would include rising grounds fitting into the grooves on the DNA, and not clefts which are the common active-site structures of enzymes. Repressor crystals and cocrystals of the repressor-operator complex will reveal the true structure.

ACKNOWLEDGMENTS

I am pleased to have the opportunity to thank Benno Müller-Hill for his constant interest, support, and encouragement during the course of this work. Special thanks are due to my past and present collaborators K. Adler, D. Bielig, H. Böhmer, E. Fanning, N. Geisler, E. Hoven, C. Murray, P. O'Conner, and I. Triesch, whose contributions to many portions of the work described herein were indispensable. I thank J. H. Miller and P. Betteridge for useful comments and suggestions. Work done in my laboratory has been supported by the Deutsche Forschungs-gemeinschaft through SFB 74.

REFERENCES

Adler, K., K. Beyreuther, E. Fanning, N. Geisler, B. Gronenborn, A. Klemm, B. Müller-Hill, M. Pfahl, and A. Schmitz. 1972. How *lac* repressor binds to DNA. *Nature* 237:322.

Alberts, B. M., F. J. Amonio, M. Jenkins, E. D. Gutmann, and F. L. Ferris. 1969. Studies with DNA-cellulose chromatography. *Cold Spring Harbor Symp. Quant. Biol.* 33:289.

Alexander, M. E., A. A. Burgum, R. A. Noall, M. D. Shaw, and K. S. Matthews. 1977. Modification of tyrosine residues of the lactose repressor protein. *Biochim. Biophys. Acta* **493**:367.

Beyreuther, K. 1975. Allosteric changes of the deoxyribonucleic acid-binding site of *lac* repressor from *Escherichia coli. Biochem. Soc. Trans.* **3**:1125.

———. 1978. Revised sequence for the *lac* repressor. *Nature* (in press).

Beyreuther, K. and B. Gronenborn. 1976. N-terminal sequence of phage *lambda* repressor. *Mol. Gen. Genet.* **147**:115.

Beyreuther, K., K. Adler, N. Geisler, and A. Klemm. 1973. The amino-acid sequence of *lac* repressor. *Proc. Natl. Acad. Sci.* **70**:3576.

Beyreuther, K., K. Adler, E. Fanning, C. Murray, A. Klemm, and N. Geisler. 1975. Amino-acid sequence of *lac* repressor from *Escherichia coli. Eur. J. Biochem.* **59**:491.

Bourgeois, S. and M. Pfahl. 1976. Repressors. *Advanc. Protein Chem.* **30**:1.

Bourgeois, S., M. Cohn, and L. E. Orgel. 1965. Suppression of and complementation among mutants of the regulatory gene of the lactose operon of *Escherichia coli. J. Mol. Biol.* **14**:300.

Calos, M. 1978. The DNA sequence for a low-level promoter of the lactose repressor gene and an "up" promoter mutation. *Nature* (in press).

Chamness, G. C. and C. D. Willson. 1970. An unusual *lac* repressor mutant. *J. Mol. Biol.* **53**:561

Chou, P. Y., A. J. Adler, and G. D. Fasman. 1975. Conformational prediction and circular dichroism studies on the *lac* repressor. *J. Mol. Biol.* **96**:29.

Coulondre, C. and J. H. Miller. 1977a. Genetic studies of the *lac* repressor. III. Additional correlations of mutational sites with specific amino acid residues. *J. Mol. Biol.* **117**:525.

———. 1977b. Genetic studies of the *lac* repressor. IV. Mutagenic specificity in the *lac I* gene of *Escherichia coli. J. Mol. Biol.* **117**:577.

Davies, J. and F. Jacob. 1968. Genetic mapping of the regulator and operator genes in the *lac* operon *J. Mol. Biol.* **36**:413.

Eshima, N., S. Fujii, and T. Horiuchi. 1972. Isolation of *lambda ind⁻* mutants. *Jpn. J. Genet.* **47**:125.

Fanning, T. G. 1975. Iodination of *Escherichia coli lac* repressor. Effect of tyrosine modification on repressor activity. *Biochemistry* **14**:2512.

Farabaugh, P. J. 1978. The sequence of the *lacI* gene. *Nature* (in press).

Files, J. G. and K. Weber, 1976. Limited proteolytic digestion of *lac* repressor by trypsin. *J. Biol. Chem.* **251**:3386.

Files, J. G., K. Weber, and J. H. Miller. 1974. Translational reinitiation: Reinitiation of *lac* repressor fragments at three internal sites early in the *lac i* of *Escherichia coli. Proc. Natl. Acad. Sci.* **71**:667.

Fowler, A. V. and I. Zabin. 1977. The amino acid sequence of β-galactosidase of *Escherichia coli. Proc. Natl. Acad. Sci.* **74**:1507.

Ganem, D., J. H. Miller, J. G. Files, T. Platt, and K. Weber. 1973. Reinitiation of a *lac* repressor fragment at a codon other than AUG. *Prog. Natl. Acad. Sci.* **70**:3165.

Geisler, N. and K. Weber. 1976. Isolation of a set of hybrid *lac* repressors made *in vitro* between normal *lac* repressor and its homogeneous tryptic core. *Proc. Natl. Acad. Sci.* **73**:3103.

————. 1977. Isolation of the amino-terminal fragment of lactose repressor necessary for DNA binding. *Biochemistry* **16**: 938.

Gilbert, W. and B. Müller-Hill. 1966. Isolation of the *lac* repressor. *Proc. Natl. Acad. Sci.* **56**: 1891.

————. 1967. The *lac* operator is DNA. *Proc. Natl. Acad. Sci.* **58**: 2415.

Gross, E. and B. Witkop. 1962. Nonenzymatic cleavage of peptide bonds: The methionine residue in bovine pancreatic ribonuclease. *J. Biol. Chem.* **237**: 1856.

Hamada, F., Y. Ohshima, and T. Horiuchi. 1973. Dissociation of the *lac* repressor into subunits. *J. Biochem.* **73**: 1299.

Holmquist, W. R. and H. Moise. 1975. Compositional nonrandomness: A quantitatively conserved evolutionary invariant. *J. Mol. Evol.* **6**: 1.

Houmard, J. and G. R. Drapeau. 1972. Staphylococcal protease: A proteolytic enzyme specific for glutamoyl bonds. *Proc. Natl. Acad. Sci.* **69**: 3506.

Jacob, F. and J. Monod. 1961. Genetic regulatory mechanisms in the synthesis of proteins. *J. Mol. Biol.* **3**: 318.

Jacob, F., R. Sussman, and J. Monod. 1962. Sur la nature du répresseur assurant l'immunité des bactéries lysogènes. *C. R. Acad. Sci.* **254**: 4214.

Jobe, A. and S. Bourgeois. 1972. The *lac* repressor-operator interaction. VII. A repressor with unique binding properties: The X86 repressor. *J. Mol. Biol.* **72**: 139.

Jobe, A., A. D. Riggs, and S. Bourgeois. 1972. *Lac* repressor-operator interaction. V. Characterization of super- and pseudo-wild type repressors. *J. Mol. Biol.* **64**: 181.

Jukes, T. H., R. Holmquist, and H. Moise. 1975. Amino acid composition of proteins: Selection against the genetic code. *Science* **189**: 50.

Kania, J. and D. T. Brown. 1976. The functional repressor parts of a tetrameric *lac* repressor-β-galactosidase chimaera are organized as dimers. *Proc. Natl. Acad. Sci.* **73**: 3529.

Laiken, S. L., C. A. Gross, and P. H. von Hippel. 1972. Equilibrium and kinetic studies of *Escherichia coli lac* repressor-inducer interactions. *J. Mol. Biol.* **66**: 143.

Lin, S.-Y. and A. D. Riggs. 1972. *Lac* repressor binding to non-operator DNA: Detailed studies and a comparison of equilibrium and rate competition methods. *J. Mol. Biol.* **72**: 671.

————. 1974. Photochemical attachment of *lac* repressor to bromodeoxyuridine-substituted *lac* operator by ultraviolet radiation. *Proc. Natl. Acad. Sci.* **71**: 947.

Matthews, K. S., H. R. Matthews, H. W. Thielmann, and O. Jardetzky. 1973. Ultraviolet difference spectra of the lactose repressor protein. *Biochim. Biophys. Acta* **295**: 159.

Miller, J. H. 1970. Transcription starts and stops in the *lac* operon. In *The lactose operon* (ed. J. R. Beckwith and D. Zipser), p. 173. Cold Spring Harbor Laboratory, Cold Spring Harbor, New York.

Miller, J. H., D. Ganem, P. Lu, and A. Schmitz. 1977. Genetic studies of the *lac* repressor. I. Correlation of mutational sites with specific amino acid residues: Construction of a colinear gene-protein map. *J. Mol. Biol.* **109**: 275.

Miller, J. H., C. Coulondre, U. Schmeissner, A. Schmitz, and P. Lu. 1975. The use of suppressed nonsense mutations to generate altered *lac* repressor molecules. In *Protein-ligand interactions* (ed. H. Sund and G. Blauer), p. 238. Walter de Gruyter, Berlin.

Müller-Hill, B. 1966. Suppressible regulator constitutive mutants in the lactose system in *Escherichia coli. J. Mol. Biol.* **15**: 374.

———. 1971. *Lac* repressor. *Angew. Chem.* **10**: 160.

———. 1975. *Lac* repressor and *lac* operator. *Prog. Biophys. Mol. Biol.* **30**: 227.

Müller-Hill, B., K. Beyreuther, and W. Gilbert. 1971. *Lac* repressor from *Escherichia coli. Methods Enzymol.* **21D**: 483.

Müller-Hill, B., L. Crapo, and W. Gilbert. 1968. Mutants that make more *lac* repressor. *Proc. Natl. Acad. Sci.* **59**: 1259.

Müller-Hill, B., G. Heidecker, and J. Kania. 1976. Repressor-galactosidase-chimaeras. In *Proceedings of the Third John Innes Symposium: Structure-function relationships of proteins* (ed. R. Markham and R. W. Horne), p. 167. Elsevier/North-Holland, Amsterdam.

Müller-Hill, B., H. V. Rickenberg, and K. Wallenfels. 1964. Specificity of the induction of the enzymes of the *lac* operon in *Escherichia coli. J. Mol. Biol.* **10**: 303.

Müller-Hill, B., B. Gronenborn, J. Kania, M. Schlotmann, and K. Beyreuther. 1977. Similarities between *lac* repressor and *lambda* repressor. In *Nucleic acid-protein recognition* (ed. H. J. Vogel), p. 219. Academic Press, New York.

Müller-Hill, B. T. Fanning, N. Geisler, D. Gho, J. Kania, P. Kathmann, H. Meissner, M. Schlotmann, A. Schmitz, I. Triesch, and K. Beyreuther. 1975. The active sites of *lac* repressor. In *Protein-ligand interactions* (ed. H. Sund and G. Blauer), p. 211. Walter de Gruyter, Berlin.

O'Gorman, R. B. and K. S. Matthews. 1977. N-bromosuccinimide modification of *lac* repressor protein. *J. Biol. Chem.* **252**: 3565.

Omenn, G. S., A. Fontana, and C. B. Anfinsen. 1970. Modification of the single tryptophan residue of staphyolococcal nuclease by a new mild oxidizing agent. *J. Biol. Chem.* **245**: 1895.

Oppenheim, A. B. and D. Noff. 1975. Deletion mapping of *trans* dominant mutations in the *lambda* repressor gene. *Virology* **64**: 553.

Oshima, Y., M. Matsuura, and T. Horiuchi. 1972. Conformational change of the *lac* repressor induced with the inducer. *Biochem. Biophys. Res. Commun.* **47**: 1444.

Perutz, M. 1970. Stereochemistry of cooperative effect in hemoglobin. *Nature* **228**: 726.

Pfahl, M. 1972. Genetic map of the lactose repressor gene (*i*) of *Escherichia coli. Genetics* **72**: 393.

Pfahl, M., C. Stockter, and B. Gronenborn. 1974. Genetic analysis of the active sites of *lac* repressor. *Genetics* **76**: 669.

Platt, T., J. G. Files, and K. Weber. 1973. *Lac* repressor. Specific proteolytic destruction of the NH_2-terminal region and loss of the deoxyribonucleic acid-binding activity. *J. Biol. Chem.* **248**: 110.

Platt, T., J. H. Miller, and K. Weber. 1970. *In Vivo* degradation of mutant *lac* repressor. *Nature* **228**: 1154.

Platt, T., K. Weber, D. Ganem, and J. H. Miller. 1972. Translational restarts: AUG reinitiation of a *lac* repressor fragment. *Proc. Natl. Acad. Sci.* **69**: 897.

Rando, R. R. 1971. Effector site labeling of the *lac* repressor. *Nat. New Biol.* **234**: 183.

Riggs, A. D. and S. Bourgeois. 1968. On the assay, isolation and characterization of the *lac* repressor. *J. Mol. Biol.* **34**: 361.

Riggs, A. D., S. Bourgeois, R. F. Newby, and M. Cohn. 1968. DNA binding of the *lac* repressor. *J. Mol. Biol.* **34**:365.

Rosenberg, J. M., O. B. Khallai, M. L. Kopka, R. E. Dickerson, and A. D. Riggs. 1977. *Lac* repressor purification without inactivation of DNA binding activity. *Nucleic Acids Res.* **4**:567.

Sams, C. F., B. E. Friedman, A. A. Burgum, D. S. Yang, and K. S. Matthews. 1977. Spectral studies of lactose repressor protein modified with nitrophenol reporter groups. *J. Biol. Chem.* **252**:3153.

Sauer, R. T. and R. Anderegg. 1978. Primary structure of the *lambda* repressor. *Biochemistry* (in press).

Schlotmann, M. 1977. "Protein-chemische Analyse von *lac* Repressoren aus *E. coli.*" Ph.D. thesis, Universität zu Köln, Köln, Germany.

Schlotmann, M. and K. Beyreuther. 1977. Some mutant *lac* repressors are specifically degraded *in vivo* during translation in *Escherichia coli. Eur. J. Biochem.* (in press).

Schlotmann, M., K. Beyreuther, N. Geisler, and B. Müller-Hill. 1975. Mutant *lac* repressors of *Escherichia coli* with altered deoxyribonucleic acid-binding properties. *Biochem. Soc. Trans.* **3**:1123.

Schmitz, A., U. Schmeissner, and J. H. Miller. 1976. Mutations affecting the quarternary structure of the *lac* repressor. *J. Biol. Chem.* **251**:3359.

Smith, J. D., K. Anderson, A. Cashmore, M. L. Hooper, and R. L. Russel. 1971. Studies on the structure and synthesis of *Escherichia coli* tyrosine transfer RNA. *Cold Spring Harbor Symp. Quant. Biol.* **35**:21.

Sommer, H., P. Lu, and J. H. Miller. 1976. *Lac* repressor. Fluorescence of the two tryptophans. *J. Biol. Chem.* **251**:3774.

Steege, D. A. 1977. 5'-Terminal nucleotide sequence of *Escherichia coli* lactose repressor mRNA: Features of translational initiation and reinitiation site. *Proc. Natl. Acad. Sci.* **74**:4163.

Thomas, R. and L. Lambert. 1962. On the occurrence of bacterial mutations permitting lysogenization by clear variants of temperate bacteriophages. *J. Mol. Biol.* **23**:277.

von Hippel, P. H., A. Revzin, C. A. Gross, and A. C. Wang. 1975. Interactions of *lac* repressor with non-specific DNA binding sites. In *Protein-ligand interactions* (ed. H. Sund and G. Blauer), p. 270. de Gruyter, Berlin.

Weber, K., T. Platt, D. Ganem, and J. H. Miller. 1972. Altered sequences changing the operator-binding properties of the *lac* repressor: Colinearity of the repressor protein with the *i*-gene map. *Proc. Natl. Acad. Sci.* **69**:3624.

Weber, K., J. G. Files, T. Platt, D. Ganem, and J. H. Miller. 1975. *Lac* repressor. In *Protein-ligand interactions* (ed. H. Sund and G. Blauer), p. 228. Walter de Gruyter, Berlin.

Willson, C., D. Perrin, M. Cohn, F. Jacob, and J. Monod. 1964. Non-inducible mutants of the regulator gene in the lactose system of *Escherichia coli. J. Mol. Biol.* **8**:582.

Wu, F. Y.-H., P. Bandyopadhyay, and C.-W. Wu. 1976. Conformational transitions of the *lac* repressor from *Escherichia coli. J. Mol. Biol.* **100**:459.

Yang, D. S., A. A. Burgum, and K. S. Matthews. 1977. Modification of the cysteine residues of the lactose repressor protein using chromophoric probes. *Biochim. Biophys. Acta* **493**:24.

lac Repressor Fragments Produced In Vivo and In Vitro: An Approach to the Understanding of the Interaction of Repressor and DNA

Klaus Weber and Norbert Geisler
Max Planck Institute for Biophysical Chemistry
D-3400 Göttingen, Federal Republic of Germany

INTRODUCTION

Lac repressor is a tetrameric molecule with two types of binding sites. One site recognizes specifically the *lac* operator DNA; the other recognizes the inducer molecule, the small sugar derivative, isopropyl-β-D-thiogalactoside (IPTG). Although the amino acid sequence of the *lac* repressor and the DNA sequence of the operator are known (Beyreuther et al. 1973; Gilbert and Maxam 1973), our understanding of the direct molecular interactions of the two macromolecules is still rather poor. Among the different approaches to this problem is one which we specifically want to stress in this paper. It is based on the existence of *lac* repressor derivatives, obtained both in vivo and in vitro, which are missing the amino-terminal part of the molecule but still show the inducer-binding activity and the tetrameric oligomerization typical of *lac* repressor. These derivatives have been found in the past to be extremely useful in studying structure and function relationship in the *lac* repressor molecule.

We first encountered the in vivo derivatives during a collaboration with J. Miller on the protein-chemical characteristics of early nonsense mutations in the *I* gene. These mutations showed negative complementation and therefore were excellent candidates for studying the phenomenon of translational reinitiation in vivo. Indeed, we found that early nonsense mutations give rise to a reinitiation of translation past the amber block. The resulting mutationally altered proteins, which were missing the amino-terminal part of the polypeptide, could still form tetramers and display unimpaired inducer binding but were devoid of DNA binding (Platt et al. 1972; Ganem et al. 1973; Files et al. 1974). These results reinforced the independently developed predictions from genetic studies (Adler et al. 1972; Miller et al. 1975) that the amino-terminal part is a necessary requirement of DNA binding but is not required for oligomerization or inducer binding.

These repressor derivatives are extremely difficult to purify, but their existence stimulated our interest in obtaining similar derivatives in vitro. The use of trypsin on native repressor has allowed us to do this (Platt et al. 1973). Over the years this "native tryptic digest" has been improved, and repressor can now be dissected into a homogeneous tetrameric core accounting for amino acid residues 60–347 and amino-terminal "head-pieces" accounting for residues 1–51 or 1–59, respectively (Geisler and Weber 1977). This native tryptic digest immediately allowed a fast and successful way to map on a protein-chemical level early mutations in the I gene and to correlate the genetic map with the protein sequence (Weber et al. 1972). The later developments on the native tryptic digest have allowed us to isolate the amino-terminal headpieces and to show that they indeed carry DNA-binding activity (Geisler and Weber 1977). Furthermore, the existence of a tetrameric, homogeneous tryptic core has invited studies on in vitro hybrids between normal and core polypeptides in order to study the problem of how many subunits of the tetrameric repressor bind simultaneously to operator DNA (Geisler and Weber 1976).

Here we summarize these experiments and try to show what predictions for structure and function relationship can be derived from a study of *lac* repressor fragments obtained in vivo and in vitro.

RESULTS

Repressor Derivatives Which Have Lost the Amino-Terminal End In Vivo: Translational Reinitiation Past a Nonsense Codon

We thought that translational reinitiation mutants might be present in a collection of spontaneous nonsense mutants because some of the mutations mapped early in the I gene but still displayed negative complementation in diploid tests with the wild-type I gene in a nonsuppressing (Su$^-$) background (Platt et al. 1972). Negatively complementing activity is assumed to result from the interaction of wild-type and mutant subunits due to the in vivo formation of mixed hybrid repressor tetramers or oligomers (Müller-Hill et al. 1968; see also below). Since the amber codon terminates translation, amber mutants that show negative complementation must reinitiate translation at a site distal to the amber codon. The resulting polypeptides must then be capable of associating with normal repressor polypeptides to form mixed hybrids. To verify this concept, we attempted to isolate the negatively complementing gene product from a variety of early amber mutants. The mutationally altered proteins showed unimpaired binding of the inducer IPTG and the tetrameric state of oligomerization typical for *lac* repressor but were unable to bind to phosphocellulose. Thus a conventional purification procedure to obtain mutationally altered proteins was very difficult (Platt et al. 1972). Purification of the mutationally altered *lac* repressors was achieved, however, by immune precipitation with antibody to native *lac* repressor followed by preparative sodium dodecyl sulfate (SDS)-polyacrylamide gel electrophoresis (Fig. 1). Although this approach allowed the isolation of only a small amount of detergent-denatured protein, it had the advantage of allowing a rapid protein-chemical characterization of the mutationally altered protein by its polypeptide chain molecular weight. Furthermore, the amino-terminal sequence of the mutationally altered protein can be directly determined from the small amount of protein recovered from the gel (Platt et al. 1972; Weiner et al. 1972). Thus the characterization of the mutationally altered *lac* repressor by polypeptide chain molecular weight and by amino-terminal sequence, together with the known wild-type amino acid sequence, allows the direct identification of the translational reinitiation site.

Our results (Platt et al. 1972; Ganem et al. 1973; Files et al. 1974) are summarized in Figure 2. The very early amber mutations, which correspond to residues 7, 12, and 17 of the normal *lac* repressor polypeptide chain, give rise to two translational restarts. The first one corresponds to valine residue 23 (π_{23}) and the second one corresponds to methionine residue 42 (π_{42}; this is the first internal in-phase AUG codon). All three early amber mutations activate π_{23} and π_{42} simultaneously. If the amber codon is moved beyond the π_{23} boundary and occurs at a

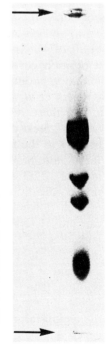

Figure 1 SDS-polyacrylamide gel electrophoresis of the antigen-antibody complex formed upon addition of anti-repressor IgG to partially purified i^{100} restart repressor (for details, see Platt et al. 1972). The top arrow marks the top of the gel and the bottom arrow indicates the dye front. The four bands (*top to bottom*) are the polypeptide chains of the heavy IgG chain (50,000 m.w.), normal lac repressor (38,000 m.w.), i^{100} mutationally altered protein (a π_{42} restart protein, 34,000 m.w.), and light IgG chain (23,000 m.w.). In this experiment 10 μg of pure *lac* repressor was added to the i^{100} protein-antibody complex.

Repressor   Restart   Proteins

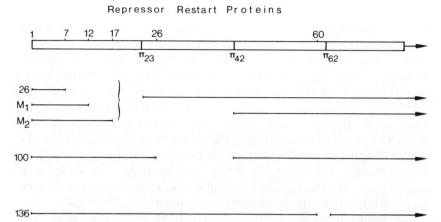

Figure 2 Diagram of polypeptide chains synthesized in strains with the early *I*-gene amber mutations 26, M_1, M_2, 100, and 136 which occur at the codons corresponding to amino acid residues 7, 12, 17, 26, and 60, respectively. π_{23}, π_{42}, and π_{62} indicate the sites of translational reinitiation of protein biosynthesis past the amber codon. This reinitiation process gives rise to the tetrameric repressor restart proteins, π_{23}, π_{42}, and π_{62}, which show unimpaired IPTG-binding activity but have no DNA-binding activity (for details, see text and Platt et al. 1972; Ganem et al. 1973; Files et al. 1974).

position corresponding to residue 26, translational reinitiation occurs only at π_{42} and no other restart polypeptides are found (Platt et al. 1972; Files et al. 1974). Amber mutations mapping beyond the π_{42} boundary, e.g., at a position corresponding to residue 60, lose the π_{42} restart, and a new initiation codon π_{62} is detected which corresponds to leucine residue 62 (Ganem et al. 1973).

The three restart *lac* repressor mutationally altered proteins π_{23}, π_{42}, and π_{62} lack the amino-terminal 23, 42, and 61 amino acid residues present in the normal repressor polypeptide chain (Fig. 2). However, all three mutationally altered proteins show unimpaired binding of the inducer IPTG and form tetramers, i.e., they sediment with a sedimentation coefficient corresponding to a molecular weight four times the value of their polypeptide chain molecular weight. In addition, the π_{42} protein can be reversibly denatured and renatured after exposure to $8\,M$ guanidine-HCl in the presence of 2-mercaptoethanol. Even more interestingly, the three restart repressors have lost the operator-binding activity and cannot bind to phosphocellulose (Platt et al. 1972), a property which is often taken as a measure of the general nonoperator DNA-binding activity of repressor (see, e.g., Müller-Hill 1975). These results show that the amino-terminal 61 residues of the repressor polypeptide chain are not necessary for either IPTG binding or tetramer formation, but that they are required either directly or indirectly (see below) for operator and nonoperator DNA binding. These conclusions agree with genetic studies which indicate that a major class of operator-binding mutations (I^{-d} mutations) mapping in the amino-terminal part of the repressor polypeptide chain do not show major changes in IPTG-binding activity (Adler et al. 1972; Pfahl 1972; Miller et al. 1975; see also Miller, this volume).

Repressor Derivatives Which Have Lost the Amino-terminal 59 Residues In Vitro: The Homogeneous Tryptic Core Obtained in a Native Digest

During our protein-chemical studies of *lac* repressor, we noticed that the protein in its native conformation showed an interesting differential sensitivity towards proteolytic attack by trypsin or chymotrypsin. When *lac* repressor was treated at 37°C in 0.1 M NH_4HCO_3 with trypsin or chymotrypsin, only a limited number of peptides were released. In an extensive study of the digestion products, we showed that trypsin released the peptides spanning the amino-terminal 59 residues, leaving a trypsin-resistant core (Weber et al. 1972; Platt et al. 1973). Later, by comparison of our data with the complete amino acid sequence of the repressor (Beyreuther et al. 1973), it was apparent that under these experimental conditions trypsin also released at least three peptides spanning the 20 carboxy-terminal residues. The residual "tryptic core" exhibited full inducer-binding activity and was predominantly in the tetrameric form (Platt et al. 1973). In addition, operator and nonoperator DNA binding was lost upon conversion of repressor to the tetrameric tryptic core (Platt et al. 1973; Lin and Riggs 1975).

A major advantage of this native tryptic digest of repressor was that it could be used to map by protein chemistry those mutations occurring in the first 59 residues. We used this system to determine the position of the mutation in seven early amber mutants of *lac* repressor, as well as the position of five I^{-d} point mutations (Weber et al. 1972; Platt et al. 1972; Ganem et al. 1973; Files et al. 1974). The unique amino-terminal sequence of the tryptic core (starting with glutamine residue 60) provided the basis for automated protein sequencing of the core polypeptide, thus allowing the localization of further amino acid exchanges beyond residue 60 of the *lac* repressor (Files and Weber 1976; Files et al. 1975; Beyreuther, this volume). Thus, approximately one-third of the repressor polypeptide chain can be easily screened for amino acid exchanges in the appropriate mutationally altered repressors. The correlation between the genetic and protein-chemical maps has been firmly established. Today, because of this correlation and because of the extremely advanced genetic mapping techniques, the majority of the mutations can be readily placed within a few amino acid residues, if not directly related to a specific amino acid residue (see Miller, this volume).

The native tryptic digest in 0.1 M NH_4HCO_3 can be made specific for the amino-terminal end by lowering the temperature to 25°C and keeping the digestion time to less than 20 minutes (Files and Weber 1976; Geisler and Weber 1976). Under these conditions it is possible to separate the "homogeneous tryptic core," which spans residues 60–347 of the repressor polypeptide, from the mixture of small tryptic peptides which account for the amino-terminal end of the chain. This homogeneous tryptic core is very similar to the π_{62} restart protein (see above). It shows unimpaired IPTG-binding activity, is fully in the tetrameric state, and can be reversibly denatured and renatured. It is devoid of operator DNA binding and has also lost nonoperator-binding activity (Lin and Riggs 1975; Geisler and Weber 1976).

Isolation of the Amino-terminal Fragment of Repressor Necessary for DNA Binding: The Repressor Headpiece

All the early variations of the native tryptic digest tried by us (Weber et al. 1972; Platt et al. 1973; Files and Weber 1976) and others (Huston et al. 1974; Beyreuther, this volume) have the shortcoming that the amino-terminal part of the repressor is digested into multiple tryptic peptides and cannot be isolated directly. Indeed, in some of the studies there is a good indication of multiple tryptic attack in this region at early times during the digest (Fig. 3) (Files and Weber 1976). In an attempt to isolate the amino-terminal 59 residues as a single polypeptide (or headpiece), we screened different digestion conditions and found that digestion in storage buffer (1 M Tris-HCl, pH 7.5, 30 or 50% in glycerol, and 0.01 M in 2-mercaptoethanol) at 25°C for several hours gave a mixture of *intact headpieces* and *homogeneous tetrameric core* (Geisler and Weber 1977). The presence of high concentrations of Tris-HCl is necessary to restrict the action of trypsin and to recover the headpieces. Separation of core and headpieces is easily achieved by gel filtration on Sephadex G-150 in 0.1 M NH_4HCO_3 (Fig. 4). This results in a headpiece preparation that is

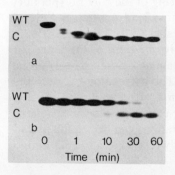

Figure 3 Time course of tryptic digestion of *lac* repressor under native conditions analyzed by SDS-polyacrylamide gel electrophoresis (10% slab gel). Buffer conditions are 0.1 M NH_4HCO_3 (*a*) and 1 M Tris-HCl (pH 7.5), 30% glycerol, 0.01 M 2-mercaptoethanol (*b*). WT and C mark the polypeptide chains of normal repressor and its homogeneous core. Note the presence of polypeptides with intermediate molecular weights early during digestion in *a* and the absence of these bands in *b* (for details, see Geisler and Weber 1977).

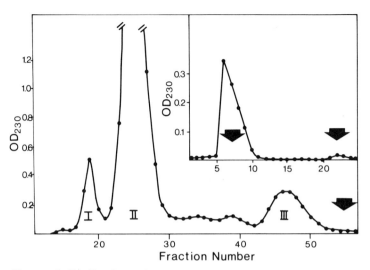

Figure 4 Purification of the repressor headpiece by chromatography on Sephadex G-150. The recovered headpiece (peak III) was further chromatographed on Sephadex G-25 (*inset*), where it appears in the void column. Peak II from the Sephadex G-150 column is the tryptic core. The arrows mark the salt and void volume of the columns (for details, see Geisler and Weber 1977).

extremely pure, as shown by the heavily overloaded gel in Figure 5. Protein-chemical characterization of the headpiece fraction showed that it contained two peptides in similar molar amounts. One peptide spanned residues 1–59 (long headpiece [LH]) and the other spanned residues 1–51 (short headpiece [SH]). However, the molar ratio of the two headpieces is not always equal, as first suspected (Geisler and Weber 1977). Recent experiments with different repressor preparations have shown that the ratio between LH and SH can vary between 1:1 and 1:3. LH and SH can also be prepared from two different mutationally altered repressors (Jovin et al. 1977). We have also shown by direct protein chemistry (Fig. 6) that the other products of the very restricted digestion in storage buffer are the homogeneous tetrameric tryptic core (accounting for residues 60–347) and an octapeptide accounting for the balance between the two headpieces (peptide T_6 accounting for residues 52–59) (Geisler and Weber 1977).

The headpieces are monomers by gel-filtration analysis and they show ordered secondary structure in circular dichroism studies (Geisler and Weber 1977). Therefore we studied the binding of the headpieces to nonoperator DNA by nitrocellulose filter binding assays. We found binding to poly[d(AT)] DNA and poly[d(As^{4}T)]. Figure 7 shows a typical binding assay for a nearly equimolar mixture of LH and SH to radioactive poly[d(A-s^{4}T)]. Specific and tight binding to operator DNA was not detected (Jovin et al. 1977).

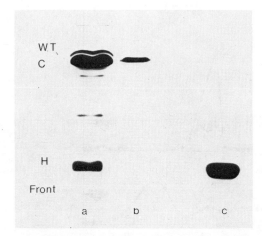

Figure 5 SDS-polyacrylamide gel electrophoresis on a 20% slab gel. (*a*) Repressor in 1 M Tris-HCl, 30% glycerol, 0.01 M 2-mercaptoethanol digested for 60 min at room temperature; (*b*) peak II from the Sephadex G-150 column (see Fig. 4); (*c*) headpiece preparation from the Sephadex G-150 column (see Fig. 4). Slots *a* and *c* are heavily overloaded to demonstrate the purity of the headpiece preparation. WT, C, and H mark the positions of repressor polypeptide, core polypeptide, and headpiece polypeptides, respectively. Note that the repressor in this experiment has not been quantitatively converted to core (for details, see Geisler and Weber 1977).

```
1                 5              10              14
Met-Lys-Pro-Val-Thr-Leu-Tyr-Asp-Val-Ala-Glu-Tyr-Ala-Gly-

15          20              25          28
Val-Ser-Tyr-Gln-Thr-Val-Ser-Arg-Val-Val-Asn-Gln-Ala-Ser-

29 30              35              40    42
His-Val-Ser-Ala-Lys-Thr-Arg-Glu-Lys-Val-Glu-Ala-Ala-Met-

43      45          50              55  56
Ala-Glu-Leu-Asn-Tyr-Ile-Pro-Asn-Arg-Val-Ala-Gln-Gln-Leu-

57     59        60              65
Ala-Gly-Lys      Gln-Ser-Leu-Leu-Ile-Gly
```

Figure 6 Amino acid sequence of the amino-terminal 65 residues of *lac* repressor (Beyreuther et al. 1973). Numbers indicate the residue number. The two arrows mark the points of cleavage by trypsin in 1 M Tris-HCl (pH 7.5), 30% in glycerol, 0.01 M 2-mercaptoethanol. The thick arrow marks the nearly quantitative cleavage at residue 59; the thin arrow marks the incomplete cleavage site at position 51. For protein-chemical characterization, the headpiece preparation (nearly equal amounts of peptides 1–59 and 1–51) was cleaved with CNBr at methionine residues 1 and 42, and the resulting soluble peptides CNBr1 (residues 43–51) and CNBr2 (residues 43–59) were recovered by fingerprinting. The tryptic peptide T6 spans amino acid residues 52–59 (for details, see Geisler and Weber 1977).

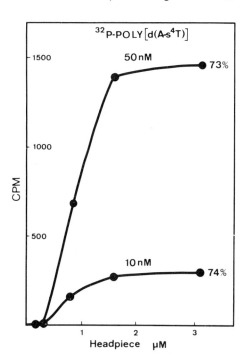

Figure 7 Binding of the head-pieces (present as a nearly equimolar mixture of SH and LH) to poly[d(A-s⁴T)]. Concentrations of nucleotides were 10 nM and 50 nM. Binding was assayed by the filter-binding procedure (Bourgeois 1971). The binding buffer contained 0.01 M Tris-HCl (pH 7.5), 0.01 M KCl, 10^{-3} M EDTA, 10^{-3} M dithiothreitol, 5% dimethylsulfoxide, 3×10^{-3} M MgCl₂, and 50 μg/ml bovine serum albumin. The reaction volume was 0.3 ml, of which 0.28 ml was filtered through Millipore AAWP nitrocellulose filters, 0.8-μm pore size and 25 mm in diameter. The reaction was performed at room temperature.

Isolation of a Set of Hybrid Repressors Made In Vitro between Normal *lac* Repressor and Its Homogeneous Tryptic Core

The availability of a homogeneous tetrameric core devoid of operator binding and the ability to renature both the homogeneous core and repressor from guanidine-HCl with high yield (Files and Weber 1976) led us to construct repressor hybrids. Denaturation and renaturation of a mixture of wild-type repressor and its homogeneous core resulted in hybrid formation (Geisler and Weber 1976). A mixture of repressor and homogeneous core was subjected to denaturation by guanidine-HCl followed by renaturation. The resulting hybrid mixture was sedimented on glycerol gradients and at least 80% of the recovered protein sedimented as a tetramer. The peak fractions containing the tetrameric repressors were pooled, freed of glycerol, and concentrated for cellogel electrophoresis. Six protein bands were resolved on the cellogel (Fig. 8) and could be recovered by elution. Aliquots of the bands B1 to B6 were characterized by polyacrylamide gel electrophoresis in the presence of sodium dodecyl sulfate to determine their polypeptide composition (Fig. 9). B1 is pure tetrameric repressor and B6 is pure tetrameric core. Fractions B2 to B5 are hybrid molecules with a decreasing number of wild-type polypeptide chains. The ratio of wild-type to core subunits is 3:1 for B2 and 1:3 for B5. The middle band is poorly resolved into B3

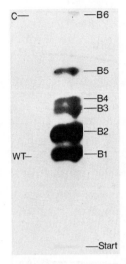

Figure 8 Electrophoretic separation on cellogel of the tetrameric hybrid mixture obtained by joint renaturation of repressor and homogeneous tryptic core from 8 M guanidine-HCl. Protein bands B1 and B6 of the hybrid set run identically with untreated repressor and core, respectively. Bands B3 and B4 are the leading and trailing part of the middle band and are usually only barely separated (for details see Geisler and Weber 1976).

and B4 and shows, for both fractions, core and repressor polypeptides in a ratio of 2:2.

The operator-binding properties of the hybrids recovered from the cellogel have been studied in preliminary binding experiments. Operator-binding curves at an operator concentration above the binding constant of normal repressor are shown in Figure 10. The determination of the half-life of the operator-hybrid complexes is given in Figure 11. Although cellogel electrophoresis induces a loss of operator DNA binding of normal repressor, the recovered B1 repressor can be considered as an internal standard for the operator-binding properties of all other hybrids, since all the hybrids have been subjected to the same treatments. By this criterion, the B2 hybrid behaves like B1 repressor both in the operator-binding curve and in the dissociation kinetics. The tryptic core B6 and the hybrid B5 show no detectable operator-binding activity. The hybrids B3 and B4 show at least a five fold reduction in operator-binding activity when compared to B1 and have reduced half-lives of 8 minutes (B3) and 15 minutes (B4). Recent experiments, however, have shown that both wild-type repressor and hybrid repressor can show subunit exchange in the native state (T. Jovin et al., unpubl.). Therefore we cannot currently

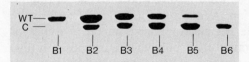

Figure 9 SDS-polyacrylamide gel electrophoresis of the hybrids B1 to B6 isolated by electrophoresis on cellogel (see Fig. 8). WT and C mark the positions of the normal and core polypeptides, respectively (for details, see Geisler and Weber 1976).

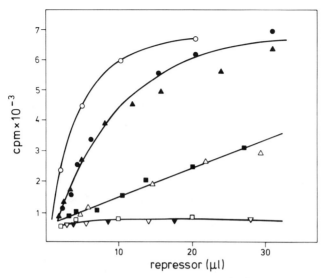

Figure 10 Binding curves of untreated wild-type repressor and hybrids to operator DNA. Reaction mixture of 1 ml contained 8×10^{-15} moles of operator and the given volumes of 1 μg/ml of repressor solutions. Symbols indicate normal repressor (○); hybrid repressors B1 (●), B2 (▲), B3 (■), B4 (△), B5 (▼), and B6 (▽); and normal repressor in the presence of isopropyl-thio-β-D-galactoside (□) (for details, see Geisler and Weber 1976).

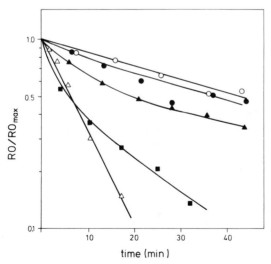

Figure 11 Rate of dissociation of hybrid repressor-operator complexes. For experimental details, see Geisler and Weber (1976). RO is the concentration of the repressor-operator complex at the given times. Symbols indicate normal repressor (○); hybrid repressors B1 (●), B2 (▲), B3 (■), B4 (△), B5 (▼), and B6 (▽).

exclude the possibility that the activity of some of the hybrids may be due to subunit exchange. Experiments now in progress are trying to distinguish between true hybrid activity and activity achieved because of reformation of wild-type repressor molecules by subunit exchange.

The procedure for making hybrids by joint denaturation and renaturation of repressor and its homogeneous tryptic core as described above is rather cumbersome and time consuming. Recently we have found a more convenient method. By shortening the digestion time of repressor with trypsin in storage buffer (1 M Tris-HCl, pH 7.5, 30% in glycerol, and 0.01 M in 2-mercaptoethanol) at 25°C (see above) full conversion to homogeneous core and headpieces is avoided (T. Jovin et al., unpubl.). When digestion is allowed to occur for only 60 minutes, incomplete conversion takes place. The protein sample is then filtered through Sephadex G-150 to remove the headpieces, and the mixture of hybrids is subjected to chromatography on double-stranded calf thymus DNA bound to cellulose. All hybrids except the core can be absorbed on the column at low ionic strength and can be eluted by a salt gradient. Since these hybrids can simply be prepared by the "restricted trypsinization of repressor in situ," their isolation is easy. Furthermore, the separation step avoids cellogel electrophoresis, which results in some damage of operator-binding activity (see above). We hope that a detailed study of these hybrids will allow a further insight into the mechanism of repressor-DNA interaction. (The details of this procedure will be given elsewhere.)

DISCUSSION

Translational Reinitiation In Vivo

The phenomenon of translational reinitiation following chain termination at a nonsense codon has been characterized by genetic and protein-chemical studies of the I gene and its product, the *lac* repressor. This in-vivo-reinitiation process occurs at a site in the same messenger RNA (mRNA) some distance past the terminator codon. So far we have identified three such sites in the early part of the mRNA coding for the first 62 amino acid residues of the repressor. Only one of these sites (π_{42}) involves a classical AUG codon; the other two involve an in vivo ambiguity of the genetic code in that the same codon can be translated into two different amino acids, depending on whether it is recognized during initiation or elongation of protein biosynthesis. These two non-AUG codons are the codons corresponding to valine residue 23 (π_{23}) and leucine residue 62 (π_{62}) of the *lac* repressor polypeptide chain. What are these codons? Studies on in vitro protein biosynthesis indicated that N-formyl methionine-dependent initiation can occur at the codons AUG and GUG, and to a lesser extent at GUA (Clark and Marker 1966; Ghosh et al. 1967). Although UUG has not been shown to act as an initiation codon in vitro, the binding of N-formylmethionyl-tRNA to ribosomes is stimulated by the trinucleotides AUG, GUG, and UUG (Clark and Marker 1966; Ghosh et al. 1967; Dube et al. 1970). These results led us to propose that the valine codon 23 (π_{23}) was GUG and the leucine codon 62 (π_{62}) was UUG (Ganem et al. 1973; Files et al. 1974). Direct nucleotide sequence analysis of the I-gene mRNA has meanwhile verified that π_{23} does indeed involve the valine codon GUG (D. A. Steege, pers. comm.). In addition, GUG has also been found to act as the initiation codon for the A-gene product of phage MS2 (Volckaert and Fiers 1973) and normal repressor (D. A. Steege, pers. comm.). To test the assumption that leucine 62 was coded by UUG, we screened a collection of amber mutants to try to detect a mutation at position 62, which would correspond to a change from UUG to UAG. Sequence studies on a repressor molecule isolated from the ultraviolet-induced amber mutant XA2 (grown on a host strain containing the tyrosine-inserting su3 suppressor) showed that this polypeptide has a tyrosine and not a leucine residue at position 62. Of the six possible leucine codons, only UUG can mutate to the amber codon UAG by a single base change, and thus the codon specifying leucine 62 must indeed be UUG (Files et al. 1975). DNA sequence analysis has further substantiated this result, since this leucine codon has been found to be UUG (W. Gilbert, pers. comm.).

How general is the phenomenon of translational reinitiation? It has been described previously for the rIIB cistron of bacteriophage T4 (Sarabhai and Brenner 1967) and the Z gene of the lac operon (Newton 1967; Michels and Zipser 1969), but direct protein-chemical identification of the restart codons was not provided in these systems. In our studies on the I gene, we have found three initiation sites within the first 62 amino acid residues. Since the sites involve not only AUG, but also GUG and UUG, we would expect translational reinitiation to be a common event for E. coli genes, and indeed recent studies on the Z gene support this assumption (D. Zipser, pers. comm.). Translational reinitiation may not be a very efficient process and may only be noticed at 5–10% of the level of normal initiation (Platt et al. 1972). However, its very existence may indeed show us a bypath mechanism for certain gene controls previously not appreciated. Are there any translational reinitiation sites past the UUG codon in position 62? We expect them, but we cannot prove their existence yet, since negative complementation can be used to detect restarts only as long as the reinitiated polypeptides form mixed hybrids with the normal repressor subunit. Also, there is a strong possibility that repressor derivatives which have lost more than the amino-terminal 62 residues may not form tetramers (see below).

One further point—the secondary structure of the messenger RNA—should be mentioned. The observation that some amber mutations activate two restarts whereas others activate only one could be related to the secondary structure of the mRNA during protein synthesis. Certain internal initiation sites may be made available to a new ribosome only after translation up to the amber block has proceeded to the extent necessary to open the regions involved in secondary structure and thereby uncovering the initiation site. In such a model the secondary structure between π_{42} and π_{62} would interfere with the reinitiation at π_{62} unless the amber block is moved very close to π_{62}. The simultaneous expression of π_{23} and π_{42} in the very early amber mutations of the I gene would suggest the absence of a significant amount of secondary structure between π_{23} and π_{42}. Internal translational initiation does not occur at the immunologically detectable levels in the wild-type I gene (Platt et al. 1972). Although this finding also could be explained by secondary structure, it is probably more likely that the translation process proceeds along the nascent mRNA, involving the internal initiation sites in elongation of protein synthesis before they have any opportunity to act as initiation sites. In this model the introduction of a nonsense codon would stop elongation prior to an internal initiation site, thereby making this site available for translational reinitiation.

Dissection of Repressor into a Homogeneous Tetrametic Core and Two Different Headpieces

Tetrameric repressor derivatives missing the amino-terminal part can be obtained in vivo as translational reinitiation products (see above) or in vitro by limited tryptic digestion of native repressor. Since 1972 (Weber et al. 1972; Platt et al. 1973) several variations have been introduced, and the native digestion of repressor has now been studied under a variety of different experimental conditions. Four main types of proteolytic attack on native repressor can be distinguished:

1. Digestion in 0.1 M NH_4HCO_3 at 37°C leads to a rapid digestion in the amino-terminal 59 residues and a slower digestion at the carboxy-terminal 40 residues. During prolonged digestion, the otherwise tetrameric core gives rise to dimer formation, although the IPTG binding remains intact (Weber et al. 1972; Platt et al. 1973; Files and Weber 1976; Beyreuther, this volume).
2. Digestion in 0.1 M NH_4HCO_3 at 25°C leads to decreased sensitivity of the repressor. By controlling the digestion time, it becomes possible to isolate a homogeneous tetrameric core accounting for residues 60–347. The amino-terminal region is digested by multiple tryptic attack and yields individual tryptic peptides (Files and Weber 1976).
3. Digestion in 0.1 M NH_4HCO_3 at 5°C for 2 hours gives rise to tetrameric core molecules with polypeptides starting at either position 52 or 60

(Huston et al. 1974) and a mixture of tryptic peptides accounting for the amino-terminal region of the *lac* repressor (N. Geisler and K. Weber, unpubl.).

4. Digestion in 1 M Tris-HCl (pH 7.5), 30% in glycerol at 25°C restricts the digestion so severely that within 1 to 2 hours only peptide bonds 51 and 59 are hydrolyzed. Thus the amino-terminal region can be isolated in the form of two headpieces, which account for residues 1–59 and 1–51, respectively. The other products are the homogeneous tryptic core (residues 60–347) and a small octapeptide accounting for the balance of residues 52–59 (Geisler and Weber 1977). The strongly reduced sensitivity of the headpieces to trypsin in 1 M Tris-HCl is not due to the fact that the headpieces remain noncovalently bound to the core until the gel-filtration step, but it reflects an inherent property of the structure of the headpieces in this buffer. Isolated headpieces are trypsin-resistant in 1 M Tris-HCl but extremely trypsin-sensitive in 0.1 M NH_4HCO_3 or 0.05 M Tris buffer (Jovin et al. 1977).

The combined results can be explained by the assumption that tetrameric repressor has different conformations under different experimental conditions and that some of these conformations can be distinguished by their differential sensitivity to trypsin. It should be noted that repressor under native conditions is not attacked by various proteases past residue 60 (Platt et al. 1973; Beyreuther et al. as cited in Müller-Hill 1975; Files and Weber 1976). Since we have now shown that the region prior to arginine 51 can be protected against proteolytic attack by trypsin or chymotrypsin, it is likely that repressor has a "weak" secondary structure, i.e., a "hinge region" between residues 50 and 60. It is interesting to note that genetic analysis has shown that some strong I^{-d} mutations are localized in this region (Adler et al. 1972; Pfahl 1972; Miller et al. 1975; Müller-Hill 1975).

The properties of the homogeneous tryptic core (Platt et al. 1973; Files and Weber 1976; Geisler and Weber 1977) and its in vivo counterpart, the third restart protein (π_{62}), have clearly established that the amino-terminal 60 residues are not necessary for IPTG binding, oligomerization, or folding of the repressor. The information for these properties clearly lies outside the amino terminus; however, for their precise localization inside the core molecule, we have only some genetic hints (Müller-Hill 1975; see Miller, this volume). The homogeneous tryptic core has been put to use for a variety of structural studies of repressor. Thus it is relatively simple to localize repressor alterations between residues 60 and 100 by automated sequence analysis of the core (Beyreuther as cited in Müller-Hill 1975; Files and Weber 1976; Beyreuther, this volume). Furthermore, the homogeneous core has been used to obtain repressor hybrids by joint renaturation of normal repressor and core after denaturation by guanidine-HCl (Geisler and Weber 1976; see below). It may also be possible that homogeneous core is much easier to crystallize than repressor due to the absence of the amino-terminal headpieces.

The DNA-binding Properties of the Amino-terminal Headpieces

The properties of the restart proteins and the homogeneous tryptic core, together with the extensive genetic analysis of operator-DNA-binding mutants, have clearly established the importance of the amino-terminal part of the repressor for both the strong and specific operator DNA binding and the weak and unspecific nonoperator DNA binding (for references, see above). Since the amino-terminal headpiece can now be isolated by severely limiting the native tryptic digest (Geisler and Weber 1977; see above), the DNA-binding properties of the amino-terminal region can be studied directly. Although these studies may fill a gap in our understanding of repressor function, currently they are difficult to interpret because of these two features:

1. The amino-terminal region was originally available only as an equimolar mixture of the peptides spanning residues 1–51 and 1–59, respectively. Thus until very recently, all our studies on DNA binding involved this mixture. We are now able to separate the two headpieces by chromatography on double-stranded calf thymus DNA bound to cellulose. The shorter headpiece (residues 1–51) binds less tightly to the column than the longer headpiece (residues 1–59), which is slightly more basic than the shorter headpiece (Jovin et al. 1977).
2. The headpieces do not show the specific operator DNA binding, but they do show the weak and unspecific nonoperator DNA binding by trapping radioactive DNA to nitrocellulose filters (Jovin et al. 1977).

The lack of operator DNA binding is not surprising, since genetic studies using negative complementation (Müller-Hill et al. 1968) and biochemical studies using repressor-core hybrids (Geisler and Weber 1976; see above) have shown that active tetrameric repressor must contain two or more normal repressor polypeptide chains. However, the results on nonspecific DNA binding are more difficult to interpret, since the interaction of basic amino acid side chains and the phosphate residues of the DNA backbone, although most likely a necessary requirement of DNA-protein interaction, will be influenced by the basicity of the protein. Thus, for instance, the stronger nonspecific DNA binding of the longer headpiece found by nitrocellulose filter assays and by DNA-cellulose chromatography could be due either to the slightly higher positive charge (the longer headpiece has 7 lysine/arginine residues and the shorter headpiece only 6; both have 5 aspartic/glutamic acid residues, 1 residue of histidine, a free amino-terminal methionine, and a negative charge at the carboxyl end) or to the fact that residues 52–59 really improve nonspecific binding as possibly suggested by the presence of several I^{-d} mutations in this region. On the other hand, these latter mutations do not seem to affect the binding of the repressor mutationally altered proteins to phosphocellulose (Müller-Hill 1975). Thus, the following preliminary results on direct headpiece-DNA interaction (Jovin et al. 1977) have to be treated with caution because of the above-mentioned difficulties.

1. The headpieces bind to phosphocellulose or to calf thymus DNA bound to cellulose. In the latter case, the peptides elute at pH 7.8 at considerably lower ionic strength than intact *lac* repressor, and the longer headpiece (LH) binds better to the column than the shorter headpiece (SH).
2. The mixture of the headpieces, as well as the individual headpiece, can trap phage DNA as well as double-stranded DNA analogs (poly[d(A-T)], poly[d(A-s⁴T)] on nitrocellulose filters. Yet, although both headpieces bind DNA quantitatively at high peptide concentrations, the required concentrations for 50% binding are 0.8 μM and 3 μM for the longer and shorter headpieces, respectively. The half-life of the complexes formed is rather small (several seconds) compared to that of the repressor (several minutes).
3. Headpieces prepared as an equimolar mixture from the repressor point mutation I^{-d} *BG2* (valine residue 9 changed to isoleucine) (Müller-Hill 1975) show a lower DNA binding than do normal headpieces. This mutationally altered repressor was previously shown to have reduced binding to phosphocellulose.
4. A variety of physicochemical techniques (ultraviolet absorption difference spectra; circular dichroism difference spectra; fluorescence spectra) show that headpieces form a defined complex with poly[d(A-s⁴T)]. These results are presented elsewhere in detail (Jovin et al. 1977). Nuclear magnetic resonance studies show that the headpieces have a defined structure, which changes upon binding to DNA (E. Grell et al., unpubl.).

Thus a variety of different techniques show direct weak interaction between the headpieces and DNA. Since intactness of the amino-terminal region of *lac* repressor has previously been shown to be a necessary requirement for nonspecific DNA binding, the simplest assumption is that the isolated monomeric headpieces retain some of their functions, i.e., nonspecific DNA binding, which they express in the tetrameric repressor. It is, however, worth mentioning that the nonspecific binding (half-lives of the complexes) is smaller for the headpieces than for repressor. It could well be that this reflects the difference in oligomerization (monomer versus tetramer) or the absence of a weak binding site (perhaps secondarily induced) in the core which has so far not been detected. In such a model the nonspecific binding of the headpieces reflects a similar binding activity typical of *lac* repressor. This binding is a prerequisite for the specific operator DNA binding, which requires the tetrameric molecule. A direct molecular interaction between the headpieces of repressor and operator DNA has now been proven by cross-linking experiments.

Outlook on the DNA-binding Site of *lac* Repressor

The number of subunits actively and simultaneously involved in DNA-repressor complex formation is still not clearly determined. There are several arguments that more than one subunit is necessary. The best argument comes from in vivo results showing that i^{-d} mutationally altered repressors are dominant over wild-type repressor (Müller-Hill et al. 1968). This phenomenon is termed "negative complementation" and is most likely due to the formation of mixed hybrid repressor tetramers in vivo. Further support comes from studies on the formation of hybrid repressors in vitro. These studies show that one normal subunit per mixed tetramer of core and wild-type subunits is not sufficient to provide activity (Geisler and Weber 1976) and that joint renaturation of two types of repressor subunits leads to repressor with operator-binding properties intermediate to those of the parental repressor species (Sadler and Tecklenburg 1976). There are several findings which favor the interpretation that *lac* repressor is still active as a dimer of two normal polypeptides in either a dimeric or tetrameric organization:

1. The mutationally altered L_1 *lac* repressor, which has an altered carboxy-terminal region due to a deletion and addition, is still able to repress at low levels in vivo, although in vitro analysis shows this repressor to be a dimer (Miller et al. 1970). The presence of a small fraction of tetramers present in vivo or in vitro cannot be excluded, especially since L_1 repressor undergoes proteolytic degradation in vivo (Platt et al. 1970). Other mutationally altered repressors which result in monomer-dimer formation have, however, been found to have no measurable DNA-binding activity (Schmitz et al. 1976).
2. Hybrid repressors have been formed by joint renaturation of repressor and core subunits after denaturation by guanidine-HCl. The resulting tetrameric hybrids have been separated by electrophoresis on cellogel and subjected to a preliminary characterization of their operator-binding activities. The results indicate that the hybrid with only one core subunit seems to act as normal repressor, whereas the hybrids with two core subunits show operator-binding activity, although strongly reduced. Thus it is possible that hybrids with only two normal repressor subunits show operator interaction, although further experiments are necessary to determine if their low binding activity is biologically significant (Geisler and Weber 1976).

3. The chimeric protein repressor–β-galactosidase obtained by fusion of the *I* and *Z* genes (Müller-Hill and Kania 1974; Kania and Brown 1976) is a tetrameric molecule containing repressor and β-galactosidase activities. Chemical cross-linking experiments have been interpreted to indicate that the repressor parts of the tetrameric protein are organized as two independent dimers on the tetrameric β-galactosidase core and that such a dimeric organization can act in operator binding (Kania and Brown 1976). Although these experiments use very different approaches and seem together rather suggestive, none of them can be taken without certain reservations. It still remains necessary to prove directly if two subunits or more interact simultaneously with the operator.

The combined genetic and biochemical evidence suggests very strongly that the headpieces of repressor are involved in both the specific operator DNA binding and the weak nonoperator DNA binding and indeed do interact directly with the DNA. However, there is no experiment which argues that the headpieces are alone responsible for the full DNA interaction of *lac* repressor. The core could readily carry a second DNA-binding site, which is either weaker or only induced after the headpiece-DNA interaction has occurred. Such a site could be crucial for the specific operator binding, and the cross-linking results of Ogata and Gilbert (pers. comm.) indicate that such a site(s) could indeed be present between residues 269 and 347 of the *lac* repressor polypeptide chain.

Note Added in Proof

We have recently found that the use of chymotrypsin or clostripain in the native digest of repressor allows the isolation of homogeneous headpieces. Chymotrypsin yields a headpiece accounting for residues 1–56. Clostripain yields a headpiece accounting for residues 1–51. (See Geisler and Weber 1978.)

ACKNOWLEDGMENT

K. W. acknowledges the pleasant and rewarding collaboration with Drs. J. Miller, T. Platt, D. Ganem, and J. G. Files in the years 1969–1975.

REFERENCES

Adler, K. K. Beyreuther, E. Fanning, N. Geisler, B. Gronenborn, A. Klemm, B. Müller-Hill, M. Pfahl, and A. Schmitz. 1972. How *lac* repressor binds to DNA. *Nature* **237**:322.

Beyreuther, K., K. Adler, N. Geisler, and A. Klemm. 1973. The amino-acid sequence of *lac* repressor. *Proc. Natl. Acad. Sci.* **70**:3576.

Bourgeois, S. 1971. Techniques to assay repressors. *Methods Enzymol.* **21:**491.

Clark, B. F. C. and K. A. Marcker. 1966. The role of N-formyl-methionyl-tRNA in protein biosynthesis. *J. Mol. Biol.* **17:**394.

Dube, S. K., P. S. Rudland, B. F. C. Clark, and K. A. Marcker. 1970. A structure requirement for codon-anti-codon interaction on the ribosome. *Cold Spring Harbor Symp. Quant. Biol.* **34:**161.

Files, J. G. and K. Weber. 1976. Limited proteolytic digestion of *lac* repressor by trypsin. *J. Biol. Chem.* **251:**3386.

Files, J. G., K. Weber, and J. H. Miller. 1974. Translational reinitiation: Reinitiation of *lac* repressor fragments at three internal sites early in the *lac i* gene of *Escherichia coli. Proc. Natl. Acad. Sci.* **71:**667.

Files, J. G., K. Weber, C. Coulondre, and J. H. Miller. 1975. Identification of the UUG codon as a translational initiation codon *in vivo. J. Mol. Biol.* **95:**327.

Ganem, D., J. H. Miller, J. G. Files, T. Platt, and K. Weber. 1973. Reinitiation of a *lac* repressor fragment at a codon other than AUG. *Proc. Natl. Acad. Sci.* **70:**3165.

Geisler N. and K. Weber. 1978. *Escherichia coli* lactose repressor. Isolation of two different homogeneous headpieces and the existence of a hinge region between residues 50 and 60 in the repressor molecule. *FEBS Lett.* **87:**215.

―――. 1976. Isolation of a set of hybrid *lac* repressors made *in vitro* between normal *lac* repressor and its homogeneous tryptic core. *Proc. Natl. Acad. Sci.* **73:**3103.

―――. 1977. Isolation of the amino-terminal fragment of lactose repressor necessary for DNA binding. *Biochemistry* **16:**938.

Ghosh, H. P., D. Söll, and H. G. Khorana. 1967. Studies on polynucleotides. LXVII. Initiation of protein synthesis *in vitro* as studied by using ribopolynucleotides with repeating nucleotide sequences as messengers. *J. Mol. Biol.* **25:**275.

Gilbert, W. and A. Maxam. 1973. The nucleotide sequence of the *lac* operator. *Proc. Natl. Acad. Sci.* **70:**3581.

Huston, J. S., W. F. Moo-Penn, K. C. Bechtel, and O. Jardetzky. 1974. Characterization of the *lac* repressor species produced by limited tryptic cleavage. *Biochem. Biophys. Res. Commun.* **61:**441.

Jovin, T. M., N. Geisler, and K. Weber. 1977. Amino-terminal fragments of *Escherichia coli lac* repressor bind to DNA. *Nature* **269:**668.

Kania, J. and D. Brown. 1976. The functional repressor parts of a tetrameric *lac* repressor-β-galactosidase chimaera are organized as dimers. *Proc. Natl. Acad. Sci.* **73:**3529.

Lin, S.-Y. and A. D. Riggs. 1975. A comparison of *lac* repressor binding to operator and to nonoperator DNA. *Biochem. Biophys. Res. Commun.* **62:**704.

Michels, C. A. and D. Zipser. 1969. Mapping of polypeptide reinitiation sites within the β-galactosidase structural gene. *J. Mol. Biol.* **41:**341.

Miller, J. H., T. Platt, and K. Weber. 1970. Strains with the promoter deletion L1 synthesize an altered *lac* repressor. In *The lactose operon* (ed. J. R. Beckwith and D. Zipser), p. 343. Cold Spring Harbor Laboratory, Cold Spring Harbor, New York.

Miller, J. H., C. Coulondre, U. Schmeissner, A. Schmitz, and P. Lu. 1975. The use of suppressed nonsense mutations to generate altered *lac* repressor molecules.

In *Protein-ligand interactions* (ed. H. Sund and G. Blauer), p. 238. Walter de Gruyter, Berlin.

Müller-Hill, B. 1975. *Lac* repressor and *lac* operator. *Prog. Biophys. Mol. Biol.* **30**:227.

Müller-Hill, B. and J. Kania. 1974. *Lac* repressor can be fused to β-galactosidase. *Nature* **249**:561.

Müller-Hill, B., L. Crapo, and W. Gilbert. 1968. Mutants that make more *lac* repressor. *Proc. Natl. Acad. Sci.* **59**:1259.

Newton, A. 1967. Effect of nonsense mutations on translation of the lactose operon of *Escherichia coli*. *Cold Spring Harbor Symp. Quant. Biol.* **31**:181.

Pfahl, M. 1972. Genetic map of the lactose repressor gene (*i*) of *Escherichia coli*. *Genetics* **72**:393.

Platt, T., J. G. Files, and K. Weber. 1973. *Lac* repressor: Specific proteolytic destruction of the NH_2-terminal region and loss of the deoxyribonucleic acid-binding activity. *J. Biol. Chem.* **248**:110.

Platt, T., J. H. Miller, and K. Weber. 1970. *In vivo* degradation of mutant *lac* repressor. *Nature* **228**:1154.

Platt, T., K. Weber, D. Ganem, and J. H. Miller. 1972. Translational restarts: AUG reinitiation of a *lac* repressor fragment. *Proc. Natl. Acad. Sci.* **69**:897.

Sadler, J. R. and M. Tecklenburg. 1976. Recovery of operator DNA binding activity from denatured lactose repressor. *Biochemistry* **15**:4353.

Sarabhai, A. and S. Brenner. 1967. A mutant which reinitiates the polypeptide chain after chain termination. *J. Mol. Biol.* **27**:145.

Schmitz, A., U. Schmeissner, J. H. Miller and P. Lu. 1976. Mutations affecting the quaternary structure of the *lac* repressor. *J. Biol. Chem.* **251**:3359.

Volckaert, G. and W. Fiers. 1973. Studies on the bacteriophage MS2. G-U-G as the initiation codon of the A-protein cistron. *FEBS Lett.* **35**:91.

Weber, K., T. Platt, D. Ganem, and J. H. Miller. 1972. Altered sequences changing the operator-binding properties of the *lac* repressor: Colinearity of the repressor protein with the *i*-gene map. *Proc. Natl. Acad. Sci.* **69**:3624.

Weiner, A. M., T. Platt, and K. Weber. 1972. Amino-terminal sequence analysis of proteins purified on a nanomole scale by gel electrophoresis. *J. Biol. Chem.* **247**:3242.

Repressor Recognition of Operator and Effectors

Mary D. Barkley
Department of Biochemistry
University of Kentucky Medical Center
Lexington, Kentucky 40506

Suzanne Bourgeois
The Salk Institute for Biological Studies
San Diego, California 92112

REPRESSOR INTERACTIONS

As predicted by Jacob and Monod (1961), negative control of the *lac* operon is accomplished by the *lac* repressor protein, the operator site on the bacterial chromosome, and small effector ligands. This paper deals with two unique attributes of the repressor protein: its ability to recognize the *lac* operator and its ability to bind inducer. The *lac* repressor (R) binds at the operator site (O) on DNA with very high affinity:

$$R + O \rightleftharpoons RO. \tag{1}$$

This simple stoichiometry reflects the observation that one repressor molecule binds one operator region.

There are two classes of ligands which affect the interaction of repressor protein and operator DNA: inducers and anti-inducers. These low-molecular-weight sugar molecules, primarily β-galactosides, can bind to repressor protein whether it is free in solution or bound to DNA. There are four sites for effector (E) per repressor tetramer, one per subunit:

$$R + 4E \rightleftharpoons RE_4. \tag{2}$$

Inducing and anti-inducing ligands interact directly with repressor protein bound to the operator, forming a ternary complex and decreasing or increasing, respectively, the affinity of repressor for operator. Binding of one inducer molecule to repressor-operator complex apparently releases the repressor from the operator:

$$RO + E \rightleftharpoons ERO \rightleftharpoons RE + O. \tag{3}$$

The binding sites on the protein for DNA and for effectors are separate sites; this is well documented by genetic evidence presented in this book and biochemical evidence discussed in this paper. However, these sites are mutually interacting: binding of effectors alters the affinity of repressor for operator, and vice versa. The interplay between the DNA- and effector-binding sites is mediated by a conformational change in repressor protein and is the substance of the regulatory mechanism.

In addition to the interaction with operator, the *lac* repressor binds with lower affinity to other base sequences in natural and synthetic DNAs. There are many nonoperator sites for repressor protein on DNA; the interaction of repressor and a single such site is written:

$$R + DNA \rightleftharpoons R - DNA. \tag{4}$$

The binding is usually insensitive to effectors.

The above four interactions have been examined extensively in vitro during the past 7 years. Before recounting the results of this work, we will describe briefly some biochemical procedures standard in investigations of the *lac* system.

METHODOLOGY

We will outline in-vitro-binding assays for the biological activities of *lac* repressor protein: DNA binding and effector binding (for reviews, see Bourgeois 1971, 1972; Müller-Hill et al. 1971). Other techniques will be described later in context. Throughout this paper, unless noted differently, "repressor" means the wild-type protein isolated from *lacI$^+$* strains or from strains which overproduce wild-type repressor (see Miller, this volume); "operator" means the operator site embedded in a large DNA molecule, such as bacteriophage DNA carrying the *lac* region (Beckwith 1970). The inducer commonly used is isopropyl-1-thio-β-D-galactoside (IPTG).

The membrane-filter technique has been especially fruitful for quantitating the binding of repressor protein and operator DNA (Riggs et al. 1970a,b,c). This assay depends on the fact that, under appropriate conditions of ionic strength (I), *lac* repressor protein adheres to nitrocellulose filters, as do many other proteins (Kihara and Kuno 1968). Moreover, radioactively labeled ligands which bind to repressor, such as sugars and DNAs, do not stick to nitrocellulose when free, but remain bound to the protein on the filter. The operator-binding assay can be adapted for use with crude preparations of repressor. Also, the repressor-operator complex immobilized on membrane filters dissociates upon washing of the filter with buffer containing inducer. The operator DNA thus released can be reclaimed. This property of the repressor protein has been exploited for purifying fragments of DNA containing the *lac* operator (Bourgeois and Riggs 1970) as well as the operator region (Gilbert 1972) away from nonoperator DNA.

The binding of repressor protein and inducer IPTG can also be determined by membrane filtration. The filter assay is most useful for rapid estimates of repressor concentrations, for example, for monitoring IPTG-binding activity during column chromatography. For quantitative measurement of IPTG binding to *lac* repressor protein, whether purified or in crude extracts, equilibrium dialysis is still the most reliable method (Gilbert and Müller-Hill 1966). Another technique, which is more sensitive than equilibrium dialysis for detecting low levels of IPTG binding, is precipitation by ammonium sulfate (Bourgeois and Jobe 1970) or by antibody (Riggs and Bourgeois 1968). However, binding constants determined by the ammonium sulfate method must be viewed with caution, since they differ significantly from the values determined by equilibrium dialysis. The antibody precipitation has been employed as the basis of a small-scale purification scheme of altered *lac* repressors for sequence analysis (Platt et al. 1972).

BINDING OF EFFECTORS

As mentioned above, effectors interact with *lac* repressor protein when it is free and when it is bound to DNA. In this section we discuss the more simple and experimentally accessible case of binding of effectors to free repressor protein, deferring consideration of the coupled effector-repressor-DNA interactions to subsequent sections.

The interaction of *lac* repressor protein and effectors has been studied with two intents: to quantitate the binding and to investigate the conformational change. The stoichiometry of binding is stated in Equation 2. In general, the reaction is characterized by a single equilibrium association constant (K_E) for the binding of ligand to a site on the protein:

$$K_E = \frac{[R'E]}{[R'][E]} \tag{5}$$

where now $[R']$ is the concentration of sites for ligand, theoretically four times the concentration of tetrameric repressor.

The binding of a wide variety of effectors to repressor has been measured by equilibrium dialysis, either directly using labeled ligand or by competition with labeled IPTG (Barkley et al. 1975). The binding constants K_E, which range from 3 M^{-1} to about $2 \times 10^6 \text{ M}^{-1}$, for a few compounds are presented in Table 1. The sugars are classified as inducers or anti-inducers by their effect on the stability of repressor-operator complex. Most of the ligands tested turned out to be inducers. The common inducer IPTG has a high affinity for repressor, $K_E = 1 \times 10^6 \text{ M}^{-1}$. The value of K_E depends somewhat on pH and ionic strength; it decreases about sixfold as the temperature increases from 4° to 40°C (Ohshima et al. 1974; Friedman et al. 1977; Butler et al. 1977). At 25°C and pH 7.6,

Table 1 Binding of repressor and repressor-operator complex to effectors

	$K_E \, M^{-1\,a}$	$^O K_E{}^b$	$K_O/^E K_O{}^c$
Inducers			
methyl-1-thio-β-D-galactoside	1.1×10^5	$(3.3 \pm 1.1) \times 10^2$	6.5×10^2
isopropyl-β-D-galactoside	$(9.9 \pm 1.5) \times 10^3$		
isopropyl-1-thio-β-D-galactoside	$(1.2 \pm 0.2) \times 10^6$	$(5.0 \pm 1.3) \times 10^3$	1×10^3
p-aminophenyl-1-thio-β-D-galactoside	$(7.6 \pm 1.7) \times 10^2$		
galactose	$(9.9 \pm 1.0) \times 10^2$		
melibiose $\left(\begin{smallmatrix} 6\text{-}O\text{-}\alpha\text{-D-galactopyranosyl-} \\ \text{D-glucose} \end{smallmatrix}\right)$	$(9.7 \pm 1.7) \times 10^3$	$(7.7 \pm 2.4) \times 10$	6×10^2
allolactose $\left(\begin{smallmatrix} 6\text{-}O\text{-}\beta\text{-D-galactopyranosyl-} \\ \text{D-glucose} \end{smallmatrix}\right)$	$(1.7 \pm 0.2) \times 10^6$		
Neutral			
o-nitrophenyl-β-D-galactoside	$(9.2 \pm 1.5) \times 10^3$		
Anti-inducers			
phenyl-β-D-galactoside	$(1.1 \pm 0.3) \times 10^3$	$(6.7 \pm 4.5) \times 10^d$	$5.6 \times 10^{-1\,d}$
o-nitrophenyl-β-D-galactoside	$(7.1 \pm 2.7) \times 10^3$	$(4.0 \pm 0.2) \times 10^{3\,d}$	$3.3 \times 10^{-1\,d}$
glucose	$(1.4 \pm 0.2) \times 10$	$(5.3 \pm 3.0) \times 10^d$	$4.9 \times 10^{-1\,d}$
lactose $\left(\begin{smallmatrix} 4\text{-}O\text{-}\beta\text{-D-galactopyranosyl-} \\ \text{D-glucose} \end{smallmatrix}\right)$	3.0 ± 1.2	$(2.2 \pm 0.3) \times 10^d$	$1.8 \times 10^{-1\,d}$

Data from Jobe and Bourgeois (1972a) and Barkley et al. (1975).

[a]K_E is the equilibrium association constant for the reaction $R' + E \rightleftharpoons R'E$, where R' is the concentration of ligand-binding sites; 0.1 M potassium phosphate buffer, pH 7.8, 10^{-3} M dithioerythritol, 10^{-3} M sodium azide, 4°C.

[b]$^O K_E$ is the equilibrium association constant for the reaction $RO + E \rightleftharpoons ORE$, calculated assuming one site for ligand on repressor bound to operator DNA. Standard conditions.

[c]$K_O/^E K_O$ is the ratio of the affinity of repressor for operator DNA in the absence of ligand to the affinity at saturation with ligand. Standard conditions.

[d]Standard conditions, except binding buffer has 0.06 M KCl, $I = 0.1$ M. As noted in the text, $^O K_E$ and $K_O/^E K_O$ are independent of ionic strength.

$\Delta G = -7.7$ kcal/mole, $\Delta H = -6.2$ kcal/mole, and $\Delta S = 5$ cal/mole deg; the enthalpy change is the main driving force for the reaction. Allolactose, the natural inducer of the *lac* operon in vivo, binds slightly more tightly than IPTG (Jobe and Bourgeois 1972a). Melibiose, the α-galactoside isomer of allolactose, binds with moderate affinity. One neutral ligand, o-nitrophenyl-β-D-galactoside (ONPG), was found that binds with moderate affinity to *lac* repressor but exerts no effect on the repressor-operator interaction. Anti-inducers are competitive inhibitors of inducer binding; presumably, they bind at the same site. The evidence that inducers and anti-inducers share a common (or partly overlapping) binding site is purely circumstantial; the arguments are three. First, the two types of effectors are chemically and structurally related compounds. Second, as just stated, their binding to *lac* repressor protein is competitive. Third, their effects on the repressor-operator interaction are simultaneously altered by mutation in the case of the i^{s}Y18 repressor to be described later (Jobe et al. 1972). Anti-inducers generally bind to repressor with low affinity. The common anti-inducer o-nitrophenyl-β-D-fucoside (ONPF) has a moderate affinity for repressor, $K_E = 7 \times 10^3\,\text{M}^{-1}$. Lactose, the substrate for β-galactosidase in vivo and itself an anti-inducer of the operon, binds with low affinity (Jobe and Bourgeois 1972b). Glucose also binds with low affinity; perhaps it represses the operon by stabilizing repressor-operator complex as well as by catabolite repression. At low temperatures, the binding of all effectors is noncooperative, indicating that the multiple ligand-binding sites on repressor are identical and independent. At 37°C, slight positive cooperativity in the binding of IPTG appears (Butler et al. 1977); under somewhat different conditions, both negative cooperativity and positive cooperativity have been observed (Ohshima et al. 1974).

The problem of the number of sites, N, for effector actually measured in equilibrium dialysis experiments has been tacitly ignored in the literature; it is assumed to be four per repressor tetramer (Müller-Hill 1971). In fact, it is some number between two and four (Ohshima et al. 1974; Butler et al. 1977). The reason for this evasion is simple: it is not clear how to account for the observations. Some investigators report a reversible change in the value of N with temperature (Oshima et al. 1974), while others find no significant change (Butler et al. 1977). Variation in the value of N between preparations of purified repressor protein is also encountered.

Besides experiments utilizing radioactive sugars, inducer binding has been studied by monitoring optical changes in the lac repressor or an attached chromophore. A shift in the fluorescence maximum of the protein (from 338 nm to 330 nm) with essentially no change in peak shape or intensity occurs in the presence of saturating concentrations of IPTG (Laiken et al. 1972). The anti-inducer glucose has no effect on the fluorescence. The spectrum is characteristic of tryptophan residues, of which there are two per repressor subunit. The fluorescence change resulting from IPTG binding involves both tryptophan residues, as deduced from spectral measurements on repressors altered by amino acid substitution at tryptophan position 201 or 220 (Sommer et al. 1976) and by chemical modification of tryptophan 220 (O'Gorman and Matthews 1977a). Titration experiments, monitoring the quenching of the protein fluorescence at 360 nm with inducer concentration, confirm the results obtained by equilibrium dialysis with regard to the affinity (Laiken et al. 1972) and the noncooperative aspect of the binding (Butler et al. 1977). However, the observed fluorescence quenching (28%) at saturation with IPTG is independent of N, the number of ligand binding sites per tetramer.

The kinetics of the IPTG-binding reaction have also been measured by monitoring changes in the protein fluorescence in stopped-flow experiments (Laiken et al. 1972; Friedman et al. 1976, 1977). The rate constants for the association and dissociation reactions have been determined; the kinetic data are consistent with the binding equilibrium of Equation 5 (Friedman et al. 1977). The association reaction is a simple bimolecular process characterized by a rate constant of about $5 \times 10^4 \, \text{M}^{-1} \text{sec}^{-1}$ at pH 8.0. The value of the rate constant is smaller than expected for a diffusion-limited reaction, and it depends slightly on pH. Equivalent results were obtained using other optical probes described below (Friedman et al. 1976). The dissociation reaction, observed after rapid dilution of repressor-IPTG complex, exhibits essentially first-order kinetics, with a rate constant of about $3 \times 10^{-1} \text{sec}^{-1}$ at pH 8.0. Equilibrium constants K_E calculated from the ratio of the rate constants are in good agreement with those obtained from equilibrium dialysis and titration experiments.

Evidence for a conformational change in *lac* repressor protein derives from several sources. A very fast, unimolecular relaxation process has been observed in temperature-jump experiments monitoring intensity changes in the fluorescence of repressor at 360 nm (Wu et al. 1976). This result suggests a rapid conformational transition between two states of repressor protein, which takes place in the absence of bound IPTG and could account for the low apparent value of the bimolecular rate constant. Additional documentation of a conformational change comes from the optical changes which occur upon binding of inducer IPTG to *lac* repressor. These include changes in the fluorescence spectrum of the protein already described (Laiken et al. 1972), in the ultraviolet absorbance spectrum of the protein (Ohshima et al. 1972; Matthews et al. 1973), and in the visible spectra of reporter groups attached to cysteine residues in the protein (Sams et al. 1977). The observed spectral changes might conceivably arise from local perturbations at the site of IPTG binding. However, the interpretation that they result from a conformational change in the repressor is strengthened by the combined data. First, anti-inducers, which presumably bind at the same site as inducers, show no effect on the fluorescence and ultraviolet spectra of repressor and show opposite effects on the visible spectra of the optically labeled repressors. Second, the groups accounting for the optical changes are at different positions in the polypeptide chain, and it is unlikely that all would be located in the IPTG-binding site. And third, as mentioned above, the spectral changes obey the same kinetics. Moreover, the kinetic data indicate that the conformational transition is rapid compared to the binding of repressor and IPTG, since only a single, bimolecular step is observed.

Besides the optical techniques, a change in conformation has been detected by differential sedimentation (Ohshima et al. 1972). The sedimentation coefficient of *lac* repressor protein increases about 3% in the presence of saturating concentrations of IPTG, suggesting that the protein molecule becomes more compact when it binds inducer. Further signs of the conformational change are manifest in the different patterns of chemical modification (Alexander et al. 1977; Yang et al. 1977; O'Gorman and Matthews 1977b) and of proteolytic cleavage (see Beyreuther, this volume) observed in the presence and absence of bound effector.

RECOGNITION OF OPERATOR

Since the binding of *lac* repressor at its operator site on DNA is the biological function of the protein, it is the subject of intensive investigation. The interaction of repressor and operator and the perturbation of that interaction by effectors have been analyzed both experimentally and theoretically. Moreover, the effects of mutational, chemical, and physical alterations in operator DNA, as well as the behavior of some repressor proteins altered by mutations, have been examined in detail. We will consider these facets of the repressor-operator interaction in this section.

Interaction of Repressor and Operator

The binding of *lac* repressor protein to operator DNA has been studied by the membrane-filter technique. So far, all the data are consistent with the bimolecular reaction of Equation 1. The equilibrium association constant (K_O) for the binding of repressor protein and operator DNA,

$$K_O = \frac{[RO]}{[R][O]} = \frac{k_a}{k_b},$$

is extremely large, about $1 \times 10^{13}\,\text{M}^{-1}$ under standard conditions ($I = 0.05\,\text{M}$, pH 7.4, 24°C) (Riggs et al. 1970c). Because of the very high affinity of repressor for operator, binding reactions are carried out at low concentrations, on the order of $10^{-12}\,\text{M}$ in both reagents. Figure 1 shows a typical binding curve. The value of the association constant K_O has been measured in equilibrium binding experiments; it agrees with the value of k_a/k_b calculated from the ratio of the rate constants from kinetic experiments. However, it is easier to detect small changes in the association constant from the more accurate kinetic measurements.

The kinetic data for the rate of formation of repressor-operator complex are plotted according to the integrated rate equation for a second-order reaction in Figure 2a. The rate constant of association (k_a) of repressor and operator (the slope of the line) is very large, about $7 \times 10^9\,\text{M}^{-1}\,\text{sec}^{-1}$ (Riggs et al. 1970a). It is only possible to determine a rate constant of this magnitude in a conventional kinetic experiment because

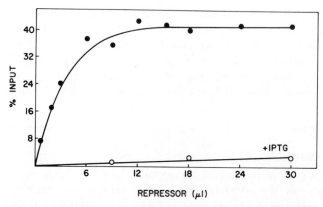

Figure 1   Binding curve for *lac* repressor and operator DNA. Aliquots of purified *lac* repressor protein and radioactively labeled λh80d*lac* DNA (1.7×10^{-11} M operator) are equilibrated in standard binding buffer ($I = 0.05$ M) at room temperature. Samples of the reaction mixture are filtered on membrane filters; the filters are washed with buffer and counted for radioactivity. The background (4%) of DNA retained by the filters in the absence of repressor has been subtracted from each point. (●) No IPTG; (○) 10^{-3} M IPTG. Standard binding buffer is 0.01 M Tris (pH 7.4), 0.01 M KCl, 0.01 M Mg $(CH_3CO_2)_2$, 10^{-4} M EDTA, 10^{-4} M dithiothreitol, 5% dimethylsulfoxide, 50 μg/ml bovine serum albumin. (Data from Riggs et al. 1970c.)

of the high affinity of repressor for operator; the time scale for the association reaction at 10^{-12} M is several minutes. A point to be noted, and to which we shall return later, is that the bimolecular rate constant k_a is at least an order of magnitude greater than the value normally expected for diffusion-limited reactions of molecules of this size.

The kinetic data for the rate of disappearance of labeled repressor-operator complex are plotted on a semilog scale in Figure 2b. The rate constant of dissociation (k_b) of repressor-operator complex (the slope of the line) is about 6×10^{-4} sec^{-1}, corresponding to a half-life ($t_{1/2}$) of about 30 minutes for the unimolecular decay process (Riggs et al. 1970a). For induction to occur as it does in the cell, without detectable lag after the addition of inducer, it is clear that the inducer molecule must accelerate the removal of repressor protein from the operator site on DNA. This fact is illustrated in Figure 2b, which shows that inducer IPTG speeds up the rate of decomposition of repressor-operator complex, and conversely, anti-inducer ONPF retards it (Riggs et al. 1970b). Since inducing and anti-inducing ligands do not alter significantly the rate of association of repressor and operator (Jobe and Bourgeois 1972c; Lin and Riggs 1972a), their effect on the rate of dissociation can be ascribed directly to a decrease or increase in the affinity of repressor for operator in the

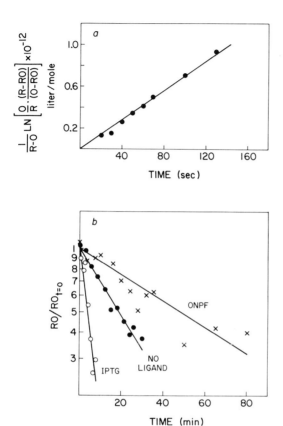

Figure 2 Kinetics of binding of *lac* repressor and operator DNA. (*a*) Rate of association of repressor and operator. At time $t = 0$, active repressor protein (2.4×10^{-12} M) and labeled λh80d*lac* DNA (1.1×10^{-12} M) are mixed; at various times *t*, samples are removed and filtered. The specific rate constant of association k_a of repressor and operator is the slope of the straight line. (Data from Riggs et al. 1970a.) (*b*) Rate of dissociation of repressor-operator complex. Repressor protein and labeled λh80d*lac* DNA are equilibrated to form labeled repressor-operator complex (8.6×10^{-12} M). At time $t = 0$, the reaction mixture is diluted tenfold into buffer containing a 50-fold excess of cold λh80d*lac* DNA, in the absence or presence of various concentrations of effecting ligand, and the rate of exchange of repressor off the labeled operator DNA onto the unlabeled operator DNA is monitored; at various times *t*, samples are removed and filtered. The specific rate constant of dissociation k_b of repressor-operator complex is the slope of the straight line. (●) No ligand; (○) 3×10^{-6} M IPTG; (x) 1.8×10^{-3} M ONPF. Standard conditions. (Data from Riggs et al. 1970b.)

presence of IPTG or ONPF, respectively. Further, these experiments establish the existence of a ternary ligand-repressor-operator complex by showing that effectors interact with repressor-operator complex; details regarding this interaction will be presented in the next section.

The effects of a variety of physical and chemical parameters on the interaction of *lac* repressor and operator DNA have also been investigated (Riggs et al. 1970a). The *lac* repressor binds to a thermodynamically stable, double-stranded structure of the operator DNA. Denaturation of the DNA destroys operator binding; the binding to operator is restored upon renaturation of the DNA. Actinomycin D inhibits the binding of repressor to operator DNA, presumably by competing with the protein for the operator site. This antibiotic, a cyclic polypeptide containing intercalative dye, binds preferentially to DNA between the base-paired sequences dG-dC, the peptide chains lying along the narrow groove of the DNA helix (Sobell 1973). The sequence of the *lac* operator contains one putative actinomycin site (see Fig. 5b). The affinity of repressor for operator is quite sensitive to ionic strength. A tenfold increase in the ionic strength of the binding buffer (from $I = 0.02$ M to $I = 0.2$ M) decreases the rate constant of association k_a about 60-fold and increases the rate constant of dissociation k_b about 5-fold, corresponding to about a 300-fold reduction in the equilibrium association constant. Increasing the negative charge on the repressor protein (isoelectric point pH 5.6) by raising the pH of the binding buffer (from pH 7.0 to pH 9.0) causes a slight reduction in the affinity of repressor for operator; the rate constant of association k_a decreases about threefold, whereas the rate constant of dissociation k_b is essentially unchanged, over this range of pH. The effect of temperature on the repressor-operator interaction, although not pronounced, is noteworthy. When the temperature is raised from 1°C to 24°C, the rate constant of association k_a increases about fourfold and the rate constant of dissociation of k_b remains constant. Thus the activation energy for the association reaction is +8.5 kcal/mole, about four times the value due to viscosity in a diffusion-limited reaction; and for the dissociation reaction, close to zero. The equilibrium constant K_O increases fourfold over this temperature range; so for the binding reaction, $\Delta H = 8.5$ kcal/mole. At 24°C and pH 7.4, $K_O = 1 \times 10^{13}$ M^{-1} and $\Delta G = -18$ kcal/mole. The entropy change, $\Delta S = 90$ cal/mole deg, is the driving force for the reaction.

Effectors

As indicated in the preceding section, the ligand-repressor-operator interaction has been investigated by membrane filtration. The data are most easily reconciled by the following simple reaction scheme:

$$R + O \underset{k_b}{\overset{k_a}{\rightleftharpoons}} RO$$

$$+ \qquad +$$

$$E \qquad E$$

$$\kappa_E \updownarrow \qquad \updownarrow {}^O\kappa_E$$

$$RE + O \underset{{}^Ek_b}{\overset{{}^Ek_a}{\rightleftharpoons}} ORE$$

As before, k_a and k_b are the rate constants of association and dissociation, respectively, of repressor and operator, where $K_O = k_a/k_b$; ${}^Ek_a$ and ${}^Ek_b$ are the effected rate constants, the rate constants of association and dissociation of repressor-ligand complex and operator.

In vivo, the differential rate of β-galactosidase synthesis displays a sigmoidal dependence on inducer concentration (Boezi and Cowie 1961; Clark and Marr 1964). Half the maximal differential rate is achieved at about 2×10^{-4} M IPTG. The sigmoidicity of the induction curve in vivo, expressed by an index analogous to a Hill coefficient of 3, is indicative of a positively cooperative process (Bourgeois 1966). Presumably, the first event in the sequence is the removal of the repressor from the operator by inducer. This is demonstrated in vitro by the equilibrium release curve in Figure 3. Here, the solid lines show the effects of various ligands on the repressor-operator binding equilibrium. The order of effectiveness of the inducers, IPTG > methyl-1-thio-β-D-galactoside (TMG) > melibiose, as inhibitors of the formation of repressor-operator complex parallels that of their capacities to induce the *lac* operon in vivo (Riggs et al. 1970b) and to bind to free repressor protein (Table 1). In this assay, anti-inducers have no visible effect. Although these experiments are a reliable measure of the relative potency of inducing ligands, the data are not suitable for quantitative treatment because the proportion of labeled complexes in the reaction mixture actually retained by the filters varies with inducer concentration.

Kinetic experiments provide a sound basis for quantitating the interaction of inducers and anti-inducers with repressor-operator complex: in particular, the measurement of the rate of dissociation as a function of concentration of effector. The effect of IPTG on the kinetics of the repressor-operator binding reaction has been investigated in detail (Barkley et al. 1975). Figure 4 shows a plot of the apparent specific rate constant of dissociation k_b(app) of repressor and operator versus IPTG concentration; the data points are the results of individual experiments, as in Figure 2b. The value of the rate constant at saturation with IPTG is the effected rate constant: ${}^Ek_b = 2 \times 10^{-1}$ sec^{-1} under standard con-

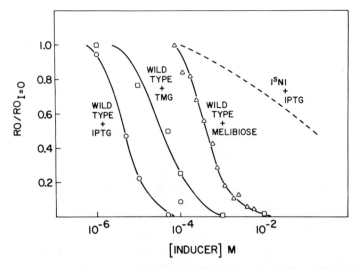

Figure 3 Effect of inducers on the repressor-operator binding equilibrium in vitro. Constant concentrations of repressor protein and operator DNA are equilibrated in the presence of various concentrations of inducing ligand, as described for Fig. 1. (——) wild-type repressor protein; (○) IPTG; (□) TMG; (△) melibiose. (Data from Riggs et al. 1970b; M. D. Barkley, unpubl.) (‒ ‒ ‒) i^{s}N1 repressor protein: IPTG. (Data from Jobe et al. 1972.)

ditions, about 1000-fold greater than in the absence of inducer. The rate constant of association of repressor protein and operator DNA is essentially the same in the presence or absence of effector: $k_a = {}^E k_a$. Thus, the equilibrium association constant ${}^E K_O$ for the binding of repressor-IPTG complex to operator DNA is about $3 \times 10^{10}\,\mathrm{M}^{-1}$. Two simple mechanisms for induction were treated mathematically: an extreme cooperative model, in which the binding of inducer causes a concerted allosteric transformation in repressor tetramer; and a noncooperative model, in which the conformational transition occurs independently in each subunit. The extreme cooperative model predicts a sigmoid curve of k_b(app) vs [IPTG], whereas the noncooperative predicts a hyperbolic curve. Since the observed plot of k_b(app) vs [IPTG] is hyperbolic, mechanisms of induction involving highly cooperative interactions between inducer sites on repressor bound to operator DNA are excluded; this result is surprising in view of the in vivo results. Also, the value of the equilibrium association constant ${}^O K_E$ for the binding of IPTG to repressor-operator complex is extracted from the plot of k_b(app) vs [IPTG] by fitting the theoretical curves to the data. Assuming one site for IPTG on repressor bound to operator DNA (solid line in Fig. 4), the affinity ${}^O K_E$ is about $5 \times 10^3\,\mathrm{M}^{-1}$.

The effects of various reaction conditions on the ternary interaction of

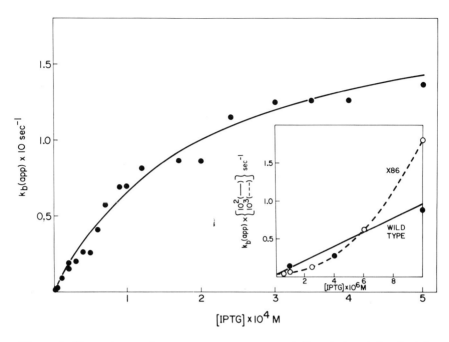

Figure 4 Dependence of apparent rate constant of dissociation k_b(app) of *lac* repressor-operator complex upon IPTG concentration. (●) Data from individual kinetic experiments with wild-type repressor protein, similar to those described for Fig. 2b. Because of the very short half-lives measured at high IPTG concentrations, the dissociation reaction is stopped precisely 30 sec prior to filtration by addition of anti-inducers (0.3 M glucose and 3×10^{-3} M ONPF). (———) Theoretical curve fit to data for wild-type repressor protein, assuming one site for IPTG. (Data from Barkley et al. 1975.) (*Insert*) Expansion of scale at low concentrations of IPTG. (○) Data from individual kinetic experiments with i^{r}X86 repressor protein. The procedure for the individual kinetic experiments is modified slightly. Purified active i^{r}X86 repressor protein and labeled λp*lac* DNA are equilibrated to form labeled i^{r}X86 repressor-operator complex (6×10^{-12} M). To reduce the extent of binding of i^{r}X86 repressor to nonoperator sites on the labeled DNA, the reaction mixture contains 2–6 μg/ml chicken blood DNA. At time $t = 0$, a 30-fold excess of cold λp*lac* DNA and various concentrations of IPTG are added; at various times t, samples are removed and filtered. Binding buffer has 0.16 M KCl, $I = 0.2$ M. (– – –) Experimental curve for i^{r}X86 repressor protein. (Data from Pfahl 1976.)

repressor protein, operator DNA, and inducer IPTG have also been investigated. The affinity $^E K_O$ of repressor-IPTG complex for operator is altered by changes in ionic strength, pH, and temperature to the same degree as is the affinity K_O of repressor for operator. The affinity $^O K_E$ of IPTG for repressor-operator complex is independent of ionic strength and temperature, and slightly dependent on pH.

The interaction of other effectors with repressor-operator complex has been similarly characterized in kinetic experiments. For all the inducers, the value of the effected rate constant ^Ek_b at saturation is the same within experimental error (Barkley et al. 1975). Thus all inducers destabilize repressor-operator complex about 1000-fold, presumably by triggering the identical conformational change in repressor protein. Anti-inducers, on the other hand, have small stabilizing effects on repressor-operator complex, at most about fivefold in the case of lactose (Jobe and Bourgeois 1972b). Table 1 contains a summary of these results. As expected from simple thermodynamic arguments, inducers bind with greater affinity to free repressor (K_E) than to repressor-operator complex (^OK_E), and conversely for the natural anti-inducers, glucose and lactose. Phenyl-β-D-galactoside and ONPF behave anomalously, apparently binding with greater affinity to free repressor than to repressor-operator complex and at the same time stabilizing repressor-operator complex two- to threefold.

Operators

The nucleotide sequence of the *lac* operator was originally deduced by Gilbert and Maxam (1973), using RNA transcripts of a DNA fragment about 27 base pairs long, which was protected from nuclease digestion by the *lac* repressor (see Fig. 5b). Subsequently, the surrounding sequence (Dickson et al. 1975), as well as the base-pair substitutions of various o^c mutated operators (Gilbert et al. 1975), was determined by methods described elsewhere in this book (see Reznikoff and Abelson). As outlined in Figure 5b, the nucleotide sequence of the operator reveals a high degree of symmetry, the function of which has been the subject of much speculation. The implications of symmetry for the interaction of repressor protein and operator DNA will be discussed later.

The affinity of *lac* repressor protein for operator DNA having various degrees of negative superhelical twist was measured in order to determine whether the binding of repressor to operator is accompanied by unwinding of the DNA helix (Wang et al. 1974). Since the release of superhelical turns in DNA is favored thermodynamically, as documented by studies of the binding of intercalative dyes (Bauer and Vinograd 1970), a protein that unwinds the duplex helix will bind with greater affinity to covalently closed, circular DNA with negative superhelical twist than it will to the identical, untwisted DNA. The angle of unwinding can be computed from the ratio of the affinities of the ligand for these two DNAs (Davidson 1972). The binding of *lac* repressor to superhelical $\lambda plac$ DNA was determined in kinetic experiments by membrane filtration. As the number of negative superhelical turns in the DNA progressed from -10 to -350, the rate constant of association (k_a) increased about fourfold and the rate constant of dissociation (k_b) decreased about threefold; the increase in the equilibrium association constant K_O was at most 14-fold. The angle of unwinding for *lac* repressor, calculated on the basis of a 26° unwinding angle for ethidium (Wang 1974), is about 90° per operator. This indicates a structural change in the operator duplex and implies that operator DNA is not in the B form when bound to *lac* repressor. However, such a small amount of unwinding is inconsistent with mechanisms of recognition involving substantial unwinding of the Watson-Crick helix by the repressor, either to form a cruciform structure (see Fig. 5d) or to expose a number of bases.

The available experimental data show considerable asymmetry in the binding of repressor and operator, first evident from the analysis of o^c mutated operators. The O^c operator constitutive mutation results in an increased basal level of expression of adjacent *lac* operon structural genes in vivo (Smith and Sadler 1971) and a decreased affinity of the mutated operator DNA for *lac* repressor in vitro (Jobe et al. 1974). The affinity is proportional to an index of constitutivity of the mutant: The more highly constitutive the o^c mutant, the lower the affinity. Figure 5b shows the base-pair substitutions and the affinities relative to wild-type operator (100), for eight o^c operators. Five of the eight substitutions are in symmetrically disposed base pairs; these mutations decrease the symmetry of the operator. However, substitutions which increase the symmetry (G-C→T-A at positions 14 and 16) also damage the operator. Moreover, repressor protein apparently interacts more strongly with the left half of the operator. Equivalent mutations (G-C→A-T at position 12 and C-G→T-A at position 24; A-T→G-C at position 15 and T-A→C-G at position 21) have a greater effect on the affinity for repressor when the substitution occurs in the left (promoter-proximal) half of the operator than when it occurs in the right half. Also, no O^c mutations resulting in high constitutivity have been found in the right half of the operator.

In addition to the *lac* operator site, there are secondary binding sites for the *lac* repressor protein on the *Escherichia coli* chromosome. The repressor has relatively high affinity for these pseudo-operators, so-called because the binding is abolished by IPTG, in contrast to the interaction with other DNA sequences. One such site has been located in the operator-proximal third of the Z gene (Reznikoff et al. 1974), and its nucleotide sequence determined (Gilbert et al. 1976b). The symmetry of the pseudo-operator is substantially reduced. However, its affinity for *lac* repressor is only 10–30-fold lower than that of wild-type operator (Reznikoff et al. 1974; Gilbert et al. 1975), comparable to that of o^c operators.

Chemical modification of operator DNA has proved fecund in elucidating more intimate details of the repressor-operator interaction. Substitution of 5-bromouracil (BrU) for thymine in *lac* operator DNA strengthens the interaction with repressor by about a factor of 10, as

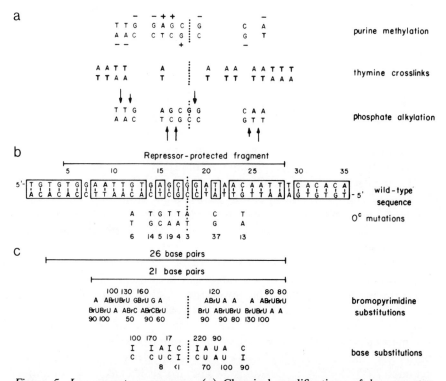

Figure 5 *Lac* operator sequence. (*a*) Chemical modifications of *lac* operator DNA. The upper portion shows the positions at which *lac* repressor inhibits (−) or enhances (+) methylation of purines by dimethyl sulfate. (Data from Gilbert et al. 1976b.) The middle portion shows the positions of the thymines at which repressor cross-links to BrU-substituted DNA upon UV irradiation. (Data from Ogata and Gilbert 1977.) The lower portion shows the positions at which repressor inhibits alkylation of phosphates by ethylnitrosourea, to a greater (long arrows) or lesser (short arrows) degree. (Data from W. Gilbert and A. Maxam, pers. comm.) (*b*) Natural *lac* operators. The upper portion shows the 35-base-pair sequence of the wild-type operator region; 28 base pairs (enclosed in boxes) are symmetric about a twofold axis (vertical dotted line). The DNA fragment protected from nuclease digestion by *lac* repressor is indicated by the solid line. (Data from Gilbert and Maxam 1973; Dickson et al. 1975.) The lower portion shows the base-pair substitutions of O^c mutations. (Data from Gilbert et al. 1975.) The numbers below the O^c sequence data are the corresponding affinities of repressor for o^c operator, expressed as a percent of the affinity for O^+ operator, for the tight-binding I^rX86 repressor protein described in the text. (Data from Jobe et al. 1974.) (*c*) Synthetic *lac* operators. The solid lines indicate 26-base-pair and 21-base-pair synthetic operators. The upper portion shows the positions of single 5-bromopyrimidine substitutions in synthetic operators; the lower portion shows the positions of single uracil and hypoxanthine substitutions. The numbers above and below the sequence data are the corresponding affinities of repressor for modified operator, expressed as a percent of the affinity for unmodified synthetic operator, for I^rX86 repressor protein. (Data from Yansura et al. 1977c; Goeddel et al. 1977c, 1978a; Goeddel et al. 1978b; M. H. Caruthers, pers. comm.)

d

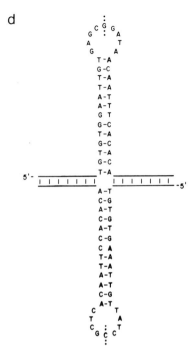

Figure 5 (continued) (*d*) Possible cruciform structure of the *lac* operator. Formation of this structure requires unwinding of the linear duplex by 3.5 helical turns.

evidenced by a tenfold decrease in the rate constant of dissociation k_b (Lin and Riggs 1972b). Ultraviolet irradiation of *lac* repressor bound to BrU-λd*lac* DNA results in photochemical attachment of the protein to the operator (Lin and Riggs 1974). The adroit application of this and other chemical probes by Gilbert and coworkers substantiates the O^c data regarding the asymmetric aspect of the repressor-operator interaction and demarcates areas of the DNA molecule in contact with repressor (Gilbert et al. 1976a,b; Ogata and Gilbert 1977). In these experiments, reactions culminating in single-strand scission of the DNA backbone are carried out on a 55-base-pair restriction fragment containing the *lac* operator, under conditions producing fewer than one break per DNA molecule. The patterns of modification in the presence and in the absence of *lac* repressor are deciphered after denaturation and gel electrophoresis of the DNA. Comparison of these patterns elucidates specific functional groups on the DNA whose modification is altered by repressor binding. The experiments show that the repressor protein either interacts with these groups in the operator or at least is in close enough contact to affect their reactivity. The results of three treatments are depicted in Figure 5a: methylation of purines with dimethyl sulfate (Gilbert et al. 1976b), cross-linking with BrU-substituted DNA (Ogata and Gilbert 1977), and alkylation of phosphates with ethylnitrosourea (W. Gilbert and A. Maxam, pers. comm.). The methylation data indicate ten contact sites in the central 17-base-pair region of the operator; seven of these are in the left half, supporting the idea based on O^c data that *lac* repressor interacts more strongly with the left half of the operator. The repressor blocks (−) methylation at seven purines, but enhances (+) it at three others, perhaps by perturbing the DNA conformation or creating an hydrophobic pocket for the reagent. Since dimethyl sulfate attacks N-7 of guanine in the major groove and N-3 of adenine in the minor groove, the methylation experiment shows that repressor makes contacts in both the major and minor grooves of the operator. The cross-linking data show 13 sites where UV-induced breakage of BrU-substituted DNA at the bromouracils is suppressed in the presence of repressor, presumably by the competing cross-linking reaction with a nearby group on the protein. This suggests that repressor makes close contacts with the thymine methyl group in the major groove of the operator at all but two of the thymines in the central 21-base-pair region and at one just outside. Although the majority of cross-linkable sites lies in the (A + T)-rich right half of the operator, the three sites where cross-linking was most frequently observed (positions 10, 11, and 15) are in the left half. The alkylation data demonstrate that repressor protects (⇓) seven phosphate groups in the central 17-base-pair region of the operator from attack by ethylnitrosourea, identifying points of contact between the protein and the phosphate backbone of the DNA. Three of the sites cluster around the middle of the operator; the other four are at symmetric positions in the symmetry blocks. The spacing of the phosphate contacts on the two strands of the DNA helix suggests that repressor binds to operator along one side of the helix.

Small DNA molecules with the nucleotide sequence of the *lac* operator have been synthesized by enzymatic joining of shorter oligodeoxyribonucleotides (Bahl et al. 1976; Yansura et al. 1977a). The oligonucleotides were prepared by chemical synthesis, using the triester (Itakura et al. 1974; Itakura et al. 1975) and diester (Goeddel et al 1977a) routes. The operator duplex has been cloned in *E. coli* on the pMB9 plasmid and shown to bind *lac* repressor in vivo (Marians et al. 1976; Heyneker et al. 1976; Sadler et al. 1977). In vitro binding studies reveal that the affinity of repressor for 21-base-pair (positions 8–28) and 26-base-pair (positions 3–28) synthetic operators is about 100-fold lower than the affinity for *lac* phage DNA (Goeddel et al. 1977b). The repressor binds well to even smaller synthetic operators; the minimal sequence required for detection in the standard assay is the central 17 base pairs (positions 10–26) (Bahl et al. 1977). The reduction in affinity is due primarily to an increase in the rate of dissociation of the complex formed with synthetic operator, since the rate of association is comparable to that observed for *lac* phage DNA.

However, if synthetic operator is carried on a plasmid DNA of molecular weight 3×10^6, the affinity is partially restored (Heyneker et al. 1976; Sadler et al. 1977). The effect of ionic strength on the binding of repressor to synthetic operator has also been examined. The binding parameters are only slightly sensitive to changes in the ionic strength of the binding buffer, in contrast to the case of *lac* phage DNA (Goeddel et al. 1977b).

In order to assess the role of particular functional groups in the interaction with *lac* repressor, Caruthers and coworkers have synthesized a host of operator analogs and determined the affinity of repressor for these modified operators (Yansura et al. 1977b; Goeddel et al. 1977c, 1978a; Goeddel et al. 1978b). Base substitutions were introduced at specific positions either by chemical synthesis of the substituted oligonucleotide or by repair synthesis using *E. coli* DNA polymerase 1. The results for operators having a single base change are summarized in Figure 5c. Replacement of thymine by 5-bromouracil (BrU) and of cytosine by 5-bromocytosine (BrC) at almost any position has minor consequences for the interaction with repressor. For operators having one bromopyrimidine, the affinity is increased (>100) or decreased (<100) less than twofold, compared to unmodified synthetic operator. In general, the effects are asymmetric, being slightly more pronounced in the left half of the operator than in the right half. There is some suggestion of symmetry in the interaction at the extremes of the symmetry blocks (positions 8, 9, 10, 11 and 25, 26, 27, 28), which is also discernible in the chemical modification data (compare Fig. 5a and Fig. 5c). However, three base substitutions, uracil for thymine at position 15 and hypoxanthine (I) for guanine at positions 16 and 17, at three O^c loci (A-T→G-C at positions 15, G-C→T-A at position 16, and C-G→T-A at position 17) cause decreases in affinity comparable to those observed for the $lacO^c$ phage DNAs (compare Fig. 5b and Fig. 5c). Apparently, loss of the thymine methyl group from the major groove at position 15 and of the guanine amino group from the minor groove at positions 16 and 17 accounts for most of the damage to these o^c operators. Removing the thymine methyl group by uracil substitution or the guanine amino group by hypoxanthine substitution at four other O^c loci (positions 12, 14, 21, and 24), as well as at three more sites (positions 19, 20, and 22), has only small effects on the affinity. Asymmetry in the interaction of repressor with the central region of the operator is especially striking here. At four symmetric positions, a modification (removal of the thymine methyl group at positions 15 and 21 or of the guanine amino group at positions 17 and 19) causes a substantial decrease in affinity when it is in the left half of the operator, but only a slight decrease or even increase in affinity when it is in the right half. The pattern of contacts derived from these studies is likewise consistent with a model of repressor binding along one side of the DNA helix, making contacts in both the major and minor grooves of the operator.

Repressors Altered by Mutations

A large number of mutants, bearing mutations in the *I* gene for *lac* repressor protein, have been isolated and classified on the basis of their genetical and biochemical properties (see Miller, this volume). This exhaustive analysis, in conjunction with the sequence work on the wild-type and repressor proteins from mutants (see Beyreuther, this volume), has generated important conclusions about structure-function relationships in the *lac* repressor. A small number of altered repressor proteins have been studied quantitatively in vitro by the techniques used for the wild-type repressor. These include 12 i^s repressors (Bourgeois and Jobe 1970; Jobe et al. 1972; Betz and Sadler 1976), three i^r repressors (Jobe and Bourgeois 1972c; Pfahl 1976; Betz and Sadler 1976; A. Schmitz et al., pers. comm.), and six tight-binding repressors (Betz and Sadler 1976). The in vitro binding characteristics of these repressors are summarized in Table 2.

The group of 12 i^s mutants (43, 44, 45, 272, 277, 2A, 14A, N1, N2, Y18, derived from a *lacI*$^+$ parental strain [Bourgeois and Jobe 1970]; 40, 41,

Table 2 Properties of mutationally altered repressors

I-gene allele	Increase in operator binding affinity[a]	Reduction in inducer binding affinity[b]	Allosteric properties[c]
I$^+$	0	0	normal
I^{s}44, 2A, 14A	0	3–9-fold	normal
I^{s}43, N2, Y18	0	>100-fold	normal
I^{s}45	0	>100-fold	altered
I^{s}40, 41	1.5-fold	60-fold	normal
I^{s}277	2-fold	>100-fold	normal
I^{s}272, N1	2–3-fold	>100-fold	altered
I^{r}X86	50-fold	2-fold	altered[d]
I^{r}B12	>10-fold	2-fold	altered[e]
I^{r}I12	40-fold	0[f]	
IB3, B11, B21, B32	3-fold	0–3-fold	normal
IB29	3-fold		altered
IB5	>10-fold	0	normal

Data from Bourgeois and Jobe (1970); Jobe et al. (1972); Jobe and Bourgeois (1972c); Pfahl (1976); Betz and Sadler (1976); and A. Schmitz et al. (pers. comm.).
[a]Estimated from the half-lives of altered repressor-operator complex, as illustrated in Fig. 2b.
[b]Determined by the ammonium sulfate precipitation technique described in the text.
[c]Defined by the equilibrium release curve illustrated in Fig. 3.
[d]Defined by the kinetic curve in Fig. 4.
[e]Biphasic dissociation kinetics in absence of IPTG; normal in presence of IPTG.
[f]Determined by equilibrium dialysis.

derived as tight-binding mutants from a wild-type *lacI*^{q} parental strain [Betz and Sadler 1976]) comprises strong i^s's (40, 41, 43, 45, 272, 277, N1, N2, Y18), which are not inducible in vivo, and weak i^s's (44, 2A, 14A), which are inducible at high concentrations of IPTG. All 12 i^s repressors show decreased affinity for inducer IPTG. The magnitude of this decrease correlates with the in vivo induction behavior of the mutants, the affinity of the repressor for IPTG being reduced only three- to ninefold for weak i^s mutants and more than 60-fold for strong i^s mutants. Seven of the i^s repressors exhibit normal affinity and five (40, 41, 272, 277, N1) exhibit slightly increased affinity for operator DNA. In most cases, the i^s repressor-operator complex responds to inducer similarly to the wild-type repressor, but with decreased affinity for IPTG; the equilibrium release curve has the same shape, only shifted to higher concentrations of IPTG. However, three strong i^s repressors (45, 272, N1) have altered allosteric properties, as evidenced by a qualitatively different shape of the equilibrium release curve (broken line in Fig. 3). From these data it is obvious that I^s mutations cannot be categorized simply as damaging the IPTG binding site of *lac* repressor, but must be divided into at least two main classes. The first class contains repressors which have only reduced affinity for inducer, otherwise behaving as wild-type repressor. The mutation in this case affects the inducer binding site only. The second class includes repressors which show tighter DNA binding and/or altered allosteric properties. The amino acid substitutions causing these effects are expected to occur in regions of the polypeptide chain which dictate the operator-binding conformation of *lac* repressor.

An intriguing class of mutants are the repressible i^r mutants; in vivo, the action of IPTG is reversed. The i^{r}X86 mutant is partially constitutive, repressible by low concentrations of inducer, and inducible by high concentrations of inducer (Chamness and Willson 1970). In vitro, the i^{r}X86 repressor has about 50-fold increased affinity for operator DNA and binds IPTG normally (Jobe and Bourgeois 1972c). It also has increased affinity for *E. coli* DNA deleted for the *lac* region (Pfahl 1976). The i^{r}X86 repressor differs somewhat from the wild-type repressor in its allosteric properties. As depicted by the broken line in Figure 4, the curve of k_b(app) vs [IPTG] is slightly sigmoidal, indicating that more than one inducer molecule is required to release i^{r}X86 repressor from the operator (Pfahl 1976). Pfahl (1976) proposed the following explanation of the in vivo behavior of this mutant, which might apply for other i^r mutants as well. In the absence of inducer, the i^{r}X86 repressor is effectively trapped at other sites on the *E. coli* chromosome and thus does not bind rapidly enough to newly synthesized operators to give full repression in a growing cell population. At low concentrations of inducer, i^r repressor is released preferentially from these sites and binds the operator site, for which it retains considerable affinity. At high concentrations of inducer, the i^{r}X86 repressor dissociates from the operator. Two other mutants exhibit similar properties, but to different degrees. The i^{r}B12 repressor, isolated with the group of tight-binding repressors described below, has roughly tenfold increased affinity for operator DNA (Betz and Sadler 1976). The i^{r}I12 repressor, isolated by reversion of a *lacI* nonsense mutation, has about 40-fold increased affinity for operator and increased affinity for λ DNA (A. Schmitz et al., pers. comm.). In a double mutant, constructed by recombination of the *I12* and *X86* mutations, these effects are amplified, resulting in a repressor protein with at least 1000-fold increased affinity for *lac* operator.

The six tight-binding mutants (derived from a wild-type *lacI^q* parental strain) show normal or slightly lower levels of *lac* enzymes in the absence of IPTG in vivo and decreased inducibility (Betz and Sadler 1976). For all of the tight-binding repressors, the affinity for operator is enhanced, generally to a small extent; the B5 repressor has tenfold increased affinity for operator, as well as increased affinity for nonoperator DNA. Five of these repressors (B3, B5, B11, B21, B32) have normal affinity for IPTG. Some of the tight-binding repressors appear to have modified allosteric properties. Saturating concentrations of IPTG accelerate the rate of dissociation of the tight-binding repressor-operator complex by only sevenfold for the B11 repressor and by 40–70-fold for three other tight-binding repressors (B5, B21, B32), as compared to about 1000-fold in the case of the wild type. The greater stability of the ternary complex accounts for the decreased inducibility in vivo.

RECOGNITION OF DNA

Besides binding very tightly to the operator site on DNA, the *lac* repressor protein binds other nucleotide sequences. The interaction of repressor and nonoperator DNA, given in Equation 4, is governed by the equilibrium association constant (K_{DNA})

$$K_{DNA} = \frac{[R-DNA]}{[R][DNA]}.$$

Here K_{DNA} is the average affinity per site and $[DNA]$ is the concentration of potential sites in nucleotides. Because of the low affinity of repressor for nonoperator DNAs and because of the multisite binding, the binding of repressor to DNA cannot be quantitated by the procedures developed to study the repressor-operator interaction. However, the equilibrium constant K_{DNA} can be measured in competition experiments on membrane filters, since the ability of unlabeled DNA to compete with labeled operator DNA for the repressor is a function of the affinity of repressor for the binding sites on the unlabeled DNA molecule. In the competition experiments, there is less than one protein molecule bound per DNA molecule; the binding constant measured is biased in the direction of the higher affinity sites. The interaction of repressor and DNA has also been investigated by physicochemical techniques. In these experiments, many repressor molecules bind to each DNA molecule; the binding constant represents the average affinity.

Electrostatic attraction between negatively charged phosphates on the DNA backbone and positively charged amino acid residues on the protein plays a major role in the interaction of repressor and DNA. In this section, we consider electrostatic effects, as well as the effects of base sequence and modification on the recognition process.

Interaction of Repressor and DNA

Two types of competition experiments have been employed to determine the affinity of repressor for DNA: equilibrium competition and rate competition (Lin and Riggs 1972a). For equilibrium competition experiments, a constant concentration of repressor protein and labeled operator DNA is equilibrated with increasing concentrations of unlabeled nonoperator DNA. Equilibrium competition curves are depicted in Figure 6a. The affinity K_{DNA} of repressor for the competing DNA relative to the affinity K_O for operator is computed from the concentration of unlabeled DNA required to reduce the amount of labeled repressor-operator complex by one-half. The equilibrium competition method requires relatively high concentrations of unlabeled DNA. The rate competition method is ten times more sensitive to the concentration of competing DNA. In these experiments the rate of association of repressor protein and labeled operator DNA is measured in the presence of a given concentration of unlabeled nonoperator DNA. The apparent rate constant of association $k_a(app)$ is smaller, since the concentration of free repressor protein is reduced due to binding to the competing DNA. Figure 6b shows the kinetics data from rate competition experiments; the apparent rate constant $k_a(app)$ is proportional to the slope of the line. The equilibrium constant K_{DNA} can be calculated from the ratio of the rate constants in the presence and absence of competing DNA, assuming that repressor is in equilibrium with nonoperator DNA during the reaction. Values for K_{DNA} obtained by the two techniques are in good agreement. For *E. coli* DNA deleted for the *lac* region under standard conditions (except that binding buffer has 3×10^{-3} M $Mg[CH_3CO_2]_2$, $I = 0.03$ M), K_{DNA} is $0.5-2 \times 10^6$ M^{-1} by equilibrium competition and $2-3 \times 10^6$ M^{-1} by rate competition.

The effects of various parameters on the binding have also been investigated by membrane filtration. The dependence of the equilibrium constant K_{DNA} upon ionic strength, pH, and temperature was measured in competition experiments (Lin and Riggs 1972a, 1975a). The affinity K_{DNA}

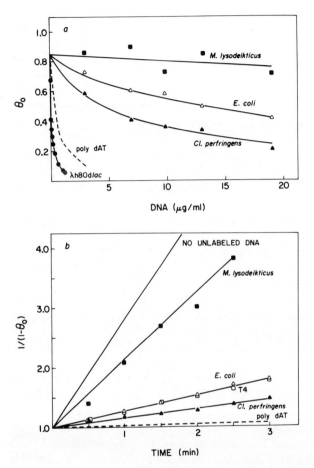

Figure 6 Competition for *lac* repressor by nonoperator DNAs. (*a*) Equilibrium competition. Aliquots of unlabeled nonoperator DNA and labeled λh80d*lac* DNA $(2.2 \times 10^{-2} \text{ M})$ are mixed, and active repressor protein $(2.2 \times 10^{-12} \text{ M})$ is added. After equilibration, samples of the reaction mixture are filtered. θ_o is the fraction saturation of labeled operator by repressor. (*b*) Rate competition. At time $t = 0$, active repressor protein $(2.2 \times 10^{-12} \text{ M})$ is added to a mixture of labeled λh80d*lac* DNA $(2.2 \times 10^{-12} \text{ M})$ and unlabeled nonoperator DNA $(0.65 \ \mu\text{g/ml})$; at various times t, samples are removed and filtered. The apparent rate constant of association $k_a(\text{app})$ of repressor and labeled operator DNA is proportional to the slope of the straight line. Unlabeled DNAs: (●) λh80d*lac*; (■) *M. lysodeikticus*; (□)T4; (▲) *Cl. perfringens*; (△) *E. coli*; (– – –) poly[(dAT)]. (———) No unlabeled DNA. Standard conditions, except binding buffer has $3 \times 10^{-3} \text{ M}$ Mg $(\text{CH}_3\text{CO}_2)_2$, $I = 0.03 \text{ M}$. (Data from Lin and Riggs 1972a.)

of repressor for DNA is slightly more dependent on ionic strength than is the affinity K_O for operator: under the above conditions, a tenfold increase in the ionic strength of the binding buffer reduces K_{DNA} about 1000-fold and K_O about 170-fold. The affinity for poly[d(AT)] decreases about sixfold as the pH is raised from 7.0 to 8.5. There is no apparent effect of temperature ($1°$–$24°C$) on the affinity for both λ DNA and poly[d(AT)]. Under conditions which abolish the binding of repressor to operator DNA, effects on the binding to unlabeled DNA obviously could not be studied by the usual competition methods. Accordingly, a technique was developed for measuring the binding of repressor to labeled nonoperator DNA directly on membrane filters (Lin and Riggs 1975b). The procedure exploits the fact that at low salt concentrations *lac* repressor protein can be photochemically attached to BrU-substituted λ DNA (Lin and Riggs 1974). In this type of experiment, actinomycin D inhibits the binding of *lac* repressor to DNA. On the other hand, the inducer IPTG does not alter the affinity of repressor for three DNAs (BrU-λ, poly[d(AT)], and poly[d(T-T-G)]:poly[d(C-A-A)]).

The average affinity of repressor for DNA has been determined by two physical methods: a boundary sedimentation technique (Revzin and von Hippel 1977) and quantitative DNA-cellulose chromatography (deHaseth et al. 1977b). In the thermodynamically rigorous sedimentation method, repressor-DNA complex is separated from free repressor protein by analytical ultracentrifugation. The free repressor concentration is measured optically, as a function of known input repressor and DNA concentrations. Analysis of the binding data yields absolute values for the equilibrium constant K_{DNA}, as well as estimates for the stoichiometry of binding and the degree of cooperativity. At 0.15 M Na^+ in phosphate buffer (pH 7.5), K_{DNA} is about 1.2×10^5 M^{-1}. One repressor molecule binds per about 24 nucleotides, in agreement with the stoichiometry found in titration experiments described below. There is no evidence of protein-protein interactions in the binding of repressor and DNA. In the chromatographic technique, repressor protein is loaded onto and eluted from a small DNA-cellulose column at constant salt concentration. For low, initial binding densities, the amount of repressor on the column decreases exponentially with washing; the free repressor concentration in the eluant is assayed fluorometrically. The equilibrium constant K_{DNA} of repressor for the column DNA is deduced from the characteristic parameter of the elution profile and the known amount of accessible DNA on the column. Although this procedure depends on a number of assumptions and judicious choice of conditions, it gives values for the binding constant which are in excellent agreement with the absolute values determined by the sedimentation technique (see Fig. 7); under the above conditions, K_{DNA} for calf thymus DNA is about 1.3×10^5 M^{-1}. The

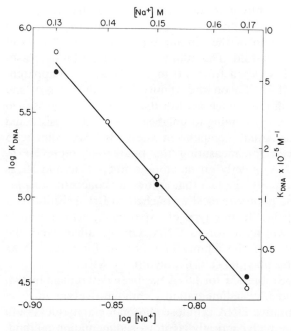

Figure 7 Dependence of equilibrium association constant K_{DNA} of *lac* repressor and nonoperator DNA upon Na^+ concentration. The number of ion pairs formed in repressor-DNA complex is proportional to the negative slope of the straight line. (●) λ DNA; boundary sedimentation technique. (Data from Revzin and von Hippel 1977.) (○) Calf thymus DNA; quantitative DNA-cellulose chromatography. (Data from deHaseth et al. 1977b corrected to pH 7.5.) Binding buffer is 0.01 M Na_2HPO_4 (pH 7.5), 1×10^{-4} M EDTA, plus NaCl to given total Na^+ concentration; 20°C.

applicability of both methods, however, is limited to values of the equilibrium constant K_{DNA} on the order of 10^4–10^6 M^{-1}.

The dependence of the binding on salt concentration, pH, and temperature has been scrutinized (Revzin and von Hippel 1977; deHaseth et al. 1977a,b). Results obtained from the physical measurements are in accord with those from membrane-filter studies, if differences in buffer composition are taken into account. As depicted in Figure 7, the equilibrium constant K_{DNA} is highly sensitive to salt concentration; K_{DNA} decreases about 20-fold as the Na^+ concentration increases from 0.13 to 0.17 M. According to the theoretical treatment described later, the number of ion pairs formed in repressor-DNA complex is proportional to the negative slope of the linear plot of log K_{DNA} vs log $[Na^+]$ (Record et al. 1976). From these data, as well as from similar data for Mg^{+2} in place of Na^+, it is estimated that the repressor-DNA interaction involves about 12 ionic interactions with the phosphate backbone (deHaseth et al.

1977a). However, at a given salt concentration (or ionic strength), the affinity of repressor for DNA is much lower when the cation is Mg^{+2}, since Mg^{+2} binds more tightly than Na^+ to DNA and thus competes more effectively with repressor for the phosphate charges. This has consequences for binding constants determined by membrane filtration in the standard buffers, which contain both K^+ and Mg^{+2}. Moreover, the choice of anion affects the affinity of repressor for DNA; replacement of Cl^- by acetate ion results in a 40-fold increase in K_{DNA} without changing the slope of the log K_{DNA} vs log $[Na^+]$ plot. The origin of this anion effect is not understood.

The repressor-DNA interaction is quite sensitive to changes in pH, but less so to changes in temperature. The equilibrium constant K_{DNA} decreases with increasing pH, about eightfold as determined by the sedimentation method over the range pH 7.2–7.6 (Revzin and von Hippel 1977) or about 18-fold as determined by DNA-cellulose chromatography over the range pH 7.8–8.4 (deHaseth et al. 1977a). Analysis of the data for hydrogen-ion effects leads to the conclusion that binding of repressor to DNA is accompanied by uptake of two protons, probably on histidines or α-amino groups. Below 30°C, there is little effect of temperature on the binding; the affinity decreases about twofold as the temperature increases from 4° to 30°C (Revzin and von Hippel 1977; deHaseth et al. 1977a). However, a greater decrease in affinity is seen at higher temperatures (deHaseth et al. 1977a). At 20°C and pH 7.5, $\Delta G = -7.3$ kcal/mole, $\Delta H = -6.0$ kcal/mole, and $\Delta S = 4.4$ cal/mole deg.

Spectroscopic techniques have also been employed to study binding of *lac* repressor to the bulk of the sites on DNA. Two notable results have come out of these experiments, namely, detection of a change in conformation of DNA upon binding of repressor and consensus regarding the stoichiometry. The circular dichroism spectra of poly[d(AT)], calf thymus DNA, and λ DNA are enhanced in the 260–280-nm region by repressor (Maurizot et al. 1974; Butler et al. 1977). The increased ellipticity of the strong DNA circular dichroism band when repressor is bound is evidence for a conformational change in the secondary structure of the DNA. The perturbed DNA spectrum is similar to the spectrum of free A-form DNA, suggesting that the spectral changes reflect tilting of some base pairs. Alternatively, the spectral changes may arise from twisting of the DNA helix. Moreover, *lac* repressor is a helix-stabilizing protein; at low ionic strength, it increases the melting temperature of poly[d(AT)] appreciably (von Hippel et al. 1975; Wang et al. 1977). The stoichiometry of the binding of repressor and DNA has been measured in titration experiments by two techniques: light scattering with poly[d(AT)] (Maurizot et al. 1974) and circular dichroism with λ DNA and poly[d(AT)] (von Hippel et al. 1975; Butler et al. 1977). In all cases, including the sedimentation results described above, one *lac* repressor binds per about 24 nucleotides. The dimensions of repressor-DNA complex obtained by electron microscopy are compatible with repressor being bound along two sides of the DNA helix (Zingsheim et al. 1977). In light of this finding, the observed stoichiometry means that the binding site on nonoperator DNA is about 24 base pairs long.

Inducer IPTG affects neither the conformational change (Maurizot et al. 1974) nor the sedimentation results (Revzin and von Hippel 1977), further testifying that the interaction of repressor and DNA is not sensitive to inducer. The binding of IPTG to repressor-DNA complex has been studied by fluorescence. The changes in the fluorescence of repressor protein upon binding of IPTG are the same in the presence or absence of DNA (von Hippel et al. 1975). This implies that *lac* repressor undergoes equivalent conformational transitions whether free in solution or bound to DNA; however, there is no concomitant change in the affinity of repressor for nonoperator DNA. Titration experiments with IPTG (Maurizot et al. 1974; von Hippel et al. 1975; Butler et al. 1977), as well as kinetic and equilibrium measurements (Friedman et al. 1977), show that inducer binds to repressor-DNA complex identically as it does to free repressor protein. These facts confirm that the binding sites on repressor for DNA and for inducer are physically distinct sites.

Effects of Base Sequence and Modification

The binding of *lac* repressor protein to a wide variety of DNAs has been characterized in competition experiments on membrane filters (Lin and Riggs 1972a, 1976; Riggs et al. 1972; Richmond and Steitz 1976; P. Lu, pers. comm.). In these studies the repressor discriminates between different DNA sequences. This is suggestive in the binding to natural DNAs where the affinity of repressor for DNA correlates roughly with the A + T content of the DNA (Lin and Riggs 1972a). Natural DNAs having a higher A + T content compete more effectively with operator, as evident in Figure 6. On a weight basis, DNA from *Clostridium perfringens* (70 mole % [A + T]) competes at least ten times better than DNA from *Micrococcus lysodeikticus* (30 mole % [A + T]). Furthermore, *lac* repressor binds to glucosylated DNAs from T2 and T4 phages with about the affinity expected on the basis of their A + T content. The extent of glucosylation of hydroxymethylcytosine residues is high: 75% for T2 DNA and 100% for T4 DNA (Georgopoulos and Revel 1971). The fact that the repressor has equal, as well as the expected, affinity for these two DNAs suggests that the interaction is not bothered by the presence of sugar groups in the major groove of DNA. Nevertheless, the interpretation that the repressor binds only to preferred, nonglucosylated sites cannot be completely rejected. No binding to ribonucleic acids could be detected. Physical studies do not reveal these differences in the average affinity of repressor for natural DNAs (Wang et al. 1977). In thermal-melting experiments, the relative ability of DNAs to compete with poly[d(AT)] for repressor is independent of A + T content. This suggests that, under the conditions of DNA excess in membrane-filter experiments, the repressor is binding at favored (A + T)-rich sequences.

Effects of base sequence on the interaction with repressor are also displayed in the binding to synthetic DNAs (Lin and Riggs 1972a; Riggs et al. 1972). The values of the equilibrium constant K_{DNA} for various DNA copolymers are listed in Table 3. These synthetic polynucleotides exhibit a range of affinities for *lac* repressor, from about $10^5 \, M^{-1}$ for poly[d(G-C)]:poly[d(G-C)] to about $5 \times 10^7 \, M^{-1}$ for poly[d(A-T)]: poly[d(A-T)] and poly[d(T-T-G)]:poly[d(C-A-A)]. The basis for the recognition process in the binding to DNA is not known. Clearly, simple base composition, A + T content, is not the only determining factor, since poly[d(A-T)]:poly[d(A-T)] binds 30 times tighter than poly-

Table 3 Binding of repressor to synthetic polynucleotides

Polymer	$K_{DNA} \, M^{-1 \, a}$	T_m (°C)	References
lac operator	$2–5 \times 10^{13}$		
d(A-T):d(A-T)	$1.5–5 \times 10^7$	60	Lin and Riggs (1972a, 1976)
d(A-U):d(A-U)	$5–7 \times 10^5$	57	Lin and Riggs (1976)
d(G-C):d(G-C)	7×10^4		Riggs et al. (1972)
d(I-C):d(I-C)	1.5×10^5		Riggs et al. (1972)
dA:dT	$5–7 \times 10^5$		Lin and Riggs (1972a)
dG:dC	$5–15 \times 10^5$		Lin and Riggs (1972a)
dI:dC	1.5×10^5		Riggs et al. (1972)
d(T-T-G):d(C-A-A)	$5–15 \times 10^{7 \, b}$		Riggs et al. (1972)
d(A-S^{4}T):d(A-S^{4}T)	2.5×10^9		P. Lu (pers. comm.)
d(A-FU):d(A-FU)	$1.5–5 \times 10^8$	59	Lin and Riggs (1976)
d(A-ClU):d(A-ClU)	$0.9–2.5 \times 10^9$	67	Lin and Riggs (1976)
d(A-BrU):d(A-BrU)	$1.2–2.5 \times 10^9$	66	Lin and Riggs (1976)
d(A-IU):d(A-IU)	$2.5–7 \times 10^9$	66	Lin and Riggs (1976)
d(A-U-HgX):d(A-U-HgX)			
X: thioglycolic acid	$1–2.5 \times 10^7$	58	Richmond and Steitz (1976)
X: β-mercaptoethanol	$3–7 \times 10^7$	56	Richmond and Steitz (1976)
X: 1-mercaptopropanediol	$0.9–2 \times 10^8$		Richmond and Steitz (1976)
X: dithiothreitol	$3–7 \times 10^8$	—^{c}	Richmond and Steitz (1976)
X: cysteamine	$1.2–3 \times 10^9$		Richmond and Steitz (1976)

[a] K_{DNA} is the equilibrium association constant for the reaction $R + DNA \rightleftharpoons R - DNA$. It is calculated relative to the association constant for operator $K_O = 2–5 \times 10^{13} \, M^{-1}$, assuming each nucleotide begins a potential binding site. Standard conditions, except binding buffer has $3 \times 10^{-3} \, M$ Mg $(CH_3CO_2)_2$, $I = 0.03 \, M$.
[b] K_{DNA} calculated assuming every third nucleotide begins a potential binding site.
[c] This DNA probably has intrastrand cross-links.

(dA):poly(dT). In the alternating copolymers, the possibility that the repressor binds to branched structures existing because of intrastrand complementarity is effectively excluded by two facts: poly[d(I-C)]: poly[d(I-C)] and poly[d(G-C)]:poly[d(G-C)] bind poorly (Riggs et al. 1972) and a cross-linked poly[d(A-U-HgX)]:poly[d(A-U-HgX)] described below binds well (Richmond and Steitz 1976). Physical measurements confirm that repressor binds more tightly to poly[d(AT)] than to natural DNAs (Revzin and von Hippel 1977; Wang et al. 1977). At 0.15 M Na^+, K_{DNA} for poly[d(AT)] is about 7×10^5 M^{-1}, roughly sixfold greater than the affinity for λ DNA. In the above studies, the affinity of repressor for nonoperator DNA varies over a relatively narrow ($\sim$500-fold) range; in all cases it is at least 10^6 orders of magnitude less than the affinity for operator DNA. However, there must exist a spectrum of DNA sites, ranging from these low-affinity sites to the high affinity observed for the particular sequence of the *lac* operator.

Effects of base modification have been probed using structural analogs of poly[d(AT)] (Lin and Riggs 1976; Richmond and Steitz 1976; P. Lu, pers. comm.). The equilibrium constants K_{DNA} for the modified copolymers are given in Table 3. These modifications can bring the affinity for nonoperator DNA sites almost as high as 10^{10} M^{-1}. The binding is strengthened dramatically by substitutions in positions 4 (S for O) and 5 (halogens for methyl) of thymine. There is only minor correlation of the binding constant with the stability of the duplex structure (T_m) in the case of the halogen-substituted analogs of poly[d(A-T)]:poly[d(A-T)]. However, the notion that *lac* repressor makes extensive contacts with nonoperator DNA bases in the major groove of the helix is refuted by the findings with poly[d(A-U-HgX)]:poly[d(A-U-HgX)]. In this polynucleotide, the methyl group of thymine is replaced by a covalently bound Hg atom and associated mercaptan X. The bulky mercaptans fill the major groove of the DNA and, in the case of dithiothreitol, cross-link the two strands. The association constants K_{DNA} for the mercuri-DNAs are large, 10^7–10^9 M^{-1}. This elegant chemical approach demonstrates that high affinity of repressor for nonoperator DNA does not require interactions in the major groove or denaturation of the DNA duplex.

MECHANISMS OF RECOGNITION

After all this, what, if anything, can we conclude about the factors important in the overall recognition process? First, recall the properties of the interaction of repressor with operator and nonoperator DNAs. The tight binding to operator and the weaker binding to nonoperator DNA sequences share these traits:

1. Sensitivity to electrostatic conditions. Increased shielding (ionic

strength) and negative charge on the protein (pH) weaken the interaction.

2. Conformational change in DNA.
3. Inhibition by actinomycin D. The antibiotic intercalates at dG-dC sequences and blocks the narrow groove of the DNA helix.
4. Effect of Br substitution in DNA. Uniform replacement of methyl by Br at the 5 position of thymine in the major groove of the DNA helix strengthens the interaction. However, in the synthetic operator, the effect of substitution at individual positions is small and variable.

Operator DNA and nonoperator DNA binding differ, however, in the following respects:

1. Effect of inducer IPTG. Inducer lowers the affinity K_O for operator DNA but, in general, does not change the affinity K_{DNA} for nonoperator DNA. The binding of repressor to nonoperator DNA is insensitive to effectors, even in the case of poly[d(T-T-G)]:poly[d(C-A-A)], which provides, in order, the sequences TTGT of four of the six bases of the symmetrical region of the *lac* operator (see Fig. 5b).
2. Temperature dependence. The affinity K_O for operator DNA increases slightly with increasing temperature, while the affinity K_{DNA} for nonoperator DNA decreases.

The size of the DNA site depends somewhat on definition. The length of the repressor-protected operator fragment is about 27 base pairs; the length of the synthetic operator is 21–26 base pairs, minimally 17 base pairs; and the length of a nonoperator DNA site is about 24 base pairs. However, the region of known O^c substitutions comprises 13 base pairs; the influence of repressor on chemical modification of operator DNA suggests that the region of contact extends 17–22 base pairs; and the effects of substitutions in the synthetic operator on the affinity for repressor encompass at least 21 base pairs.

The arrangement of *lac* repressor on DNA is not known, although there is some evidence pertaining to the geometry of the complex. As discussed in this paper, the pattern emerging from the chemical-modification and base-substitution studies suggests that repressor binds along one side of the operator duplex. The electron microscopic evidence showing that more than one repressor molecule can occupy the same stretch of nonoperator DNA is in keeping with the model of one-sided binding. However, it is not known how many subunits of the protein make contact with the DNA, operator or otherwise (see Weber and Geisler, this volume). In studies with hybrid repressors composed of normal and tryptic core (lacking the N-terminal fragment necessary for **DNA** binding) (see Beyreuther; Weber and Geisler; both this volume) subunits, more than one normal subunit per tetramer is required for binding to operator DNA (Geisler and Weber 1976). Comparing the size of the operator site, about 60–90 Å long, with the dimensions of the tetramer, about 80–90 Å square, from electron microscopy on single molecules (Ohshima et al. 1975; Zingsheim et al. 1977), it seems likely that the operator accommodates one repressor molecule. In this situation, at least two subunits could interact with the operator. The N-terminal headpiece fragments, which possess ordered secondary structure, bind to nonoperator DNA with an apparent stoichiometry of one headpiece per about 24 nucleotides (Geisler and Weber 1977; Jovin et al. 1977). Although 24 base pairs is a maximum estimate for the size of the binding site, this finding might mean that only one repressor subunit is involved in binding to DNA. Preliminary evidence indicates that the headpiece makes essentially the same contacts with *lac* operator as does tetrameric repressor (R. Ogata and W. Gilbert, pers. comm.). As far as the number of DNA binding sites per repressor tetramer is concerned, the conclusion from the repressor-operator binding studies described in this paper is that *lac* repressor has a single site for DNA (Eq. 1). However, this does not rule out the possibility of more than one DNA binding site, only one of which is detectable by the membrane-filter technique. Structural data for both the solution (Ohshima et al. 1975) and microcrystalline (Steitz et al. 1974) forms of the protein indicate that the repressor molecule possesses at least twofold rotational symmetry, consistent with the existence of two DNA binding sites per tetramer.

This leads us to consider the role of symmetry in the recognition process. Given the symmetric aspect of the operator DNA sequence and the considerable potential for symmetry in the *lac* repressor protein, a tetramer of identical subunits, the question naturally arises. In the absence of X-ray structural data, we can only enumerate various possibilities. Either the repressor-operator interaction exploits the component symmetries, or it does not make use of them. If not, then there are two modes of binding consistent with the facts mentioned above. In the first, two subunits of the repressor make contacts with operator DNA. The interaction is asymmetric because the symmetries of repressor and operator do not match. In the second, only one subunit contacts the DNA, necessarily asymmetrically. This alternative is not excluded by the results for hybrid repressors, since the requirement of a second normal subunit in the tetramer for binding to operator may be a conformational or environmental one. The available experimental data from studies with altered operators described in a preceding section reveal asymmetry in the interaction of repressor and operator. Nevertheless, the more appealing notion is that symmetry does play a role. In this case, two subunits are symmetrically disposed along DNA, making contacts with the operator. The symmetry of the interaction is imperfect, though, partly because the nucleotide sequence of the operator is not totally symmetric and possibly because the repressor and operator symmetries are not completely congruent, or some combination of the two. The evidence that the repressor interacts more strongly with the left half of the operator leads to a testable prediction. If symmetry is an important factor in the repressor-operator interaction, then improving the symmetry of the operator so that the right half is made to resemble more closely the left half (A-T→C-G at positions 20 and 22) should result in a "super-operator," with higher affinity for repressor than wild-type operator. The requisite nucleotide sequence could be generated either synthetically or genetically. An operator mutant which appears to be a likely candidate for carrying a mutation of this type has been isolated (Pfahl and Bourgeois 1976).

Electrostatic effects on protein–nucleic acid interactions have received theoretical attention recently. Using a general thermodynamic treatment based on polyelectrolyte theory (Manning 1969, 1972) and assuming no specific anion effects, Record et al. (1976) calculated the number of ion pairs formed between ligand and polynucleotide from the known dependence of the equilibrium constant on salt concentration. Knowledge of the electrostatic contribution to the binding energy permits evaluation of the nonelectrostatic component. For *lac* repressor, the interactions with operator as well as nonoperator DNA have been interpreted in light of this theory and were found to differ significantly with respect to their electrostatic properties (deHaseth et al. 1977a; Record et al. 1977). As described in a preceding section, binding of repressor and nonoperator DNA involves formation of about 12 ion pairs coupled with uptake of two protons. The overall association reaction is entropically driven by the release of cations from DNA upon binding of repressor. This suggests that the attractive forces in the binding of repressor to nonoperator DNA sequences are mostly electrostatic. The repressor-operator binding data described above (Riggs et al. 1970a) have also been analyzed, after adjustment for the presence of both monovalent (K^+) and divalent (Mg^{++}) cations in the binding buffer. The estimated number of ion pairs in the repressor-operator complex is about eight, or four fewer ionic interactions than in repressor-DNA complexes. Alkylation experiments described in a preceding section have identified seven phosphate contact sites in operator DNA, in support of the estimated eight ion pairs. As expected for the repressor-operator interaction, the nonelectrostatic component of the binding energy is substantial, about 9 kcal/mole of favorable free energy at 24°C. Under standard conditions, about half of the overall free energy change is an entropic contribution from cation release.

A number of detailed models for protein–nucleic acid interactions have been proposed. Sung and Dixon (1970) have constructed a model for histone binding to DNA, in which they demonstrated that the major groove of DNA in the B conformation readily accommodates an α-helical structure of the amino-terminal region of the protein. An analogous model has been suggested for *lac* repressor (Adler et al. 1972). Carter and Kraut (1974) have constructed a model for the complementary binding of helical antiparallel β-polypeptide ribbons in the minor groove of double-stranded RNA. The RNA helix assumes a hybrid form between the A and A' conformations; hydrogen bonds form between the ribose 2'-hydroxyls and the peptide carbonyl oxygens. The 2'-hydroxyl group, present in RNA but absent in DNA, plays an important role in the precise complementarity between the RNA and polypeptide double helices. Mimicking this model is another model for binding to DNA in the B conformation (Church et al. 1977). Here, unusual hydrogen bonds form between deoxyribose 3'-oxygens and alternate peptide amides; most amino acid side groups on the inside of the β-ribbon could interact with DNA bases in the minor groove without distortion of the backbone conformation. Besides these models for backbone interactions, a model for unambiguous recognition of base pairs in both the major and minor grooves of double-helical nucleic acids has been presented (Seeman et al. 1976). In this model, formation of two hydrogen bonds between recognition sites on the bases and amino acid side chains is necessary for unique identification of a given base pair.

The role of both the major and minor grooves in the recognition of DNA by *lac* repressor is becoming apparent. The minor groove is mentioned by the fact that actinomycin D inhibits the interaction with both operator and nonoperator DNAs. However, it is conceivable that intercalation of the dye abolishes the binding by distorting the DNA structure. As for the major groove, the affinity of repressor for uniformly halogen-substituted operator and nonoperator DNAs is decidedly enhanced. On the other hand, blocking the major groove has no deleterious effect on nonoperator DNA binding. Chemical-modification studies suggest that repressor makes contacts mainly in the minor groove of nonoperator DNA (Kolchinsky et al. 1976). In contrast, chemical-modification and base-substitution studies of the repressor-operator interaction indicate that the repressor makes contacts with DNA bases in both grooves of the helix. Again, a significant difference in the interaction of repressor with operator and nonoperator DNA sequences is evident. Recognition of nonoperator DNA apparently utilizes the minor groove, perhaps via backbone hydrogen bonds as in the model described above. Variations in the affinity may reflect subtleties of the duplex structure or charge distribution. Recognition of operator DNA involves both the major and minor grooves, probably via hydrogen bonds with the DNA bases as well. Potential recognition sites at specific positions in the 21-base-pair operator sequence have been identified (Goeddel et al. 1978a). These data suggest that hydrophobic interactions contribute to the stability of the repressor-operator complex.

We end the comparison of the interactions of repressor with operator and nonoperator DNAs with a general comment, and a word of caution, about specificity. The specificity, or relative preference, of *lac* repressor for operator over nonoperator DNA is conveniently defined as the ratio of the respective association constants K_O/K_{DNA} (Lin and Riggs 1975a). Under the conditions of the membrane-filtration experiments, where there is less than one repressor per DNA molecule, the effective affinity of a nonoperator DNA site is the product of the number of sites and the intrinsic affinity. Thus a large number of low-affinity sites will compete with the operator for repressor just as well as a small number of high-affinity sites. Considering the example of *E. coli* DNA under physiological conditions, $K_O/K_{DNA} \simeq 10^8$ on a molar basis, or $\simeq 4 \times 10^6$ on a weight basis. In the *E. coli* genome, the 2×10^5-fold weight excess of nonoperator DNA over operator means the actual specificity is $4 \times 10^6 / 2 \times 10^5 \simeq 20$. In fact, experiments with *E. coli* minicells demonstrate that in vivo more than 90% of the repressor molecules are bound to the *E. coli* chromosome (Kao-Huang et al. 1977). Although the specificity of *lac* repressor for *lac* operator is high, it is finite. It should be apparent, then, that the ability to detect binding of protein to specific DNA sequences in vitro will be affected by binding at other sites and will depend on the relative effective affinities of the protein for the specific sequence and the rest of the sites on the DNA. In addition to the consequences for in vivo regulation (see Reznikoff and Abelson, this volume), binding to nonoperator DNA may play an integral role in the repressor's quest for operator.

The experimental results for the repressor-operator interaction described in a preceding section highlight two remarkable features, namely, the very tight binding of repressor and operator and the rapidity with which the repressor protein finds the operator site on DNA. A logical question is whether the interaction achieves its extraordinary specificity through a mechanism in which the repressor protein binds to an unusual DNA structure. Several models for the recognition process have been presented. One type includes models in which DNA base pairs in the operator region are disrupted, the repressor reading the sequence of the exposed bases. Gierer (1966) has proposed a cruciform model for specific repressor-operator interactions, for which the twofold symmetry of the operator sequence is a prerequisite. Alternate models are those in which the operator region is fully base-paired, the repressor reading the base sequence in the grooves of the helix. Along these lines are the general models for the interaction of polypeptides with double-stranded RNA or DNA mentioned above, and of proteins with kinked DNA helices (Crick and Klug 1975), as well as a novel look at the features revealed by helical arrangement of operator DNA sequences (O'Neill 1976).

The question of whether the binding of *lac* repressor protein to operator DNA unwinds the duplex helix was resolved by the experiments with superhelical DNA. The small amount of unwinding measured precludes the possibility that the repressor protein promotes the formation of looped-out structures in the operator DNA. However, the unwinding experiments do not address the question of whether the operator exists in a hairpin or other partially single-stranded structure in a stable state in the absence of repressor. It is highly unlikely that such a structure would be more stable than the fully paired duplex. Assuming the helix state to be favored thermodynamically over the cruciform state, von Heijne and Blomberg (1976) have treated a kinetic model for the helix-cruciform transition. The mean lifetimes calculated for the cruciform state are quite short, inconsistent with the notion that cruciforms persist in a metastable state. Moreover, the facts that the operator sequence does not contain any mismatched or modified bases, that the 27-base-pair operator fragment has a T_m of 67°C in 0.15 M NaCl, 0.015 M Na citrate (Gilbert and Maxam 1973), and that repressor binds with high affinity to the chemically synthesized 21- and 26-base-pair operators all argue that the DNA is double-stranded.

Crick and Klug (1975) have postulated another type of unusual DNA structure, in which the double-stranded helix executes right-angle turns. These kinks in the DNA helix can be constructed by unstacking one base pair and unwinding the duplex helix by about 25°. The base sequences near a kink would be more exposed than they would be in a linear stretch of DNA. The authors speculate that when *lac* repressor binds to the operator site on DNA, the double helix becomes kinked in four places, thus accounting for the 90° unwinding measured. Although there is no further experimental evidence attesting to the existence of kinks in DNA, and no reason on theoretical grounds to recommend kinking over smooth bending of the double helix (Kuhn and Thürkauf 1961; M. Levitt as cited in Finch et al. 1977), the idea is tantalizing. Electron microscopy results do not lend much support to this hypothesis in the case of the repressor-operator interaction (Hirsch and Schleif 1976). In positively stained electron micrographs of 203-base-pair restriction fragments of DNA containing the *lac* promoter-operator region, the naked DNA does not appear kinked. The mean length of the DNA is shortened less than 2% when repressor is bound to the operator. In a large, 800-base-pair restriction fragment, the DNA shows only a slightly increased tendency to bend at the site of repressor binding.

O'Neill (1976) has scrutinized the base sequence of the *lac* and λ operators, which are "cast" on an DNA helix. In the two-dimensional representation of the helix, a "face" sequence of 3 base pairs visible in the major or minor groove alternates with a backbone sequence of 2 base pairs hidden at the half-turns. The twofold rotational symmetry of the *lac* operator seen in the linear array (Fig. 5b) persists in the helical representation. O'Neill proposes that a 6-base-pair face sequence in the left half of the operator (positions 9, 12, 13, 14, 17, and 18), which also occurs in the λ operator, is the recognition sequence for repressors. This sequence appears inverted in the right half of the *lac* operator, generating an 11-base-pair face sequence. Of these 11 base pairs, five correspond to known O^c loci and the rest appear to interact weakly with *lac* repressor (see Fig. 5).

The intriguing problem of explaining the very fast rate of association of *lac* repressor and operator DNA has elicited several mechanisms for facilitated diffusion. The enhancement of the rate constant k_a over the value for a diffusion-limited reaction calculated from the von Smoluchowski equation has been ascribed to a variety of processes: long-range electrostatic attraction, reduction in dimensionality of diffusion, and direct transfer of repressor protein between DNA binding sites. In the latter two cases, the binding of repressor to the operator site is visualized as a two-step process: the protein first binds to DNA and then searches the DNA molecule for the operator. Adam and Delbrück (1968) have pointed out that diffusion reaction rates can be accelerated by reduction of dimensionality. The model for the association of repressor and operator consists of three-dimensional diffusion of the repressor to a DNA molecule, followed by one-dimensional diffusion along the DNA chain. Richter and Eigen (1974) have performed a theoretical treatment for the diffusion of a sphere (repressor) toward a rod (DNA) under the influence of an electric field. In this case, the two-step process is contracted to a single step by extending the effective range of the operator to the average distance a repressor molecule diffuses along DNA before dissociating. On the basis of their equations, they reached two conclusions. First, electrostatic attraction between the repressor protein and the operator site on DNA is not the essential rate-enhancing mechanism. They showed that dissociation rates should be much more sensitive to ionic strength than are association rates, the reverse of what is observed for the repressor-operator interaction. Electrostatic forces are deemed important because of the unusual sensitivity of the rate constant of association k_a to ionic strength. However, the electrostatic effects are probably exerted indirectly through the dissociation rate of the non-operator DNA binding. Second, they estimate the size of the DNA target required to account for the observed rate of association k_a to be about 1000 Å or 300 base pairs.

Berg and Blomberg (1976, 1977) have given a more explicit rendition of this model without electrostatic forces. Here, the DNA molecule is taken to be a long cylinder or random coil with an operator site embedded in it. They consider the coupled three- and one-dimensional diffusions of a particle (repressor) outside and along the entire chain. The solution of this problem yields the complete time course of the association reaction in terms of molecular parameters which can be evaluated by comparison with experiment. They found that the rate constant k_a depends indirectly on ionic strength via its dependence on the equilibrium constant K_{DNA} for the nonoperator binding. The computed value of about $10^{-9}\,cm^2\,sec^{-1}$ for the one-dimensional diffusion constant is clearly much smaller than the presumed value of $5 \times 10^{-7}\,cm^2\,sec^{-1}$ for the three-dimensional diffusion constant.

An alternative mechanism for the searching process via direct transfer of the *lac* repressor from site to site on the DNA has been proposed (Bresloff and Crothers 1975; von Hippel et al. 1975). This model would imply transitional binding of two DNA sites by the repressor protein. A direct-transfer process has been invoked to explain the binding kinetics of the intercalative dye ethidium (Bresloff and Crothers 1975). The advantage of this mechanism is that it allows a faster path for the ligand to seek a preferred binding site than mechanisms requiring dissociation to free ligand. For a direct-transfer process to function as a rate-enhancing mechanism at dilute concentrations ($10^{-12}\,M$ operator or $30\,ng/ml$ *lac* phage DNA), one must postulate intramolecular transfer events within the domain of a single DNA molecule. Thus, the rate constant of association k_a should be a function of the effective DNA concentration, that is, of the length of the DNA (von Hippel et al. 1975).

There is little experimental evidence bearing directly on either of these hypothetical mechanisms for facilitated diffusion. It is not known whether *lac* repressor has a second potential binding site for DNA, as required by the direct-transfer model. The prediction of both models that the rate constant k_a should decrease for small operator DNA fragments below a certain size has not been adequately tested. However, there are some data that are suggestive. For sonicated operator DNA fragments about 1000–2000 base pairs long, the equilibrium constant K_O (Bourgeois and Riggs 1970) and the rate constant of dissociation k_b (Gilbert 1972) are the same as for the whole phage DNA, indicating that the rate constant of association k_a is not lowered for DNA pieces of that size. As mentioned in a preceding section, for 21- and 26-base-pair synthetic operators, the value of the rate constant k_a is about the same as that for high-molecular-weight operator DNA under standard conditions, or about fivefold lower if the increased mobility of the synthetic operator is taken into account. The fact that the rate constant k_a is essentially independent of ionic strength is expected if nonoperator DNA binding plays a role in the searching process. However, a "free" operator site is not quite the same entity as an operator site embedded in DNA. Deeper understanding of the various aspects of the recognition mechanism clearly necessitates more structural information and physical experimentation.

ACKNOWLEDGMENTS

We thank all the scientists who made unpublished data and manuscripts available to us. We also thank A. D. Riggs for discussions during preparation of this manuscript. Work in our laboratories is supported by the National Institutes of Health.

REFERENCES

Adam, G. and M. Delbrück. 1968. Reduction of dimensionality in biological diffusion processes. In *Structural chemistry and molecular biology* (ed. A. Rich and N. Davidson), p. 198. Freeman, San Francisco.

Adler, K., K. Beyreuther, E. Fanning, N. Geisler, B. Gronenborn, A. Klemm, B. Müller-Hill, M. Pfahl, and A. Schmitz. 1972. How *lac* repressor binds to DNA. *Nature* **237**:322.

Alexander, M. E., A. A. Burgum, R. A. Noall, M. D. Shaw, and K. S. Matthews. 1977. Modification of tyrosine residues of the lactose repressor protein. *Biochim. Biophys. Acta* **493**:367.

Bahl, C. P., R. Wu, J. Stawinsky, and S. A. Narang. 1977. Minimal length of the lactose operator sequence for the specific recognition by the lactose repressor. *Proc. Natl. Acad. Sci.* **74**:966.

Bahl, C. P., R. Wu, K. Itakura, N. Katagiri, and S. A. Narang. 1976. Chemical and enzymatic synthesis of lactose operator of *Escherichia coli* and its binding to lactose repressor. *Proc. Natl. Acad. Sci.* **73**:91.

Barkley, M. D., A. D. Riggs, A. Jobe, and S. Bourgeois. 1975. Interaction of effecting ligands with *lac* repressor and repressor-operator complex. *Biochemistry* **14**:1700.

Bauer, W. and J. Vinograd. 1970. Interaction of closed circular DNA with intercalative dyes. II. The free energy of superhelix formation in SV40 DNA. *J. Mol. Biol.* **47**:419.

Beckwith, J. R. 1970. *Lac*: the genetic system. In *The Lactose Operon* (ed. J. R. Beckwith and D. Zipser), p. 5. Cold Spring Harbor Laboratory, New York.

Berg, O. G. and C. Blomberg. 1976. Association kinetics with coupled diffusional flows. Special application to the *lac* repressor-operator system. *Biophys. Chem.* **4**:367.

———. 1977. Association kinetics with coupled diffusion. An extension to coiled-chain macromolecules applied to the *lac* repressor-operator system. *Biophys. Chem.* **7**:33.

Betz, J. L. and J. R. Sadler. 1976. Tight-binding repressors of the lactose operon. *J. Mol. Biol.* **105**:293.

Boezi, J. A. and D. B. Cowie. 1961. Kinetic studies of β-galactosidase induction *Biophys. J.* **1**:639.

Bourgeois, S. 1966. "Sur la nature du répresseur de l'opéron lactose d'*Escherichia coli.*" Ph.D. thesis, University of Paris.

———. 1971. Techniques to assay repressors. *Methods Enzymol.* **21D**:491.

———. 1972. Methods for studying protein-nucleic acid interaction. *Acta Endocrinol Suppl.* **168**:178.

Bourgeois, S. and A. Jobe. 1970. Superrepressors of the *lac* operon. In *The lactose operon* (ed. J. R. Beckwith and D. Zipser), p. 325. Cold Spring Harbor Laboratory, Cold Spring Harbor, New York.

Bourgeois, S. and A. D. Riggs. 1970. The *lac* repressor-operator interaction. IV. Assay and purification of operator DNA. *Biochem. Biophys. Res. Commun.* **38**:348.

Bresloff, J. L. and D. M. Crothers. 1975. DNA-ethidium reaction kinetics: Demonstration of direct ligand transfer between DNA binding sites. *J. Mol. Biol.* **95**:103.

Butler, A. P., A. Revzin, and P. H. von Hippel. 1977. Molecular parameters characterizing the interaction of *Escherichia coli lac* repressor with non-operator DNA and inducer. *Biochemistry* **16**:4757.

Carter, C. W., Jr. and J. Kraut. 1974. A proposed model for interaction of polypeptides with RNA. *Proc. Natl. Acad. Sci.* **71**:283.

Chamness, G. C. and C. W. Willson. 1970. An unusual *lac* repressor mutant. *J. Mol. Biol.* **53**:561.

Church, G. M., J. L. Sussman, and S. H. Kim. 1977. Secondary structural complementarity between DNA and proteins. *Proc. Natl. Acad. Sci.* **74**:1458.

Clark, D. J. and A. G. Marr. 1964. Studies on the repression of β-galactosidase in *Escherichia coli. Biochim. Biophys. Acta* **92**:85.

Crick, F. H. C. and A. Klug. 1975. Kinky helix. *Nature* **255**:530.

Davidson, N. 1972. Effect of DNA length on the free energy of binding of an unwinding ligand to a supercoiled DNA. *J. Mol. Biol.* **66**:307.

deHaseth, P. L., T. M. Lohman, and M. T. Record, Jr. 1977a. Nonspecific interaction of *lac* repressor with DNA: An association reaction driven by counterion release. *Biochemistry* **16**:4783.

deHaseth, P. L., C. A. Gross, R. R. Burgess, and M. T. Record, Jr. 1977b. Measurement of binding constants for protein-DNA interactions by DNA cellulose chromatography. *Biochemistry* **16**:4777.

Dickson, R. C., J. Abelson, W. M. Barnes, and W. S. Reznikoff. 1975. Genetic regulation: The *lac* control region. *Science* **187**:27.

Finch, J. T., L. C. Lutter, D. Rhodes, R. S. Brown, B. Rushton, M. Levitt, and A. Klug. 1977. Structure of nucleosome core particles of chromatin. *Nature* **269**:29.

Friedman, B. E., J. S. Olson, and K. S. Matthews. 1976. Kinetic studies of inducer binding to lactose repressor protein. *J. Biol. Chem.* **251**:1171.

———. 1977. Interaction of *lac* repressor with inducer. Kinetics and equilibrium measurements. *J. Mol. Biol.* **111**:27.

Geisler, N. and K. Weber. 1976. Isolation of a set of hybrid *lac* repressors made in vitro between normal *lac* repressor and its homogeneous tryptic core. *Proc. Natl. Acad. Sci.* **73**:3103.

———. 1977. Isolation of the amino-terminal fragment of lactose repressor necessary for DNA binding. *Biochemistry* **16**:938.

Georgopoulos, C. P. and H. R. Revel. 1971. Studies with glucosyl transferase mutants of the T-even bacteriophages. *Virology* **44**:271.

Gierer, A. 1966. Model for DNA and protein interactions and the function of the operator. *Nature* **212**:1480.

Gilbert, W. 1972. The *lac* repressor and the *lac* operator. In *Polymerization in biological systems* (ed. G. E. W. Wolstenholme and M. O'Connor), p. 245. Associated Scientific Press, Amsterdam.

Gilbert, W. and A. Maxam. 1973. The nucleotide sequence of the *lac* operator. *Proc. Natl. Acad. Sci.* **70**:3581.

Gilbert, W. and B. Müller-Hill. 1966. Isolation of the *lac* repressor. *Proc. Natl. Acad. Sci.* **56**:1891.

Gilbert, W., J. Majors, and A. Maxam. 1976a. How proteins recognize DNA sequences. In *Organization and expression of chromosomes. Life Sciences Research Report 4* (ed. V. G. Allfrey et al.), p. 167. Heyden and Son, London.

Gilbert, W., A. Maxam, and A. Mirzabekov. 1976b. Contacts between the *lac* repressor and DNA revealed by methylation. In *Control of ribosome synthesis. Alfred Benson Symposium IX* (ed. N. O. Kjeldgaard and O. Maaløe), p. 139. Academic Press, New York.

Gilbert, W., J. Gralla, J. Majors, and A. Maxam. 1975. Lactose operator sequences and the action of *lac* repressor. In *Protein-ligand interactions* (ed. H. Sund and G. Blauer), p. 193. Walter de Gruyter, Berlin.

Goeddel, D. V., D. G. Yansura, and M. H. Caruthers. 1977a. Studies on gene control regions. I. Chemical synthesis of lactose operator deoxyribonucleic acid segments. *Biochemistry* **16**:1765.

———. 1977b. Binding of synthetic lactose operator DNAs to lactose repressors. *Proc. Natl. Acad. Sci.* **74**:3292.

———. 1977c. Studies on gene control regions. VI. The 5-methyl of thymine, a *lac* repressor recognition site. *Nucleic Acids Res.* **4**:3039.

———. 1978a. How *lac* repressor recognizes *lac* operator. *Proc. Natl. Acad. Sci.* (in press).

Goeddel, D. V., D. G. Yansura, C. Winston, and M. H. Caruthers. 1978b. Studies on gene control regions. VII. The effect of 5-bromouracil substituted *lac* operators on the *lac* operator-*lac* repressor interaction. *J. Mol. Biol.* (in press).

Heyneker, H. L., J. Shine, H. M. Goodman, H. W. Boyer, J. Rosenberg, R. E. Dickerson, S. A. Narang, K. Itakura, S.-Y. Lin, and A. D. Riggs. 1976. Synthetic *lac* operator DNA is functional in vivo. *Nature* **263**:748.

Hirsh, J. and R. Schleif. 1976. High resolution electron microscopic studies of genetic regulation. *J. Mol. Biol.* **108**:471.

Itakura, K., N. Katagiri, and S. A. Narang. 1974. Synthesis of lactose-operator gene fragments by the improved triester method. *Can. J. Chem.* **52**:3689.

Itakura, K., N. Katagiri, S. A. Narang, C. P. Bahl, K. Marians, and R. Wu. 1975. Chemical synthesis and sequence studies of deoxyribooligonucleotides which constitute the duplex sequence of the lactose operator of *Escherichia coli. J. Biol. Chem.* **250**:4592.

Jacob, F. and J. Monod. 1961. Genetic regulatory mechanisms in the synthesis of proteins. *J. Mol. Biol.* **3**:318.

Jobe, A. and S. Bourgeois. 1972a. *Lac* repressor-operator interaction. VI. The natural inducer of the *lac* operon. *J. Mol. Biol.* **69**:397.

———. 1972b. *Lac* repressor-operator interaction. VIII. Lactose is an anti-inducer of the *lac* operon. *J. Mol. Biol.* **75**:303.

———. 1972c. The *lac* repressor-operator interaction. VII. A repressor with unique binding properties: The X86 repressor. *J. Mol. Biol.* **72**:139.

Jobe, A., A. D. Riggs, and S. Bourgeois. 1972. *Lac* repressor-operator interaction. V. Characterization of super- and pseudo-wild-type repressors. *J. Mol. Biol.* **64**:181.

Jobe, A., J. R. Sadler, and S. Bourgeois. 1974. *Lac* repressor-operator interaction.

IX. The binding of *lac* repressor to operators containing O^c mutations. *J. Mol. Biol.* **85**:231.

Jovin, T. M., N. Geisler. and K. Weber. 1977. Amino-terminal fragments of *Escherichia coli lac* repressor bind to DNA. *Nature* **269**:668.

Kao-Huang, Y., A. Revzin, A. P. Butler, P. O'Connor, D. W. Noble, and P. H. von Hippel. 1977. Nonspecific DNA binding of genome-regulating proteins as a biological control mechanism: Measurement of DNA-bound *Escherichia coli lac* repressor in vivo. *Proc. Natl. Acad. Sci.* **74**:4228.

Kihara, H. K. and H. Kuno. 1968. Microassay of protein with nitrocellulose membrane filters. *Anal. Biochem.* **24**:96.

Kolchinsky, A. M., A. D. Mirzabekov, W. Gilbert, and L. Li. 1976. Preferential protection of the minor groove of non-operator DNA by *lac* repressor against methylation by dimethyl sulfate. *Nucleic Acids Res.* **3**:11.

Kuhn, W. and M. Thürkauf. 1961. Biegungsdeformation elastischer Stäbe durch die Wärmebewegung. *Z. Elektrochem.* **65**:307.

Laiken, S. L., C. A. Gross, and P. H. von Hippel. 1972. Equilibrium and kinetic aspects of *Escherichia coli lac* repressor-inducer interactions. *J. Mol. Biol.* **66**:143.

Lin, S.-Y. and A. D. Riggs. 1972a. *Lac* repressor binding to non-operator DNA: Detailed studies and a comparison of equilibrium and rate competition methods. *J. Mol. Biol.* **72**:671.

———. 1972b. *Lac* operator analogues: Bromodeoxyuridine substitution in the *lac* operator affects the rate of dissociation of the *lac* repressor. *Proc. Natl. Acad. Sci.* **69**:2574.

———. 1974. Photochemical attachment of *lac* repressor to bromodeoxyuridine-substituted *lac* operator by ultraviolet radiation. *Proc. Natl. Acad. Sci.* **71**:947.

———. 1975a. The general affinity of *lac* repressor for *E. coli* DNA: Implications for gene regulation in procaryotes and eucaryotes. *Cell* **4**:107.

———. 1975b. A comparison of *lac* repressor binding to operator and to non-operator DNA. *Biochem. Biophys. Res. Commun.* **62**:704.

———. 1976. The binding of *lac* repressor and the catabolite gene activator protein to halogen-substituted analogues of poly[d(A-T)]. *Biochim. Biophys. Acta* **432**:185.

Manning, G. S. 1969. Limiting laws and counterion condensation in polyelectrolyte solutions. I. Colligative properties. *J. Chem. Phys.* **51**:924.

———. 1972. On the application of polyelectrolyte "limiting laws" to the helix-coil transition of DNA. I. Excess univalent cations. *Biopolymers* **11**:937.

Marians, K. J., R. Wu, J. Stawinski, T. Hozumi, and S. A. Narang. 1976. Cloned synthetic *lac* operator DNA is biologically active. *Nature* **263**:744.

Matthews, K. S., H. R. Matthews, H. W. Thielmann, and O. Jardetzky. 1973. Ultraviolet difference spectra of the lactose repressor protein. *Biochim. Biophys. Acta* **295**:159.

Maurizot, J.-C., M. Charlier, and C. Hélène. 1974. *Lac* repressor binding to poly[d(A-T)]. Conformational changes. *Biochem. Biophys. Res. Commun.* **60**:951.

Müller-Hill, B. 1971. *Lac* repressor. *Angew. Chem.* **10**:160.

Müller-Hill, B., K. Beyreuther, and W. Gilbert. 1971. *Lac* repressor from *Escherichia coli*. *Methods Enzymol.* **21D**:483.

Ogata, R. and W. Gilbert. 1977. Contacts between the *lac* repressor and thymines in the *lac* operator. *Proc. Natl. Acad. Sci.* **74**:4973.

O'Gorman, R. B. and K. S. Matthews. 1977a. Fluorescence and ultraviolet spectral studies of *lac* repressor modified with N-bromosuccinimide. *J. Biol. Chem.* **252**:3752.

———. 1977b. N-bromosuccinimide modification of *lac* repressor protein. *J. Biol. Chem.* **252**:3565.

Ohshima, Y., T. Horiuchi, and M. Yanagida. 1975. Structure of the *lac* repressor studied by negative staining. *J. Mol. Biol.* **91**:515.

Ohshima, Y., M. Matsuura, and T. Horiuchi. 1972. Conformational change of the *lac* repressor induced with the inducer. *Biochem. Biophys. Res. Commun.* **47**:1444.

Ohshima, Y., T. Mizokoshi, and T. Horiuchi. 1974. Binding of an inducer to the *lac* repressor. *J. Mol. Biol.* **89**:127.

O'Neill, M. C. 1976. Similarities in the helical sequences of the repressor-binding sites in the *lac* and λ operators. *Nature* **260**:550.

Pfahl, M. 1976. *Lac* repressor-operator interaction: Analysis of the X86 repressor mutant. *J. Mol. Biol.* **106**:857.

Pfahl, M. and S. Bourgeois. 1976. Isolation of pseudo revertants of *lacOᶜ* mutants: Selection system for superoperator mutations. *J. Bacteriol.* **128**:257.

Platt, T., K. Weber, D. Ganem, and J. H. Miller. 1972. Translational restarts: AUG reinitiation of a *lac* repressor fragment. *Proc. Natl. Acad. Sci.* **69**:897.

Record, M. T., Jr., P. L. deHaseth, and T. M. Lohman. 1977. Interpretation of monovalent and divalent cation effects on the *lac* repressor-operator interaction. *Biochemistry* **16**:4791.

Record, M. T., Jr., T. M. Lohman, and P. deHaseth. 1976. Ion effects on ligand-nucleic acid interactions. *J. Mol. Biol.* **107**:145.

Revzin, A. and P. H. von Hippel. 1977. Direct measurement of association constants for the binding of *Escherichia coli lac* repressor to non-operator DNA. *Biochemistry* **16**:4769.

Reznikoff, W. S., R. B. Winter, and C. K. Hurley. 1974. The location of the repressor binding sites in the *lac* operon. *Proc. Natl. Acad. Sci.* **71**:2314.

Richmond, T. J. and T. A. Steitz. 1976. Protein-DNA interaction investigated by binding *Escherichia coli lac* repressor protein to poly[d(A·U-HgX)]. *J. Mol. Biol.* **103**:25.

Richter, P. H. and M. Eigen. 1974. Diffusion controlled reaction rates in spheroidal geometry. Application to repressor-operator association and membrane-bound enzymes. *Biophys. Chem.* **2**:255.

Riggs, A. D. and S. Bourgeois. 1968. On the assay, isolation, and characterization of the *lac* repressor. *J. Mol. Biol.* **34**:361.

Riggs, A. D., S. Bourgeois, and M. Cohn. 1970a. The *lac* repressor-operator interaction. III. Kinetic studies. *J. Mol. Biol.* **53**:401.

Riggs, A. D., S. Lin, and R. D. Wells. 1972. *Lac* repressor binding to synthetic DNA's of defined nucleotide sequence. *Proc. Natl. Acad. Sci.* **69**:761.

Riggs, A. D., R. F. Newby, and S. Bourgeois. 1970b. *Lac* repressor-operator interaction. II. Effect of galactosides and other ligands. *J. Mol. Biol.* **51**:303.

Riggs, A. D., H. Suzuki, and S. Bourgeois. 1970c. *Lac* repressor-operator interaction. I. Equilibrium studies. *J. Mol. Biol.* **48**:67.

Sadler, J. R., M. Tecklenburg, J. L. Betz, D. V. Goeddel, D. G. Yansura, and M. H. Caruthers. 1977. Cloning of chemically synthesized lactose operators. *Gene* 1:305.

Sams, C. F., B. E. Friedman, A. A. Burgum, D. S. Yang, and K. S. Matthews. 1977. Spectral studies of lactose repressor protein modified with nitrophenol reporter groups. *J. Biol. Chem.* 252:3153.

Seeman, N. C., J. M. Rosenberg, and A. Rich. 1976. Sequence-specific recognition of double helical nucleic acids by proteins. *Proc. Natl. Acad. Sci.* 73:804.

Smith, T. F. and J. R. Sadler. 1971. The nature of lactose operator constitutive mutations. *J. Mol. Biol.* 59:273.

Sobell, H. M. 1973. The stereochemistry of actinomycin binding to DNA and its implications in molecular biology. *Prog. Nucleic Acid Res. Mol. Biol.* 13:153.

Sommer, H., P. Lu, and J. H. Miller. 1976. *Lac* repressor: Fluorescence of the two tryptophans. *J. Biol. Chem.* 251:3774.

Steitz, T. A., T. J. Richmond, D. Wise, and D. Engelman. 1974. The *lac* repressor protein: Molecular shape, subunit structure, and proposed model for operator interaction based on structural studies of microcrystals. *Proc. Natl. Acad. Sci.* 71:593.

Sung, M. T. and G. H. Dixon. 1970. Modification of histones during spermiogenesis in trout: A molecular mechanism for altering histone binding to DNA. *Proc. Natl. Acad. Sci.* 67:1616.

von Heijne, G. and C. Blomberg. 1976. Kinetic aspects of the DNA helix-cruciform transition. *J. Theor. Biol.* 63:347.

von Hippel, P. H., A. Revzin, C. A. Gross, and A. C. Wang. 1975. Interaction of *lac* repressor with non-specific DNA binding sites. In *Protein-ligand interactions* (ed. H. Sund and G. Blauer), p. 270. Walter de Gruyter, Berlin.

Wang, A. C., A. Revzin, A. P. Butler, and P. H. von Hippel. 1977. Binding of *E. coli lac* repressor to non-operator DNA. *Nucleic Acids Res.* 4:1579.

Wang, J. C. 1974. The degree of unwinding of the DNA helix by ethidium. I. Titration of twisted PM2 DNA molecules in alkaline cesium chloride density gradients. *J. Mol. Biol.* 89:783.

Wang, J. C., M. D. Barkley, and S. Bourgeois. 1974. Measurements of unwinding of *lac* operator by repressor. *Nature* 251:247.

Wu, F. Y.-H., P. Bandyopadhyay, and C.-W. Wu. 1976. Conformational transitions of the *lac* repressor from *Escherichia coli*. *J. Mol. Biol.* 100:459.

Yang, D. S., A. A. Burgum, and K. S. Matthews. 1977. Modification of the cysteine residues of the lactose repressor protein using chromophoric probes. *Biochim. Biophys. Acta* 493:24.

Yansura, D. G., D. V. Goeddel, and M. H. Caruthers. 1977a. Studies on gene control regions. II. Enzymatic joining of chemically synthesized lactose operator deoxyribonucleic acid segments. *Biochemistry* 16:1772.

Yansura, D. G., D. V. Goeddel, D. L. Cribbs, and M. H. Caruthers. 1977b. Studies on gene control regions. III. Binding of synthetic and modified synthetic *lac* operator DNAs to lactose repressor. *Nucleic Acids Res.* 4:723.

Zingsheim, H. P., N. Geisler, F. Mayer, and K. Weber. 1977. Complexes of *Escherichia coli lac*-repressor with non-operator DNA revealed by electron microscopy: Two repressor molecules can share the same segment of DNA. *J. Mol. Biol.* 115:565.

The *lac* Promoter

William S. Reznikoff
Department of Biochemistry
College of Agricultural and Life Sciences
University of Wisconsin
Madison, Wisconsin 53706

John N. Abelson
Department of Chemistry
University of California-San Diego
LaJolla, California 92037

INTRODUCTION

The *lac* promoter is a region of DNA required for the initiation of transcription of the *lac* operon (Jacob et al. 1964; Scaife and Beckwith 1967; Miller 1970; Reznikoff 1972; Dickson et al. 1975). The nucleotide sequence of the promoter contains the information necessary for the specific interaction of two proteins with the DNA. These proteins are RNA polymerase and a positive stimulatory protein, the catabolite gene activator protein, CAP (also termed CRP and CGA protein in other chapters of this volume). It is currently believed that transcription initiation occurs by the following general process. CAP in the presence of adenosine 3′,5′-monophosphate (cyclic [c]AMP) binds to a site in the promoter. The binding of the CAP–cAMP complex stimulates the productive interaction of RNA polymerase with the promoter such that, if the four ribonucleoside triphosphates are present, a *lac* mRNA transcript will be initiated (de Crombrugghe et al. 1971; Eron and Block 1971). This interaction of RNA polymerase with the promoter may be a complex process involving several steps such as the specific loose binding of RNA polymerase to the closed helix (formation of the "closed complex"), the generation of a region of localized denaturation (formation of the "open" or "rapid start complex"), and the initiation of the transcript (Chamberlin 1974).

A complete understanding of the structure of the promoter and an analysis of how specific changes in the structure alter one or more of the reactions mentioned above may yield some insight as to how the various steps in the RNA polymerase–*lacP* interaction occur and how the CAP–cAMP complex stimulates this interaction. In this paper we present the current information about the genetic and nucleotide sequence structure of the *lac* promoter. Then we describe in some detail what is known about the two specific protein-DNA recognition reactions and how variations in the promoter structure alter these reactions. We also investigate the possibility of additional factors playing a role in *lac* transcription initiation and present a general model for this process.

GENETICS

The promoter has been defined by three classes of point mutations and by several deletions, most of which were isolated and described by J. Beckwith and his colleagues. These are diagrammatically described in Figure 1, and some of them are located exactly in the promoter sequence shown in Figures 4, 5, and 6. The class-I and class-II point mutations are *cis*-dominant mutations which decrease the level of *lac* operon expression (Scaife and Beckwith 1967; Hopkins 1974). As shown by some representative in vivo experiments in Table 1, these mutations effect this depression of *lac* expression by different means. Class-I mutations decrease the response of the *lac* promoter to the presence of the CAP–cAMP complex because, as described later, the CAP–cAMP complex has a lower affinity for the *lac* promoter variants which contain class-I mutations. The class-II mutations appear from these data to act primarily by depressing the ability of RNA polymerase to interact productively with *lacP*, although some of them also alter the response to the CAP–cAMP complex. We shall see that some but not all of these class-II mutations actually lower the affinity of RNA polymerase for the *lac* promoter. As indicated in Figure 1, the class-I mutations are located in the left-hand side of the promoter, and the class-II mutations map between the class-I mutations and the operator (Beckwith et al. 1972; Hopkins 1974).

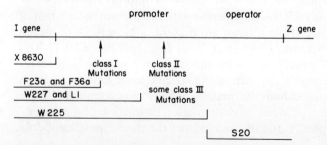

Figure 1 The *lac* regulatory elements. The *lac* promoter has been genetically defined by a series of point mutations and deletions which include: class-I point mutations which define the CAP–cAMP complex target site, class-II point mutations which define the RNA polymerase target site, a series of *tonB* deletions which remove the *I* gene and varying amounts of *lacP*, and the *S20* deletion which removes all of *lacO* but leaves *lacP* intact (Miller et al. 1970; Eron et al. 1970; Beckwith et al. 1972; Arditti et al. 1973; Hopkins 1974; Dickson et al. 1975; Mitchell et al. 1975).

Table 1 Expression of *lacP* mutations in *crp⁺cya⁺* and *crp⁻cya⁻* genetic backgrounds

	β-Galactosidase activities		Ratio of activities
lacP Genotype	*crp⁺ cya⁺*	*crp⁻ cya⁻*	
Wild type	100.00	2.0	50
P⁻L157 (class II)	6.2	0.12	50
P⁻L241 (class II)	7.1	0.26	30
P⁻L305 (class II)	7.5	0.6	10
P⁻L8 (class I)	6.0	2.0	3

Expression is indicated as the amount of β-galactosidase produced in the presence of IPTG with the values normalized to the P^+, crp^+, cya^+ value = 100. (Data from Hopkins 1974.)

It has been possible to isolate a third class of promoter mutations (class-III, sometimes called P^r or P^s mutations) which facilitate *lac* expression in the absence of the CAP–cAMP complex. This has been accomplished by two techniques: isolating Lac⁺ mutants in a *crp⁻* (lacking CAP) and/or *cya⁻* (lacking adenyl cyclase) background or by isolating second-site revertants of class-I mutations (Silverstone et al. 1970; de Crombrugghe et al. 1971; Arditti et al. 1973; W. S. Reznikoff and K. Thornton, unpubl.). These mutations presumably act by facilitating the interaction of RNA polymerase with *lacP*.

A variety of deletions have also been useful in defining the *lac* promoter. Several deletions which enter the promoter region from the left-hand side (as shown in Fig. 1) delineate the location of the CAP–cAMP complex interaction site. Miller and coworkers (1970) isolated deletion *X8630* which removes the entire *I* gene but does not alter *lac* promoter activity. Thus it defines the left-hand side of the CAP–cAMP interaction site (Miller et al. 1970; Dickson et al. 1975). The deletion *L1*, which has the phenotype of a very strong class-I mutation (Beckwith et al. 1972), defines the approximate boundary between the CAP–cAMP complex interaction site and the region required for RNA polymerase interaction. The *L1* deletion covers all known class-I mutations and thus probably eliminates the entire CAP–cAMP complex interaction site (Scaife and Beckwith 1967; Beckwith et al. 1972). The *L1* deletion recombines with all tested class-II mutations and does not alter the in vivo CAP–cAMP-independent transcription of *lacP*; therefore, it presumably does not remove any nucleotides essential for the RNA polymerase–*lacP* recognition reaction (Beckwith et al. 1972; Hopkins 1974). Other deletions which remove part or all of the CAP–cAMP interaction site but not the RNA polymerase interaction site include *F23a*, *F36a*, and *W227*. A similar deletion which extends still further (removing sequences necessary for RNA polymerase interaction) is *W225* (Mitchell et al. 1975). Finally, Eron et al. (1970) have described a deletion called *S20*, which enters the controlling element region from the *Z* side and removes a substantial portion of the *lac* operator. This deletion still permits *lacY* gene expression. Presumably no essential portion of the promoter has been removed by this deletion. Thus *S20* defines the right-hand side of the promoter (Eron et al. 1970; Reznikoff et al. 1974; Dickson et al. 1975).

The Sequence of the *lac* Promoter

The entire nucleotide sequence of the wild-type *lac* promoter has been determined, as well as the sequence changes found in a variety of promoter mutations. Initially the sequence was determined through an indirect approach by Dickson et al. (1975). RNA copies of the *lacP-O* region were synthesized and purified by a technique schematically presented in Figure 2. The essential steps in this approach included (1) The generation of a read-through copy of *lacP-O* utilizing transcripts initiated downstream at a bacteriophage promoter, and (2) the purification of the *lacP-O* RNA by two cycles of DNA-RNA hybridization using DNA molecules which carry *lac* DNA in opposing orientations and which contain deletions defining the *Z*-gene and *I*-gene sides of the region.

The many sequences consistent with the data produced by the analysis of the *lacP-O* RNA were reduced to a single sequence by analyzing RNA coded for by the opposite strand. This RNA was generated by an analogous procedure. The basic sequence of the promoter and operator region is shown in Figure 3. Recently, Gilbert and Maxam and their coworkers have confirmed the results of this indirect sequence approach by a direct DNA sequencing method.

In addition to the wild-type promoter, the changes generated by a variety of point mutations and an extended deletion, *L1*, have been defined exactly and the endpoints of some other deletions have been approximately located. An enlargement of the promoter sequence and the known mutations is presented in Figure 4. To date, the sequencing results confirm most of the conclusions from previously known genetic results, i.e., all class-I point mutations fall under the *L1* deletion, the class-II mutations map between the *L1* deletion and the operator, the class-I mutations *L8* and *L37* are at the same site, the class-I mutations *L8* and *L29* are at different sites, and the *UV5* class-III mutation maps between *L8* and the operator (Beckwith et al. 1972; Hopkins 1974; Dickson et al. 1975, 1977; Gilbert 1976). The one discrepancy between the genetic data and the sequence data is that the sequence data indicated that the *L8* and *L29* sites were inverted vis-à-vis the operator from the order originally proposed (Beckwith et al. 1972; Dickson et al. 1977).

① In vitro transcription of λ p <u>lac</u> 5 DNA

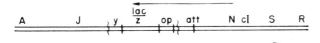

② Hybridization to r strand of λp<u>trp</u>/<u>lac</u> X8555 DNA

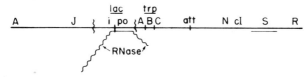

③ Hybridization to *l* strand of λ p<u>trp</u>-<u>lac</u> DNA

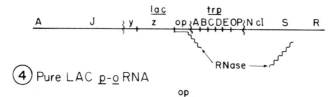

④ Pure LAC <u>p-o</u> RNA

op.

Figure 2 Synthesis and isolation of *lacP-O* RNA. An RNA copy of the *lacP-O* region was generated in vitro for sequencing purposes by the following protocol. RNA was transcribed utilizing a λ*plac* 5 DNA template under conditions where the *lacP-O* region was copied by read-through transcription. The *lacP-O* RNA was purified by two sequential hybridizations to separated strands of *lac* transducing phage DNAs. The specific *lac* transducing phage DNAs used contained deletions defining the *I*-gene and *Z*-gene sides of *lacP-O* and had the *lac* region in opposite orientations. The detailed procedure is described by Dickson et al. (1975) and Barnes et al. (1975).

Details of the CAP–cAMP Target Site

From this genetic and sequence information alone, we can draw several conclusions about what regions of the DNA are important for the binding of the CAP–cAMP complex to the *lac* promoter. The endpoints of the *X8630* and *L1* deletions suggest that the CAP–cAMP complex recognizes a sequence residing in a region between positions −87 and −49 shown in Figures 3 and 4. The point mutations specifically indicate that this complex must "see" positions −57 and −66; moreover, these two positions are arranged around a center of symmetry (Dykes et al. 1975; Dickson et al. 1977; A. Maxam and W. Gilbert, pers. comm.) located

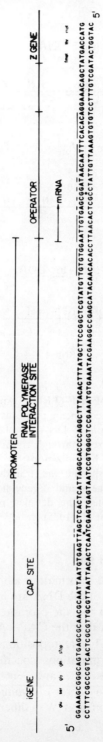

Figure 3 The *lacP-O* sequence. The complete sequence of *lacP-O*, as well as the C terminus of *lacI* and the N terminus of *lacZ*, is presented.

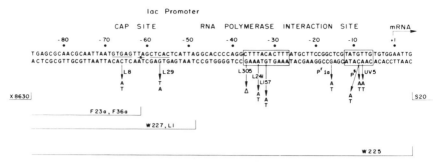

Figure 4 The *lac* promoter sequence. The details of the *lacP* sequence as defined by deletions *X8630* and *S20* are presented in addition to the locations of the point mutations determined as of January 10, 1978, the proposed symmetry element in the CAP site, and the regions of similarity with other promoters in the RNA polymerase interaction site (Schaller et al. 1975; Pribnow 1975a,b; Dickson et al. 1975, 1977; Gilbert 1976; Seeburg et al. 1977; W. S. Reznikoff, unpubl.).

between positions −61 and −62, suggesting that the CAP–cAMP complex recognizes the symmetrical sequence between positions −55 and −68.

These conclusions have been confirmed through a variety of biochemical experiments performed by Majors (1975a and pers. comm.). The first question addressed was, Can specific DNA binding of the CAP–cAMP complex be demonstrated and, if so, how is this binding affected by class-I mutations? Majors found that by using reasonably small restriction fragments (≈200 nucleotide pairs long) one could show specific cAMP-dependent binding of CAP to the *lac* promoter by means of a filter-binding assay (this observation was independently confirmed by Mitra et al. [1975]) and that this binding was not found when the same restriction fragment contained the *L8* or *L1* class-I mutations.

Recently it has become possible to probe for certain "contacts" between DNA-binding proteins and G residues and A residues in the DNA using a modification of the DNA-sequencing technique described by Maxam and Gilbert (1977). The first step in the generation of specific phosphodiester cleavages at the site of A or G residues is the modification of these nucleosides with dimethyl sulfate to yield 3-methyladenine and 7-methylguanine, respectively. If the methylation reaction is carried out in the presence of a specific DNA-binding protein, unique adenine and guanine residues may fail to be methylated. This suggests that there are informational contacts between the protein and the specific A residues in the narrow groove and/or the specific G residues in the broad groove. When Majors performed this experiment using the CAP–cAMP complex and *lacP-O* DNA, he achieved the result shown in Figure 5a. The G residues at positions −68, −66, −57, and −55 were not methylated (suggesting that the CAP–cAMP complex had points

(a) lac CAP SITE

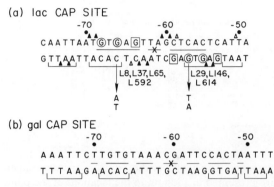

(b) gal CAP SITE

Figure 5 The CAP site. The sequences of the *lac* CAP site (*a*) and the *gal* CAP site (*b*) are presented along with the proposed symmetry elements and the known *lac* class-I promoter mutation changes (Musso et al. 1977; Dickson et al. 1977). The effect on methylation by dimethyl sulfate of the *lac* CAP-site G residues by prior binding of the CAP–cAMP complex is indicated by circles and squares: (O) methylation is blocked for the indicated residues; (□) methylation is enhanced (J. Majors, pers. comm.). No effect on the methylation of A residues was detected. Contacts between CAP and the phosphate groups on *lacP* DNA, as determined by which phosphotriester bonds block CAP–cAMP binding in the ethyl nitrosourea experiment, are indicated as follows: (▲) Completely missing species; (△) partially missing species. Similarities shared by the two sequences are indicated with brackets.

of contact with the DNA at these locations), whereas the G residues at positions −63, −59, and −53 had enhanced methylation (J. Majors, pers. comm.). A related method for defining contact points involves the methylation of the *lacP* DNA prior to the addition of the CAP–cAMP complex and then the catching of the protein-DNA complexes on nitrocellulose filters. The DNA retained on the filters is then examined by electrophoresis on 20% polyacrylamide gels. Using this approach, it was determined that DNAs with 7-methylguanine at positions −68 and −55 were not retained on the filter (presumably because they did not bind to the CAP–cAMP complex), whereas methylation at positions −71, −70, −66, and −57 resulted in reduced retention of the DNA on the filter (J. Majors, pers. comm.).

Finally, Majors (pers. comm.) used the chemical probe ethyl nitrosourea to look for contacts between the CAP–cAMP complex and the phosphate groups on *lacP* DNA. A preparation of end-labeled *lacP* DNA was exposed to ethyl nitrosourea such that each molecule was, on average, ethylated once to yield an alkali-labile phosphotriester bond. This DNA was mixed with CAP + cAMP and passed through a nitrocellulose filter. The retained DNA fragments were analyzed by standard electrophoresis on a 20% polyacrylamide gel after alkaline cleavage of the phosphotriester bonds. Any missing species suggested that an ethyl moiety on that particular phosphate blocked the binding of the CAP–cAMP complex. These important phosphate groups are indicated with triangles in Figure 5a.

The results of these chemical-modification experiments suggest two structural features of the CAP-DNA interaction: (1) CAP binds in a symmetrical fashion (as suggested by the genetics), and (2) CAP binds on only one side of the helix (J. Majors [pers. comm.] has noted that all important sites of chemical modification can be seen from one side of CPK model).

One other CAP–cAMP-dependent promoter, the *gal* promoter, has been defined in considerable detail (Musso et al. 1977; de Crombrugghe and Pastan, this volume). The similarities between the CAP-site sequences in these two systems are shown in Figure 5 and are as follows. The two CAP sites are approximately in the same location vis-à-vis the mRNA start sites, and one can see in this region of the *gal* promoter a symmetry element containing the four G-residue contact points mentioned above. However, this symmetry element has slightly different dimensions than the one in the *lac* promoter, and a mutation of one of the presumed contact G residues in the *gal* promoter (at position −66) has been found which does not appear to alter the CAP–cAMP stimulation of *gal* expression. In addition to these similarities involving the symmetry element, there are other sequences between −75 and −50 (for *lac*; −75 to −48 for *gal*) which are identical. It is not known how or if these sequences play a role in the interaction of the CAP–cAMP complex with the *lac* and *gal* promoters.

The sequence between −70 and −50 for another CAP–cAMP-sensitive promoter—the *araBAD* promoter—has also been determined (R. Schleif, pers. comm.; G. Wilcox, pers. comm.), but no sequence similar to that found in the *lac* or *gal* CAP sites is discernible.

Details of the RNA Polymerase Interaction Site

By examining the genetic and sequence data displayed in Figures 4 and 6, one can also reach some conclusions as to what sequence information plays a role in the RNA polymerase–*lacP* interaction. The total information involved probably lies between positions −48 (the end of *L1*) and +5 (the approximate beginning of *S20*). Positions −37, −34, and −32 (the sites of mutations *L305*, *L241*, and *L157*) must play a role in the specific interaction of RNA polymerase with *lacP*, whereas the nucleotide pairs at positions −16 (site of *P^{r}1a*), −9 (site of *P^s* and *UV5*), and −8 (site of *UV5*) influence the CAP–cAMP-independent interaction of RNA polymerase with *lacP* (Dickson et al. 1975; Gilbert 1976; W. S. Reznikoff, unpubl.). The sequence shows no extended (>5 nucleotide pairs long)

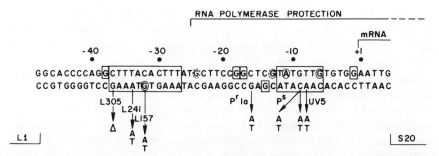

Figure 6 The RNA polymerase interaction site. The sequence of the region bounded by the deletions *L1* and *S20* is shown, with the known mutations and similarities with other promoters indicated as described in Fig. 4. The furthest extent of leftward protection from pancreatic DNase by RNA polymerase is shown (J. Gralla, pers. comm.; Gilbert 1976), as well as the effect on methylation of A and G residues by formation of the RNA polymerase–*lacP* open complex: (◌) partial inhibition; (○) complete inhibition; (□) stimulation of methylation (L. Johnsrud, pers. comm.).

symmetry elements. There is an unusual distribution of GC-rich and AT-rich sequences (high GC from −48 to −37 and from −24 to −13, high AT from −36 to −25).

One approach to analyzing the structure of the *lac* promoter–RNA polymerase interaction site is to compare its sequence with that of other promoters. The nucleotide sequences (from position −50 to +1) of several promoters recognized by *Escherichia coli* RNA polymerase are presented in Figures 7 and 8. Any comparison is limited by considerations such as the fact that some promoters also contain recognition sites for other sequence-specific proteins (such as λP_L, λP_{RM}, λP_R, $\lambda imm^{434}P_R$, $\lambda imm^{434}P_{RM}$, and *trpP*). Nonetheless, some interesting similarities and differences can be seen. Most promoters (26 of 29 presented) are greater than 50% AT. The *lac* promoter is an exception to this generalization, containing 24 AT base pairs. Other exceptions are the *lacI*-gene promoter (a weak promoter in vivo and in vitro) and the tRNA^Tyr promoters (which are weak in vitro). Most promoters have an asymmetrical distribution of purines and pyrimidines on their two strands (19 of 29 are pyrimidine-rich on the antisense strand displayed in Fig. 7; the *lac* promoter antisense strand is 60% pyrimidine-rich; the *I*-gene promoter is, however, only 48% pyrimidine-rich on its antisense strand).

There are, in addition, two specific regions which show similarities between different promoters. The 7-base-pair regions from position −6 to −12 in *lacP* are similar to the sequence TATRATR which, as previously pointed out by Pribnow (1975a,b) and Schaller et al. (1975), is present with slight variations in sequence and exact location in most other promoters. The mutation *UV5*, which enhances CAP–cAMP-independent

```
        -50       -40       -30       -20       -10       +1
         .         .         .         .         .         .

lac        TAGGCACCCCAGGCTTTACACTTTATGCTTCCGGCTCGTATGTTGTGTGGA

lacI       GACACCATCGAATGGCGCAAAACCTTTCGCGGTATGGCATGATAGCGCCCG

gal        ATTTATTCCATGTCACACTTTTCGCATCTTTGTTATGCTATGGTTATTTCA

araBAD     AGCGGATCCTACCTGACGCTTTTTATCGCAACTCTCTACTGTTTCTCCATA

araC       TTTCTGCCGTGATTATAGACACTTTTGTTACGCGTTTTTGTCATGGCTTTG

trp        TCTGAAATGAGCTGTTGACAATTAATCATCGAACTAGTTAACTAGTACGCA

tRNA tyr   TTCTCAACGTAACACTTTACAGCGGCGCGTCATTTGATATGATGCGCCCCG
     1&2

λP         TTATCTCTGGCGGTGTTGACATAAATACCACTGGCGGTGATACTGAGCACA
  L

λP         CTAACACCGTGCGTGTTGACTATTTTACCTCTGGCGGTGATAATGGTTGCA
  R

λP         CAACACGCACGGTGTTAGATATTTATCCCTTGCGGTGATAGATTTAACGTA
  RM

λP         TACCTCTGCCGAAGTTGAGTATTTTTGCTGTATTTGTCATAATGACTCCTG
  O

λP '       TTAACGGCATGATATTGACTTATTGAATAAAATTGGGTAAATTTGACTCAA
  R

λc17       TGGTGTATGCATTTATTTGCATACATTCAATCAATTGTTATAATTGTTATC

i434P      CAAGAAAAACTGTATTTGACAAACAAGATACATTGTATGAAATACAAGAAA
    R

i434P      TTTGTCAAATACAGTTTTTCTTGTGAAGATTGGGGGTAAATAACAGAGGTG
    RM

fd X       CTCTTAATCTTTTTGATGCAATTCGCTTTGCTTCTGACTATAATAGACAGG

fd II      ACAAAACATTAACGTTTACAATTTAAATATTTGCTTATACAATCATCCTG

fd IIb     GTTTGAATCTTTGCCTACTCATTACACCGGATGTACTTAAAATATATG

fd VIII    TGATACAAATCTCCGTTGTACTTTGTTTCGCGCTTGGTATAATCGCTGGG

ØX174 A    AAATAACCGTCAGGATTGACACCCTCCCAATTGTATGTTTTCATGCCTCCA

ØX174 B    GCCAGTTAAATAGCTTGCAAAATACGTGGCCTTATGGTTACAGTATGCCCA

ØX174 D    GAGATTCTCTTGTTGACATTTTAAAAGAGCGTGGATTACTATCTGAGTCCG

SV40       GAATGCAATTGTTGTTGTTAACTTGTTTATTGCAGCTTATAATGGTTACAA
```

Figure 7 Promoter sequences. The antisense strands of the promoters are indicated with all of them aligned with the residue equivalent to the mRNA start point at +1. The proposed regions of similarity are underlined. References for the sequences are: *lac* (Dickson et al. 1975); *lacI* (Calos 1978); *gal* (Musso et al. 1977); *araBAD* (B. Smith and R. Schleif; L. Greenfield and G. Wilcox; both pers. comm.); *araC* (B. Smith and R. Schleif; L. Greenfield and G. Wilcox; both pers. comm.) (the start point in this case is deduced from the location of RNA polymerase bound to the site [Hirsh and Schleif 1976], the length of *araC* transcripts from a defined template, and the structure of the sequence [R. Schleif, pers. comm.]); *trp* (Bennett et al. 1976); tRNA$_{1,2}^{Tyr}$ (Sekiya et al. 1976); λP_L (Maniatis et al. 1974); λP_R (Maniatis et al. 1975; Walz and Pirrotta 1975); λP_{RM} (Ptashne et al. 1976; Scherer et al. 1977); $\lambda C17$ (Rosenberg et al. 1978 and this volume, and, with minor differences, A. Walz and V. Pirrotta, pers. comm.); $\lambda imm^{434}P_R$ and P_{RM} (V. Pirrotta, pers. comm.); fd$X$ (Schaller et al. 1975; Sugimoto et al. 1975b); fdII (H. Schaller, pers. comm.); fdIIb (H. Schaller, pers. comm.); fdVIII (Takanami et al. 1976); ϕX174 *A*, *B*, and *D* (Sanger et al. 1977); and SV40 (Dhar et al. 1974).

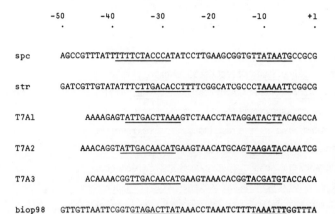

Figure 8 Additional promoter sequences. The antisense strands of six additional promoter sequences are presented as described for Fig. 7. References for these sequences are: *spc* and *str* (L. Post et al., pers. comm.); T7-*A1* (U. K. Siebenlist, pers. comm.); T7-*A2* and T7-*A3* (Pribnow 1975a,b; U. K. Siebenlist, pers. comm.); and *biop*98 (T. Otsuka and J. Abelson, unpubl.).

lac transcription, alters this 7-base-pair sequence so that it completely fits the proposed TATRATR sequence. One promoter which does not appear to contain this sequence is the *trp* promoter. As also noticed by Seeburg et al. (1977), the sequence between sites −37 and −27 is similar to the comparable region in many other promoters. This is also indicated in Figure 7. This region contains several known promoter mutations (λP_L^-*sex1* [Kleid et al. 1976], λP_{RM}*116* [Meyer et al. 1975], *lacP*−*L241* and *lacP*−*L305* [Dickson et al. 1975], *lacP*−*L157* [W. S. Reznikoff, unpubl.]). It is not clear from the available data what the prototypic sequence is for this region. For example, one would predict from the properties of *lacP*−*L305* that a G residue in position 1 of this sequence should have a negative effect on the relevant site-specific reaction, and yet several promoters have G in this site (e.g., fd*II*, λP_L, λP_R, λP_O, SV40, ϕX174D, and *trp*). It is possible that G is acceptable in this location when found in conjunction with another G in the fourth position. Another curious fact is that portions of this approximate sequence are found in a reiterated form in several promoters (e.g., it is found five times in the *gal* promoter). An interesting exception is the case of the *I*-gene promoter. It contains no obviously related sequence in this region, yet the existence of an I^q mutation at position −35 which enhances promoter activity (Calos 1978) indicates that this region is indeed important in recognition by RNA polymerase of the *I*-gene promoters.

The RNA polymerase–*lacP* interaction has been studied in a variety of biochemical experiments. The *lac* mRNA start site has been determined in vitro for both the *UV5* and wild-type promoters. The majority of *lac* mRNA molecules initiate with an A residue corresponding to position 1; the remainder initiate with the G residue corresponding to position -1 (Maizels 1973; Gilbert 1976; Majors 1975b; L. Maquat, unpubl.).

A simple model is that distinct segments of the promoter sequence contribute to the informational contacts required for specific steps in the RNA polymerase–*lacP* interaction. For instance, one part of the sequence might be read during closed-complex formation, another part during the conversion of the closed complex to the open complex, and still another part for the initiation event. One particular experiment which sheds some light on this question is the protection experiment performed by J. Gralla (pers. comm.; Gilbert 1976). RNA polymerase was allowed to form an open complex with the *UV5 lac* promoter and then unprotected DNA was digested with pancreatic DNase. The remaining complex (consisting of RNA polymerase and the 43-base-pair fragment partially indicated in Fig. 6) was stable but, once dissociated, could not reform. These results are in general agreement with those found in similar experiments performed with other promoter systems (fd, T7-*A2*, T7-*A3*, and P_R (Schaller et al. 1975; Sugimoto et al. 1975a; Pribnow 1975a,b; Walz and Pirrotta 1975) and could be interpreted to mean that all of the RNA polymerase–DNA contacts necessary for *maintenance* of the open complex are between positions -24 and $+19$, although other contacts outside of this region (presumably before -24) facilitate the *formation* of the open complex. This observation is in general agreement with the fact that *lacP⁻* mutations located at -34 and -37 prevent formation of the open complex (Reznikoff 1976; L. Maquat, unpubl.).

This protected complex is capable of initiating correct transcripts, suggesting that the information required for initiation once the open complex is formed is also found in the -24 to $+19$ region. However, no data exist on the efficiency of transcription initiation from such a complex; thus one cannot conclude that sites outside this region do not directly influence the initiation event. In fact, the properties of the mutation *L157* (see below) suggest this as a distinct possibility.

In spite of these results, recent experiments by Okamoto et al. (1977) and H. Schaller (pers. comm.) again raise the question of the importance of the sequence prior to -24. Takanami (Okamoto et al. 1977) used the *Hha*I site in the fd*VIII* promoter (the G3 promoter in the Takanami nomenclature) to fuse the -18 through $+212$ region to four different *Hha*I fragments. These chimeric fragments were examined for their RNA-polymerase-binding capacity and their initiation potential. All of these molecules did bind polymerase and would code for transcripts. A possible conclusion from these experiments is that the fd*VIII* promoter belongs to a class of promoters in which the region prior to -18 does not play a critical role in the recognition process. However, these assays were qualitative in nature (did binding and initiation occur or not? no quantitative values or kinetics were presented) and, fortuitously, the three chimeras which qualitatively gave the best binding also have the fdVIII promoter fragment fused to DNAs which have generated a sequence in the −40 to −30 region similar to other promoters. L. Maquat (unpubl.) has performed a similar experiment with the *lac* system. An *Alu* fragment carrying the *UV5* promoter was cut at the *Hpa*II site (−17 to −20) and fused to itself so that the following divergent structure was generated: +36←−−20→+36. Such a chimeric molecule does serve as a template, but transcription initiation occurs at a much slower rate than found with the intact *UV5 Alu* fragment. The −18→+36 *UV5 Hpa*II-*Alu* fragment does not serve as a template.

The informational contacts between RNA polymerase and *lacP UV5* DNA in the open complex have also been studied in dimethyl sulfate protection experiments performed by L. Johnsrud (pers. comm.). The results are described in Figure 6. A striking observation is that the G residue at −32 (the same position as the *L157* mutation) is protected from dimethyl sulfate by RNA polymerase. One is forced to the conclusion that polymerase maintains this contact while in the open complex, although this region is sensitive to the action of pancreatic DNase. Other contacts discovered by Johnsrud are at positions −6, −11, −13, and −24 as indicated in Figure 6. These sites are different from those of any mutations analyzed to date. Two of the strong contacts (−6 and −11) fall within the sequence similarity noted by Pribnow (1975a,b) and Schaller et al. (1975), reinforcing the notion that this region is important in the RNA polymerase–*lacP* interaction. No contacts were noticed beyond the start site, which agrees with the suggestion, from the properties of deletion S20, that this region does not play an informational role in the binding of RNA polymerase to *lacP*. At least five G residues were seen to have their methylation by dimethyl sulfate enhanced by RNA polymerase. These are also shown in Figure 6. One might consider that the enhanced methylation at position −1 results from unwinding necessary for the initiation event (L. Johnsrud, pers. comm.).

A final means of studying the relationship of different parts of the sequence to different steps in the RNA polymerase–*lacP* interaction is the analysis of how different class-II and class-III mutations affect these reactions. The assays used examined these effects on the formation and stability of the open complex (presumably reflecting requirements for both closed and open complex formations) and on the transcription initiation reaction. Qualitative binding assays were first reported by Reznikoff (1976) in which RNA polymerase was incubated for 30 minutes with a *Hin*d restriction digest of φ80p*lac* DNAs containing various promoter mutations. The nonspecific complexes were dissociated with a heparin challenge, the complexes were collected on nitrocellulose filter paper, the complexed restriction fragments were released with an SDS treatment, and the resulting fragments were displayed on polyacrylamide gels. Subsequently, L. Maquat (unpubl.) performed similar experiments which quantitatively examined the rate of formation of the RNA polymerase–*lac* promoter open complex by varying the time of heparin addition and by quantitating the amount of *lacP* DNA on the gels relative to internal standards. In addition, both L. Maquat (unpubl.) and J. Majors (pers. comm.) have utilized a transcription assay in which the template activity of a small restriction fragment (usually the *Hae*III fragment) carrying various genetic versions of *lacP* was analyzed. (J. Majors analyzed *lacP⁺*, *Pˢ*, and *L8-UV5*, and L. Maquat studied *LacP⁺*, *L8-UV5*, *Pʳ1a*, *Pʳ9*, *Pʳ111*, and *P⁻L157*.) The interaction of RNA polymerase with the fragment was terminated at different times by the addition of heparin along with the four ribonucleoside triphosphates, and the resulting transcripts were quantitated by polyacrylamide gel electrophoretic analysis. These experiments indicated that the properties of all *lac* promoter mutations, with the interesting exception of *P⁻L157*, could be explained as resulting from alterations in the rate of formation of the open complex. The results of these experiments for various promoters relative to the wild-type *lac* promoter are as follows:

1. The class-II mutations *L241* and *L305* prevent formation of the open complex.
2. The deletion *S20* does not alter the rate of formation of the open complex.
3. The class-III mutations enhance the rate of formation of the open complex. The order of promoters according to their rates of open-complex formation in the filter-binding assay is *UV5-Pʳ109-Pʳ111-Pʳ1a-Pʳ104-Pʳ2C-S20*. This is exactly the same order that is found for in vivo expression in the absence of CAP and cAMP. The initiation assays also rank promoters as would be predicted from in vivo results.
4. The class-II mutation *L157* appears to bind at least as well as the wild-type promoter, but in the transcription assay little RNA product is found. Thus *L157* appears to inhibit initiation (or causes frequent termination of transcription after incorporation of less than five ribonucleotides). Presumably *L157* acts by inhibiting some conformational change of the RNA polymerase on the DNA (it is not known whether RNA polymerase is situated at exactly the same site when bound to *L157* DNA as is the case for *UV5* DNA) or a change in RNA polymerase itself. The $\lambda P_L sex1$ mutation appears to be a similar sequence change (a C/G→A/T transversion at site −31 in an $^{ACA}_{TGT}$ sequence) (Kleid et al. 1976) and it would be of interest to examine what effect it has on binding as opposed to initiation.

CAP–cAMP Stimulation of *lac* Transcription Studied In Vitro

The transcription assay developed by J. Majors (pers. comm.) and by L. Maquat (unpubl.) has also been used to study the CAP–cAMP stimulation of *lac* transcription. The basic observations may be summarized as follows:

1. CAP–cAMP stimulates expression of the wild-type *lac* promoter 5- to 20-fold. CAP also stimulates expression from all tested class-III mutationally altered templates including *L8-UV5* (J. Majors 1975b and pers. comm.; L. Maquat, unpubl.).
2. CAP–cAMP enhances the association rate and decreases slightly the dissociation rate of the RNA polymerase–*lacP* open complex (J. Majors, pers. comm.; L. Maquat, unpubl.).
3. CAP–cAMP abolishes the sensitivity to different Mg^{++} concentrations during the binding reaction for the wild-type and P^s promoters (J. Majors, pers. comm.).
4. CAP–cAMP at high concentrations or at normally stimulatory concentrations in the absence of the CAP site will inhibit transcription initiation from class-III mutants (L. Maquat, unpubl.).

A result of these experiments which is not consistent with the in vivo results is that the CAP–cAMP stimulation of the wild-type promoter fragment never yields a rate of association or a final yield of transcript equivalent to that found with the *L8-UV5* or P^s fragments without CAP–cAMP stimulation (J. Majors, pers. comm.; L. Maquat, unpubl).

How Does the Repressor Block Transcription?

Current information indicates that, although RNA polymerase and the *lac* repressor may specifically recognize distinct nonoverlapping sequences, the binding of the two proteins constitutes mutually exclusive events. Therefore, the repressor is believed to act by preventing the formation of the RNA polymerase–*lacP* open complex.

The genetic results which suggest that the recognition sequences are separate are shown in Figures 4 and 6 of this chapter and in Figure 5 of Barkley and Bourgeois (this volume). The most operator-proximal promoter mutation known is *UV5*, which is located at positions −8 and −9; the most promoter-proximal operator mutation known is located at site +5 (numbering as in Figs. 4 and 6). Chemical probe experiments suggest much closer contact points. The repressor-operator cross-linking experiments described by Ogata and Gilbert (1977) indicate that the repressor contacts the thymine at +1, which is complementary to the first ribonucleotide of the in vitro transcript. The RNA polymerase–promoter dimethyl sulfate protection experiments summarized in Figure 6 show that polymerase enhances methylation of the guanine at position −1 and prevents methylation of the guanine at position −6 (L. Johnsrud, pers. comm.).

The mutually exclusive nature of the binding of the two proteins was first suggested by the pancreatic DNase protection experiments. The repressor protects a sequence (−3 to +21) (Gilbert and Maxam 1973) which is located almost entirely within the RNA-polymerase-protected sequence (−24 to +19) (J. Gralla, pers. comm.; Gilbert 1976). This model was confirmed by transcription and filter-binding studies utilizing purified restriction fragments (Majors 1975b; Reznikoff 1976). The repressor does not disengage prebound RNA polymerase, and RNA polymerase will not form an open complex in the presence of the repressor.

Are Other Factors Involved?

So far we have assumed that the participants involved in the initiation of *lac* transcription include RNA polymerase holoenzyme, the *lac* promoter, the four ribonucleoside triphosphates, and the modulating factors CAP (plus cAMP) and the repressor (plus inducer). In fact, purified systems including only these components do appear to function in a qualitatively appropriate fashion. However, there exist data which suggest that "magic spot" (ppGpp) and perhaps one or more additional protein factors may enhance the initiation of *lac* transcription.

The nucleotide ppGpp was first implicated as a stimulatory factor in *lac* transcription by in vitro experiments examining *lac*-DNA-directed β-galactosidase synthesis (de Crombrugghe et al. 1971; Yang et al. 1974). It was determined that ppGpp stimulates β-galactosidase synthesis and that this stimulation occurs at the level of transcription initiation due to the results of experiments utilizing "uncoupled" in vitro systems (where transcription occurs in the absence of amino acids and translation occurs in the presence of rifampicin or with purified mRNA) (Kung et al. 1974; Yang et al. 1974; Reiness et al. 1975) and as a result of *lac* mRNA production measurements in crude systems (de Crombrugghe et al. 1971; Aboud and Pastan 1975). The in vivo relevance of these studies is now being examined (P. Primakoff, pers. comm.). No enhancement of *lac* transcription by ppGpp has been detected in the purified RNA polymerase–*lacP* DNA transcription system (L. Maquat, unpubl.).

Evidence for the possible existence of additional protein factors involved in *lac* transcription initiation comes in part from the work of H. Weisbach and his collaborators. This group is fractionating the complex DNA-dependent β-galactosidase synthesis system into individual purified components and is starting with the known purified components and adding fractions of the crude system to look for stimulatory responses. From these two approaches, some new protein factors have been identified, at least one of which appears to act at the level of transcription initiation (Kung et al. 1974). No in vivo evidence yet exists which shows a requirement for this or other additional protein factors in *lac* transcription initiation.

Mutations in RNA Polymerase

In 1972, Silverstone et al. described the isolation of the *alt* mutations. These mutations have two pleiotropic phenotypes: they are temperature-sensitive for growth and, at permissive temperatures, they phenotypically suppress defects in the CAP–cAMP system. An *alt cya* or *alt crp* double mutant expresses the *lac* operon three- to fivefold more frequently at 30°C than is observed in a *cya* or *crp* single mutant. Recent work by Travers et al. (1978) and Burgess and his coworkers (pers. comm.) has shown that the *alt* mutations are in the structural gene for the sigma subunit of RNA polymerase. Thus, alterations in sigma modify the in vivo affinity of RNA polymerase for the *lac* and other CAP–cAMP-sensitive promoters.

A Model for the Initiation of *lac* Transcription

In light of the information described above, we now feel that the initiation of *lac* transcription can be best described by a model similar to that presented by Pribnow (1975a,b) and Gilbert (1976). The model envisions the following steps:

1. RNA polymerase forms a loose but specific complex with the *lac* promoter using nucleotide-sequence information found in the region from site −34 to −37. This complex could be termed a "closed complex" (Chamberlin 1974) or a "recognition complex" (Pribnow 1975b).
2. RNA polymerase forms a tight "open complex" (Chamberlin 1974) using primarily the sequence information found at −6 through −12. It is the formation of this complex which is the rate-determining step for the wild-type *lac* promoter and which is influenced by the CAP–cAMP complex, class-III promoter mutations, and possibly by magic-spot and other ancillary factors (similar ideas have been expressed previously for this and other promoter systems). This event can be termed "entry."

The CAP–cAMP complex might act via a protein-protein interaction with RNA polymerase (Gilbert 1976) or by subtly altering the conformation of the DNA via telestability (Burd et al. 1975; Dickson et al. 1975) to alter the rate of open-complex formation.

A mechanism which invokes a telestability-type stimulation is attractive in that this stimulation might mimic the alteration in DNA structure caused by class-III mutations and agents which are presumed to stimulate transcription initiation by destabilizing the DNA (glycerol, dimethyl sulfoxide, negative superhelical twists, elevated temperatures, etc.); however, there is no evidence from the methylation experiments that the CAP–cAMP complex does alter the structure of the DNA sufficiently to be detected 42 base pairs away. A prediction of this model is that every *crp*⁻ mutation can be explained by a failure to make a CAP molecule which binds specifically to DNA.

CAP might influence the "entry" of RNA polymerase by a protein-protein interaction if, for example, the entry step involved conformational changes in both the polymerase and the DNA, with the equilibria for both reactions lying somewhat to the left. Any event which facilitated either conformational change might drive the total reaction to completion. Predictions of the CAP–RNA polymerase interaction model are that CAP should make contact with RNA polymerase and that some *crp*⁻ mutations should affect this RNA polymerase contact site. Alternatively, one should be able to isolate some mutations in RNA polymerase which have a Crp⁻ phenotype, that is, which alter the CAP contact site on RNA polymerase.

3. RNA polymerase initiates the *lac* message.

The RNA polymerase–*lacP* contact at site −32 might optimally align RNA polymerase in the open complex (and thus participates in step 2 above) or might actually stimulate initiation by facilitating a conformational change in RNA polymerase (thereby playing a part in step 3 above). The location of *L157* raises the possibility that a simple linear distribution of sequential recognition sites in the promoter will be found to be an oversimplification.

We have modified our past idea on where entry occurs (from the −37 to −26 interval to the −12 to −6 region) due to considerations such as the following:

1. Mutations which affect the entry process would be expected to map in or near the region involved in the process (those in the region would presumably supply specific informational content for the reaction, whereas those located nearby might alter the general structure of the DNA). Class-III mutations are those believed to affect the entry process—they facilitate open-complex formation. Only three class-III mutations have been sequenced so far; two of them lie within the −12 to −6 region and one lies 4 base pairs away. None of them lie in the GC-rich region from −48 to −37 or in the region from −37 to −26 which the previous model would have predicted. Clearly, we need to obtain sequence information about other class-III mutations. An

additional prediction of the previous model is that one should be able to isolate deletions which end in the −48 to −37 region and which stimulate CAP–cAMP-independent *lac*-specific transcription. None have been found, although they have not been looked for extensively.

2. The class-II promoter mutations *L305* and *L241* display a property which we previously found confusing, that is, in addition to altering the ability of RNA polymerase to recognize the promoter, they also reduce the ability of CAP to stimulate the RNA polymerase–*lacP* interaction (Hopkins 1974; see Table 1). This property is exactly what one would expect if one assumed that in the wild-type promoter the conversion of the closed complex to the open complex was the rate-limiting step (the step affected by CAP binding) and that in the mutants carrying *L305* and *L241* closed-complex formation became rate-limiting. Thus, these two mutations would define not the "entry site" but rather a previous "recognition site."

3. Finally, the *gal* promoter sequence gives no evidence of the alternating GC- and AT-rich blocks found in *lacP*, yet one would presume that the CAP-stimulated mode of *gal* transcription occurs in a manner analogous to that for *lac*.

Further understanding of how the *lac* promoter functions will be aided by generating a collection of mutant *lac* promoters which contain alterations at each of the sites in the *lac* promoter sequence, followed by detailed analyses of whether each change alters the CAP-DNA interaction, the formation of the RNA polymerase–*lacP* closed complex, the entry step, or the initiation event. We would also like to find out whether CAP does contact RNA polymerase when bound to the DNA. Finally, the role of any additional factors must still be elucidated.

ACKNOWLEDGMENTS

W. S. R. is the recipient of the Harry and Evelyn Steenbock Career Development Award. The previously unpublished research work by W. S. R. and Lynne Maquat was supported by grant GM-19670 from the National Institutes of Health and by funds from the Wisconsin Alumni Research Foundation. J. A. was a recipient of grant PCM-74-21089 from the National Science Foundation. We thank Lorraine Johnsrud and John Majors for communicating to us their unpublished results and for their comments on the manuscript.

REFERENCES

Aboud, M. and I. Pastan. 1975. Activation of transcription by guanosine 5′-diphosphate, 3′-diphosphate, transfer ribonucleic acid, and a novel protein from *Escherichia coli*. *J. Biol. Chem.* **250:**2189.

Arditti, R., T. Grodzicker, and J. Beckwith. 1973. Cyclic adenosine monophosphate-independent mutants of the lactose operon of *Escherichia coli. J. Bacteriol.* **114:**652.

Barnes, W. M., W. S. Reznikoff, F. R. Blattner, R. C. Dickson, and J. Abelson. 1975. The isolation of RNA homologous to the genetic control elements of the lactose operon. *J. Biol. Chem.* **250:**8184.

Beckwith, J., T. Grodzicker, and R. Arditti. 1972. Evidence for two sites in the *lac* promoter region. *J. Mol. Biol.* **69:**155.

Bennett, G. N., M. E. Schweingruber, K. D. Brown, C. Squires, and C. Yanofsky. 1976. Nucleotide sequence of region preceding *trp* mRNA initiation site and its role in promoter and operator function. *Proc. Natl. Acad. Sci.* **73:**2351.

Burd, J., R. Wartell, J. B. Dodgson and R. D. Wells. 1975. Transmission of stability (telestability) in deoxyribonucleic acid. *J. Biol. Chem.* **250:**5109.

Calos, M. 1978. The promoter of the lactose repressor gene: The DNA sequence for a low level promoter and an up promoter mutation. *Nature* (in press).

Chamberlin, M. 1974. The selectivity of transcription. *Annu. Rev. Biochem.* **43:**721.

de Crombrugghe, B., B. Chen, M. Gottesman, H. Varmas, M. Emmer, and R. Perlman. 1971. Regulation of *lac* mRNA synthesis in a soluble cell-free system. *Nat. New Biol.* **230:**37.

Dhar, R., S. Weissman, B. Zain, J. Pan, and A. Lewis, Jr. 1974. The nucleotide sequence preceding an RNA polymerase initiation site on SV40 DNA. II. The sequence of the early strand transcript. *Nucleic Acids Res.* **1:**595.

Dickson, R. C., J. N. Abelson, W. M. Barnes, and W. S. Reznikoff. 1975. Genetic regulation: The *lac* control region. *Science* **182:**27.

Dickson, R. C., J. Abelson, P. Johnson, W. S. Reznikoff, and W. M. Barnes. 1977. Nucleotide sequence changes produced by mutations in the *lac* promoter of *Escherichia coli. J. Mol. Biol.* **111:**65.

Dykes, G., R. Bambara, K. Marians, and R. Wu. 1975. Statistical significance of primary structural features found in DNA-protein interaction sites. *Nucleic Acids Res.* **2:**327.

Eron, L. and R. Block. 1971. Mechanism of initiation and repression of *in vitro* transcription of the *lac* operon of *Escherichia coli. Proc. Natl. Acad. Sci.* **68:**1828.

Eron, L., J. Beckwith, and F. Jacob. 1970. Deletion of translational start signals in the *lac* operon of *E. coli.* In *The lactose operon* (ed. J. R. Beckwith and D. Zipser), p. 353. Cold Spring Harbor Laboratory, Cold Spring Harbor, New York.

Gilbert, W. 1976. Starting and stopping sequences for the RNA polymerase. In *RNA polymerase* (eds. R. Losick and M. Chamberlin), p. 193. Cold Spring Harbor Laboratory, Cold Spring Harbor, New York.

Gilbert, W. and A. Maxam. 1973. The nucleotide sequence of the *lac* operator. *Proc. Natl. Acad. Sci.* **70:**3581.

Hirsh, J. and R. Schleif. 1976. Electron microscopy of gene regulation: The L-arabinose operon. *Proc. Natl. Acad. Sci.* **73:**1518.

Hopkins, J. D. 1974. A new class of promoter mutations in the lactose operon of *Escherichia coli. J. Mol. Biol.* **87:**715.

Jacob, F., A. Ullmann, and J. Monod. 1964. Le promoteur, élément génétique necessaire a l'expression d'un opéron. *C. R. Acad. Sci.* **258:**3125.

Kleid, D., Z. Humayun, A. Jeffrey, and M. Ptashne. 1976. Novel properties of a restriction endonuclease isolated from *Haemophilus parahaemolyticus*. *Proc. Natl. Acad. Sci.* **73**:293.

Kung, H., N. Brot, C. Spears, B. Chen, and H. Weissbach. 1974. *In vitro* transcription and translation of the *lac* operon. *Arch. Biochem. Biophys.* **160**:168.

Maizels, N. 1973. The nucleotide sequence of the lactose messenger ribonucleic acid transcribed from the UV5 promoter mutant of *E. coli*. *Proc. Natl. Acad. Sci.* **70**:3585.

Majors, J. 1975a. Specific binding of CAP factor of *lac* promoter DNA. *Nature* **256**:672.

———. 1975b. Initiation of *in vitro* mRNA synthesis from the wild-type *lac* promoter. *Proc. Natl. Acad. Sci.* **72**:4394.

Maniatis, T., A. Jeffrey, and D. Kleid. 1975. Nucleotide sequence of the rightward operator of phage lambda. *Proc. Natl. Acad. Sci.* **72**:1184.

Maniatis, T., M. Ptashne, B. G. Barrell, and J. Donelson. 1974. Sequence of a repressor binding site in the DNA of bacteriophage lambda. *Nature* **250**:394.

Maxam, A. and W. Gilbert. 1977. A new method for sequencing DNA. *Proc. Natl. Acad. Sci.* **74**:560.

Meyer, B., D. Kleid, and M. Ptashne. 1975. λ Repressor turns off transcription of its own gene. *Proc. Natl. Acad. Sci.* **72**:4785.

Miller, J. H. 1970. Transcription starts and stops in the *lac* operon. In *The lactose operon* (ed. J. R. Beckwith and D. Zipser), p. 353. Cold Spring Harbor Laboratory, Cold Spring Harbor, New York.

Miller, J. H., W. S. Reznikoff, A. E. Silverstone, K. Ippen, E. R. Signer, and J. R. Beckwith. 1970. Fusions of the *lac* and *trp* regions of the *Escherichia coli* chromosone. *J. Bacteriol.* **104**:1273.

Mitchell, D., W. Reznikoff, and J. Beckwith. 1975. Genetic fusions defining *trp* and *lac* operon regulatory elements. *J. Mol. Biol.* **93**:331.

Mitra, S., G. Zubay, and A. Landy. 1975. Evidence for the preferential binding of the catabolite gene activator protein (CAP) to DNA containing the *lac* promoter. *Biochem. Biophys. Res. Commun.* **67**:857.

Musso, R., R. DiLauro, M. Rosenberg, and B. de Crombrugghe. 1977. Nucleotide sequence of the operator-promoter region of the galactose operon of *Escherichia coli*. *Proc. Natl. Acad. Sci.* **74**:106.

Ogata, R. and W. Gilbert. 1977. Contacts between the *lac* repressor and thymine in the *lac* operator. *Proc. Natl. Acad. Sci.* **74**:4973.

Okamoto, T., K. Sugimoto, H. Sugisaki, and M. Takanami. 1977. DNA regions essential for the function of a bacteriophage fd promoter. *Nucleic Acids Res.* **4**:2213.

Pribnow, D. 1975a. Nucleotide sequence of an RNA polymerase binding site at an early T7 promoter. *Proc. Natl. Acad. Sci.* **72**:784.

———. 1975b. Bacteriophage T7 early promoters: Nucleotide sequences of two RNA polymerase binding sites. *J. Mol. Biol.* **99**:419.

Ptashne, M., K. Backman, M. Z. Humayun, A. Jeffrey, R. Maurer, B. Meyer, and R. T. Sauer. 1976. Autoregulation and function of a repressor in bacteriophage lambda. *Science* **194**:156.

Reiness, G., H.-L. Yang, G. Zubay, and M. Cashel. 1975. Effects of guanosine tetraphosphate on cell-free synthesis of *Escherichia coli* ribosomal RNA and other gene products. *Proc. Natl. Acad. Sci.* **72**:2881.

Reznikoff, W. S. 1972. The operon revisited. *Annu. Rev. Genet.* **6**:133.

————. 1976. Formation of the RNA polymerase-*lac* promoter open complex. In *RNA polymerase* (ed. R. Losick and M. Chamberlin), p. 441. Cold Spring Harbor Laboratory, Cold Spring Harbor, New York.

Reznikoff, W. S., R. B. Winter, and C. K. Hurley. 1974. The location of the repressor binding sites in the *lac* operon. *Proc. Natl. Acad. Sci.* **71**:2314.

Rosenberg, M., D. Court, D. L. Wulff, H. Shimatake, and C. Brady. 1978. The relation between function and DNA sequence in an intercistronic regulatory region in phage λ. *Nature* (in press).

Sanger, F., G. M. Air, B. G. Barrell, N. L. Brown, A. R. Coulson, J. C. Fiddes, C. A. Hutchison III, P. M. Slocombe, and M. Smith. 1977. Nucleotide sequence of bacteriophage ϕX174 DNA. *Nature* **265**:687.

Scaife, J. and J. Beckwith. 1967. Mutational alteration of the maximal level of *lac* operon expression. *Cold Spring Harbor Symp. Quant. Biol.* **31**:403.

Schaller, H., C. Gray, and K. Herrmann. 1975. Nucleotide sequence of an RNA polymerase binding site from the DNA of bacteriophage fd. *Proc. Natl. Acad. Sci.* **72**:737.

Scherer, G., G. Hobom, and H. Kössel. 1977. DNA base sequence of the P_o promoter region of phage λ. *Nature* **265**:117.

Seeburg, P., C. Nusslein, and H. Schaller. 1977. Interaction of RNA polymerase with promoters from bacteriophage fd. *Eur. J. Biochem.* **74**:107.

Sekiya, T., T. Takeya, R. Contreras, H. Kupper, H. G. Khorana, and A. Landy. 1976. Nucleotide sequences at the two ends of the *E. coli* tyrosine tRNA genes and studies on the promoter. In *RNA polymerase* (ed. R. Losick and M. Chamberlin), p. 455. Cold Spring Harbor Laboratory, Cold Spring Harbor, New York.

Silverstone, A. E., R. R. Arditti, and B. Magasanik. 1970. Catabolite-insensitive revertants of *lac* promoter mutations. *Proc. Natl. Acad. Sci.* **66**:773.

Silverstone, A. E., M. Goman, and J. G. Scaife. 1972. *alt.*: A new factor involved in the synthesis of RNA by *Escherichia coli. Mol. Gen. Genet.* **118**:223.

Sugimoto, K., T. Okamoto, H. Sugisaki, and M. Takanami. 1975a. The nucleotide sequence of an RNA polymerase binding site on bacteriophage fd DNA. *Nature* **253**:410.

Sugimoto, K., H. Sugisaki, T. Okamoto, and M. Takanami. 1975b. Studies on bacteriophage fd DNA. III. Nucleotide sequence preceding the RNA start site on a promoter-containing fragment. *Nucleic Acids Res.* **2**:2091.

Takanami, M., K. Sugimoto, H. Sugisaki, and T. Okamoto. 1976. Sequence of promoter for coat protein gene of bacteriophage fd. *Nature* **260**:297.

Travers, A. A., R. Buckland, M. Goman, S. F. J. LeCrice, and J. G. Scaife. 1978. A mutation affecting the sigma subunit of RNA polymerase changes transcriptional specificity. *Nature* (in press).

Walz, A. and V. Pirrotta. 1975. Sequence of the P_R promoter of phage lambda. *Nature* **254**:118.

Yang, H.-L., G. Zubay, E. Urm, G. Reiness, and M. Cashel. 1974. Effects of guanosine tetraphosphate, guanosine pentaphosphate, and β-γ methyl-guanosine pentaphosphate on gene expression of *Escherichia coli in vitro. Proc. Natl. Acad. Sci.* **71**:63.

Genetic Fusions of the *lac* Operon: A New Approach to the Study of Biological Processes

Phillip Bassford, Jonathan Beckwith, Michael Berman,*
Edith Brickman, Malcolm Casadaban,† Leonard Guarente,
Isabelle Saint-Girons,‡ Aparna Sarthy, Maxime Schwartz,‡
Howard Shuman, and Thomas Silhavy
Department of Microbiology and Molecular Genetics
Harvard Medical School
Boston, Massachusetts 02115

INTRODUCTION

The lactose operon represents one of the best worked-out systems of gene expression and regulation. The extent to which the details of *lac* operon control have been elaborated depended, in good part, on aspects of lactose metabolism which make it a particularly easy system to analyze. These include a sensitive and rapid assay for β-galactosidase, a number of different indicator media for distinguishing phenotypes of mutant strains, and an ability to select both forward and reverse mutations in the operon and in the regulatory gene (see Beckwith 1970 for a review of most of these; see also Hopkins 1974).

The most important aspect of lactose metabolism which distinguishes it from most other biochemical pathways and contributes to its ease of analysis is the nature of lactose itself. Since lactose is a disaccharide, glucose-1-4-β-D-galactose, substituted derivatives with various moieties replacing the glucose can be synthesized which will have affinity for one or another component of the system. For instance, one of the indicator media used includes 5-bromo-4-chloro-3-indolyl-β-D-galactoside (XG), which is a substrate for β-galactosidase. When hydrolyzed, this compound forms a blue dye, thus providing a sensitive test for the presence of β-galactosidase activity. Since XG is not an inducer of the *lac* operon, it can be used to distinguish inducible from constitutive strains, as well as to discriminate between strains which produce high and low levels of β-galactosidase, in general, and to detect plaque-forming transducing phages which carry the *lacZ* gene.

Present addresses: *Department of Biology, Brown University Providence, Rhode Island 02912; †Department of Medicine, Stanford University School of Medicine, Palo Alto, California 94305; ‡Institut Pasteur, 25, rue du Docteur Roux, Paris 15^e, France.

The technical principles and approaches used in studying the lactose operon are not directly applicable to most other regulatory systems because they rely on the particular nature of lactose. In some cases, direct selections for regulatory mutants are available with chemical analogs of substrates, intermediates, or end products of a pathway (e.g., the arabinose operon [Englesberg et al. 1965] and the tryptophan operon [Cohen and Jacob 1959]). In certain pathways, direct selections for forward mutations in structural genes of an operon have been developed (e.g., the galactose operon [Adhya and Shapiro 1969] and the arabinose operon [Englesberg et al. 1962]). However, no system combines the variety of features which have facilitated progress in understanding *lac* operon regulation. One way to overcome this technical barrier to a more accessible analysis of other regulatory systems is to create a situation in which it is possible to monitor the expression of a particular gene or operon via the expression of the *lac* operon genes themselves. This can be done by generating *genetic fusions* of the *lac* operon genes, *lacZ* and *lacY*, to the genes of interest.[1]

GENE FUSIONS

The concept of using gene fusions of *Escherichia coli* genes as a way to facilitate genetic analysis first appeared when Jacob et al. (1965) described fusions of the *lacY* gene to the *purE* operon. Strains carrying such fusions exhibited purine control of the synthesis of the galactoside permease, the product of *lacY*. These fusions were obtained on an F' plasmid carrying both the *lac* and *purE* genes, which are located close to one another on the *E. coli* chromosome. At this point, the ability to generate fusions between *lac* and other genes was limited to those genes close to the *lac* operon. Subsequently, other analogous cases of gene fusions have been explored in which the fused genes ordinarily lie close to one another on the chromosome. These include *ara-leu* (Kessler and Englesberg 1969), *gal-bio* (Ketner and Campbell 1974), and *arg-rpo* (Errington et al 1974) fusions.

However, the limitation on the fusion approach—that the genes in question be close to one another—was removed, at least conceptually, with the development of a technique for transposing the *lac* genes to other positions on the bacterial chromosome (Cuzin and Jacob 1964). For instance, in one case the *lac* operon was transposed to a chromosomal position close to the *trp* operon. Ordinarily these two operons lie quite

[1]Genetic symbols: *lac, ara, gal, mal, glp*—genes determining the catabolism of lactose, arabinose, galactose, maltose, and glycerol, respectively; *leu, bio, arg, trp, thr,* and *pur*—genes determining the biosynthesis of leucine, biotin, arginine, tryptophan, threonine, and purine, respectively; *rpo*—gene coding for RNA polymerase subunits; *tyrT*—gene coding for tyrosine tRNA; *phoA*—gene coding for alkaline phosphatase; *rel*—gene coding for a protein involved in guanosine tetraphosphate synthesis.

far apart on the chromosome. Between the *trp* and *lac* loci in this transposition strain lies the *tonB* locus which determines the sensitivity to bacteriophages φ80 and T1 (Fig. 1). Selection for *tonB* mutations in such a strain occasionally yields deletions of the *tonB* locus which extend into the *lac* region on the one hand and into the *trp* region on the other. In this way, for instance, derivatives can be isolated in which the *lacY* gene is fused to the *trp* operon and is thus put under the control of the *trp* regulatory system (Fig. 1, class I) (Beckwith et al. 1967; Miller et al. 1970). A further important step in the fusion approach was the development of techniques which allowed the detection of fusion strains in which all of the structural genes of the *lac* operon (*Z*, *Y*, and *A*) were intact and fused to the *trp* operon (Fig. 1, class II) (Reznikoff and Beckwith 1969; Reznikoff et al. 1969; Mitchell et al. 1975). Such strains exhibited a Lac⁺ phenotype when the *trp* operon was expressed constitutively due to a mutation in the repressor gene for the *trp* operon, *trpR*.

Strains carrying fusions between the *trp* and *lac* operons, while proving useful for studying the *lac* operon, have also permitted new approaches to the analysis of the *trp* operon. Such fusions have been used for the following *trp* operon studies: (1) isolation of *trp* regulatory mutants (Reznikoff and Thornton 1972); (2) in vitro studies of the *trp* operon, resulting in detection of the repressor for this system (Zubay et al. 1972); and (3) determination that the termination signal for *trp* operon transcription lies outside of the last structural gene, *trpA* (Mitchell et al. 1976).

Recently we have used a variation of the fusion approach to analyze in more detail the transcription termination signal at the end of the *trp* operon, t_{trp}. Ordinarily, transcription termination signals at the end of operons are difficult to analyze genetically, since mutations in them have no effect on the expression of the operon of which they are a part. However, such termination signals could be studied if the effects on adjacent genes of transcriptional read-through past such signals could be measured. This approach was used to study t_{trp}. Strains were isolated which carried *tonB* deletions extending into the *lac* promoter at one extremity, but which did not extend into t_{trp} at the other (Fig. 1, class III). These strains are Lac⁻ due to deletion of *lacP* and do not exhibit a Lac⁺

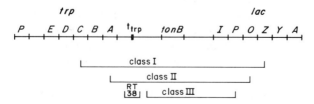

Figure 1   Fusions of the *lac* and *trp* operons.

phenotype even when a *trpR⁻* mutation is introduced. The t$_{trp}$ represents a barrier to read-through transcription into the *lac* operon. These strains can then be used to select mutant derivatives in which the termination at t$_{trp}$ is reduced or eliminated, thus permitting read-through transcription into the *lac* operon, and a Lac⁺ phenotype. This selection has been used to detect mutations in t$_{trp}$ (Fig. 1, RT38) (Guarente and Beckwith 1978). In addition, selection of Lac⁺ derivatives of class-III deletion strains (in a *trpR⁻* background) has yielded mutations in the structural gene for rho protein, a protein known to play a role in bacteriophage λ transcription termination and in bacterial operon polarity. These results show that rho protein also plays a role in the termination of transcription of bacterial operons (Guarente et al. 1977).

Gene fusions have also proved useful in the study of bacteriophage λ. Since bacterial genes can be incorporated into the λ chromosome when transducing phages are formed, such phages can be used to isolate fusions between the bacterial and phage genes. In one case, fusions of the *trp* operon to a λ operon allowed a better understanding of the function of λ *N*-gene product (Franklin 1974). In a second case, fusions of the *lac* operon to a λ operon controlled by the λ *N* gene allowed in vitro detection of the *N*-gene product, using β-galactosidase synthesis as an assay for its activity (Epp and Pearson 1976). Finally, the structural gene for the λ repressor was fused to the *lac* operon. Strains carrying such fusions produced large amounts of the λ repressor, since the synthesis of this protein was now under the control of the very active *lac* promoter (Gronenborn 1976). This latter example illustrates the usefulness of the gene fusion technique for isolating strains which produce large amounts of proteins, ordinarily seen in only small amounts.

HYBRID PROTEINS AS A RESULT OF GENE FUSIONS

The useful feature of most of the *lac* fusion strains described so far is that a conveniently assayable *lac* operon gene product has been put under the control of another regulatory system. In many of these fusions, e.g., *purE-lacY* or *trp-lacY*, the endpoints of the deletion which generate the fusions lie within structural genes of the two operons (Fig. 2). Presumably, in many cases, hybrid proteins are produced by what is, in essence, the construction of a hybrid gene. True hybrid proteins would only be produced when the phase of reading of the hybrid gene is the same as that of the two original genes. Since the selection or screening procedures which yielded these strains did not involve a selection for activity of either fused gene product, in most cases, it is unlikely that the hybrid protein will have these activities. However, in some cases, such hybrid proteins might be antigenically related to the original proteins. The appearance of hybrid genes which produce active protein products might be limited by

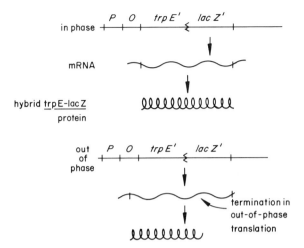

Figure 2   Gene fusions.

the essentiality of the amino- or carboxy-terminal amino acid sequence of a particular protein. However, more and more cases are being reported where removal of one or the other end of a protein does not eliminate enzymatic activity (Yourno et al. 1970; Jackson and Yanofsky 1974; Müller-Hill and Kania 1974; Ino et al. 1975; Mitchell et al. 1976).

The amino-terminal portion of β-galactosidase is not essential for enzymatic activity. A deletion, M15 (or XA21), was isolated which removes amino acids 11–42 from the protein and codes for an inactive product (Accolla and Celada 1976) (Fig. 3). However, in the presence of antibody to the enzyme, β-galactosidase activity is restored. The enzymatic activity can also be restored to *lacZ* gene products missing an amino-terminal sequence by fusing them to the amino-terminal sequence of many other proteins. This was first shown by Müller-Hill and Kania (1974) in the following way. A strain was constructed which carried a *lacI* mutation (I^q), which caused overproduction of repressor protein, and a *lacZ* ochre mutation (*U118*) (corresponding to amino acid 17 in the protein) which resulted in termination of protein synthesis early in the gene (Fig. 3). Selection for Lac$^+$ revertants of this strain yielded back-mutations, ochre suppressor mutations, and *deletions which fused the* lacZ *gene to the* lacI *gene*. Such deletions removed the protein-chain termination signal at the end of *lacI*, the chain initiation signal at the

Figure 3 Fusions of the *lacZ* and *lacI* genes. The *U118* mutation has been shown to alter the codon for amino acid 17 in β-galactosidase (Zabin et al. 1978).

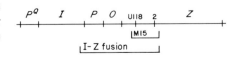

beginning of *lacZ*, and the *lacZ U118* termination signal. The substitution of varying extents of the amino-terminal sequence of the *lac* repressor for the missing amino-terminal sequence of β-galactosidase was apparently sufficient to allow β-galactosidase activity. In one case, the hybrid protein had both repressor and β-galactosidase activity.

As discussed below, the findings of Müller-Hill and Kania (1974) provided a novel approach to studying several biological questions. Again, however, the formation of hybrid, enzymatically active β-galactosidase proteins depended on the proximity of *lac* to the gene of interest, in this case, *lacI*. What was required was a method for permitting ready fusion of *lacZ*, either intact or with a deleted terminus, to any other gene on the bacterial chromosome. What follows is a description of a new approach to isolating such fusions and the logic which led to it.

A GENERAL METHOD FOR FUSING THE *lac* OPERON TO OTHER GENES

Transposition of *lac* to Predetermined Positions

Let us consider a hypothetical operon which includes gene *X*, to which we wish to fuse the *lacZ* and *lacY* genes. One possible first step is to transpose the *lac* region to a site close to or within the gene *X*. (Ordinarily, this cannot be conveniently done for most regions of the chromosome by previously described techniques.) If genetic homology exists between the two regions, then it should be possible to select for recombination events which generate the appropriate transposition. Since there usually is no extensive homology between any two regions chosen at random (Fig. 4a), these events will be very rare. Therefore, it is necessary to generate that homology. This can be accomplished by the insertion of

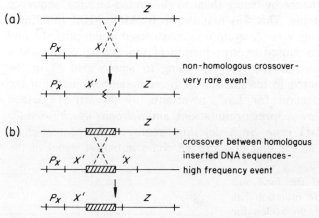

Figure 4 Mechanisms for transposition of the *lac* operon. Arrows indicate direction of transcription.

identical segments of DNA into the two regions, near or in gene X and in the *lac* operon (Fig. 4b). Given genetic homology between the two regions, recombination events may occur at a reasonable frequency.

Several methods exist for inserting DNA sequences in the chromosome. These include isolation of insertion sequence mutations, translocation of antibiotic resistance markers, insertion of the bacteriophage Mu-1 chromosome, and insertion of the bacteriophage λ genome at different positions on the chromosome (all reviewed in Bukhari et al. 1977). Casadaban (1976a) chose to use bacteriophage Mu-1 as a tool for simplifying gene fusion technology. The following is a description of this approach.

Bacteriophage Mu-1 is a temperate phage which upon lysogenization inserts its genome $(28 \times 10^6$ daltons) at random around the bacterial chromosome. A significant percentage of Mu-1 lysogens are auxotrophic due to insertion of the Mu-1 genome into a gene for a biosynthetic pathway (Taylor 1963). Thus it is possible, using appropriate selection or screening procedures, to detect Mu-1 insertions in or near a gene of interest (e.g., gene X and *lac*). In addition, the approaches exist for detecting Mu-1 insertions in essential genes (Nomura and Engbaek 1972). Once strains have been isolated which carry the Mu-1 genome in or near gene X and in or near *lac*, a genetic cross can be performed (Fig. 4b) which will result in the production of recombinants in which *lac* has been transposed close to gene X. To facilitate crosses of this type, a λ transducing phage was constructed which carried the *lac* region and one end of the Mu-1 genome (Fig. 5a). The only genetic homology that exists between such a λ phage (missing its *att* site[2]) and the chromosome of strains which carry the Mu-1 genome in gene X and are deleted for the *lac* region (Fig. 5b) is in the gene-X region. Selection for lysogens after infection of such strains with this special λ phage yields strains with *lac* integrated near gene X (Fig. 5c). In order to facilitate selection for fusions, the *lac* operon carried on the λ genome is missing its promoter region and is therefore inactive.

Fusion of *lacZ* to Gene *X*

The steps just described bring *lac* and gene X close together, but do not fuse them. What prevents transcription initiated at P_x from proceeding into the *lac* operon is the long sequence of Mu-1 DNA which must contain at least one barrier to continued transcription (Fig. 5c). The last step in generating the fusions is the removal of such barriers. The initial use of a Mu-1 phage which is thermoinducible makes this step possible. Strains carrying the structure indicated in Figure 5c can be used to select

[2]Attachment site on the chromosome for a temperate bacteriophage.

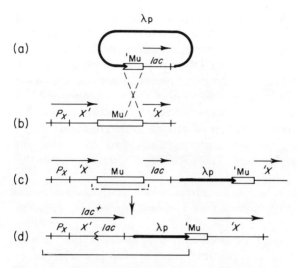

Figure 5 Steps leading to fusion of the *lac* operon to other bacterial genes. Arrows indicate direction of transcription.

for Lac⁺ revertants which are also thermoresistant. A single mutational event which can generate such revertants is a deletion which removes those genes of Mu-1 lethal to the cell and, at the same time, removes all barriers to transcription in the Mu-1 genome. It is this approach which has been used successfully to fuse the *lac* operon to a number of different bacterial genes.

In Table 1 we have listed the fusions of the *lac* operon isolated in this laboratory so far using this technique. (These are all examples of fusions in which the *lacZ* gene is intact.)

In addition, fusions have been isolated between the *lac* and *argA* genes by Eckhardt (Eckhardt 1977; Kelker and Eckhardt 1977). In each case the synthesis of β-galactosidase exhibits the regulation expected for the promoter to which it has been fused. For instance, fusions of *lacZ* to the *ara* operon result in strains in which β-galactosidase synthesis is induced by the presence of arabinose in the growth media (Table 2). In our laboratory such fusions can be isolated within approximately 1 month, using genes where the detection of Mu-1 insertions is easily achieved.

Employing this approach, fusions have been isolated in which an intact *lacZ* structural gene is brought under the control of a new promoter. The β-galactosidase protein which is produced by such fusion strains is identical with that produced by a wild-type Lac⁺ strain. We call such fusion strains *operon fusions*. In contrast, we can use the same general approach to isolate strains which produce β-galactosidase molecules whose amino-terminal sequence has been replaced by the amino-terminal sequence of another protein. This can be done by incorporating the *lacZ*

Table 1 Fusions of the *lac* operon to other bacterial genes or operons using the Casadaban (1976a) technique

Gene or operon fused to	Regulation of β-galactosidase observed	References
ara operon	induced by arabinose	Casadaban (1976a)
araC gene	repressed by the *araC* gene product and glucose	Casadaban (1976b)
leu operon	repressed by leucine	Casadaban (1976a)
malA operon	induced by maltose	Silhavy et al. (1976)
Both *malB* operons (see Fig. 7)	induced by maltose	Silhavy et al. (1976, 1977), P. Bassford (unpubl.)
thr operon	repressed by threonine	I. St.-Girons (unpubl.)
phoA gene	repressed by inorganic phosphate	A. Sarthy (unpubl.)
tyrT	increases with faster growth rates	M. Berman (1977)
glpT gene	induced by glycerol	T. J. Silhavy et al. (unpubl.)

U118 mutation onto the λ*plac* Mu phage before initiating the sequence of steps leading to selection for fusions (Fig. 6). Using this phage derivative, the ultimate selection for Lac⁺ colonies at 42°C yields strains in which the early portion of the *lacZ* gene (including the *U118* site) has been removed

Table 2 Induction of β-galactosidase by arabinose in *ara-lac* fusion strains

	β-Galactosidase units	
Fusion	L(+)-arabinose	L(−)-arabinose
1	1100	0.45
2	2600	0.28
3	830	12.0
4	400	1.1
5	1900	9.4
6	250	7.0
7	390	1.2
8	610	0.29

These data are representative examples of the data obtained by Casadaban (1976a). Units of activity are described in that paper.

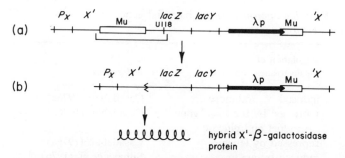

Figure 6 Steps leading to the formation of hybrid proteins between β-galactosid-ase and other bacterial proteins. Arrows indicate direction of transcription.

and replaced by a portion of a nearby gene as with the *lacI-lacZ* fusions of Müller-Hill and Kania (1974). Such strains produce hybrid β-galac-tosidase molecules and are termed *protein fusions*.

USES OF *lac* FUSIONS

Fusions of the *lac* operon using this technique have been employed to study certain regulatory problems which heretofore had appeared relatively intractable. Several examples follow.

Regulation of the *araC* Gene

The study of gene regulation is most easily done with genes whose products have a readily assayable product, such as an enzyme. Regulatory genes usually code for products whose sole function is to control the activity of another gene or genes. In addition, the products of regulatory genes are usually made in very low amounts. In some cases the only assay for a regulatory gene product is an in vitro measure of gene regulation. Such an assay is relatively tedious and not very sensitive. Thus, to study the question of whether a regulatory gene is itself regulated can be extremely difficult.

The technique of gene fusion has been employed to circumvent such problems in studying regulatory genes. By causing the synthesis of β-galactosidase to come under the control of the promoter for a regulatory gene, such an analysis is made possible. One regulatory gene of particular interest is the *araC* gene which codes for a positive control factor for the arabinose operon. Casadaban (1976b) has used the Mu fusion technique described above to construct *araC-lacZ* fusions. New regulatory features of the *araC* gene were discovered using β-galactosid-ase activity as a measure of *araC* gene promoter function. Introduction into such a fusion strain of an F′ episome carrying a wild-type *araC* gene resulted in a repression of β-galactosidase synthesis. These results show that the *araC* gene controls its own synthesis via a negative control mechanism. Further, β-galactosidase was subject to catabolite repression in *araC-lacZ* fusions, suggesting that the *araC* gene is under positive control by the CAP-cAMP complex.

The Use of Gene Fusions to Isolate New Classes of Regulatory Mutants

Constitutive Mutations of the malT *Regulatory Gene*

In many regulatory systems no procedures exist for selecting certain classes of regulatory mutants. Such is the case for the *malT* gene which controls in a positive fashion the synthesis of proteins involved in maltose utilization in *E. coli* (Schwartz 1967). In the arabinose system, where positive control also operates, mutations have been detected in the *araC* gene (*araC^c* mutations) which render the arabinose operon constitutive. Strains carrying *araC^c* mutations were selected as variants resistant to the anti-inducing effects of D-fucose (Englesberg et al. 1965). A similar selection does not exist for *malT^c* mutations. However, since fusions of the *lac* genes to each of the *mal* operons exist, it becomes possible to use growth on lactose to select for regulatory effects on the maltose system. In particular, a *malA-lac* fusion has been used. Strains carrying such fusions will be unable to grow on lactose, unless the *mal* genes are induced. Among mutants derived from such strains which are able to use lactose as a carbon source are those with mutations which map in the *malT* gene and which result in constitutive expression of the *mal* genes. These are by definition presumed to be *malT^c* mutations (M. Debarbouillé, H. A. Shuman, T. J. Silhavy, and M. Schwartz, pers. comm.).

The existence of fusions for each of the *mal* operons allows selections for mutants which have altered controlling elements for each operon separately. Again, prior to the construction of *mal-lac* fusions, these mutants could not be selected.

Promoter Mutations of a Stable RNA Gene

Certain aspects of the regulation of stable RNA synthesis have been clarified in the last few years. The nature of the *rel* gene product and a role for guanosine tetraphosphate in this regulation have been established (Nomura et al. 1974). However, further elaboration of how transcription of stable RNA genes is regulated has been stymied by the limitation in doing genetic studies on such genes. The fusion of the *lac* genes to a stable RNA gene provides many of the selection and screening tools of the *lac* operon for the study of the latter system. Such fusions have been isolated between the *lac* genes and the *tyrT* or *supF* (previously termed *su3*) gene, the structural gene for a tyrosine tRNA (Berman 1977). This tRNA gene has been particularly well studied since mutations in it give rise to one of the suppressors of amber (UAG) codons (Smith 1973). However, no regulatory mutations affecting the transcription of this tyrosine tRNA gene have been defined. Using the *lac-tyrT* fusions, mutations have been characterized which, in all probability, alter the *tyrT* promoter region (Berman 1977). These mutations result in a lowered level of *lac* expression in the fusions, and when incorporated by recombination into a wild-type suppressor gene (*supF⁺*), they result in a lowered level of amber suppression. By selecting for lowered or raised levels of *lac* expression in such fusions, it should be possible to detect both linked and unlinked mutations which alter *tyrT* regulation.

Use of β-Galactosidase–Repressor Hybrid Proteins

As mentioned above, a series of strains have been isolated in which an amino-terminal portion of β-galactosidase has been replaced by an amino-terminal sequence of the *lac* repressor protein (Müller-Hill and Kania 1974). Among such hybrid proteins are some which retained both β-galactosidase and repressor activity. These results indicated that linking together domains of different proteins leads to functioning hybrid proteins. Such a process may well have been important in evolution. Cross-linking studies with the proteins provided the first evidence that repressor could be active as a dimer. In addition, such hybrids allowed analysis of the nonspecific DNA binding site at the amino terminus of the repressor (Müller-Hill et al. 1976, 1977; Kania and Müller-Hill 1977; Heidecker and Müller-Hill 1977).

β-Galactosidase as a Label for Membrane and Periplasmic Proteins

We have employed the gene fusion technique to study the mechanism of protein transport in bacteria. Proteins are found in several different cellular locations in bacteria, including the cytoplasm, the cytoplasmic membrane, the periplasmic space, and the outer membrane. In particular, we are interested in analyzing the components of genes or the proteins they code for which determine the ultimate locations of different proteins. One way to approach this question is to generate a series of strains which produce fragments of particular proteins (e.g., by using nonsense mutations) and then determine the location of each of the fragments. However, it is usually difficult to detect such protein fragments. To overcome this problem, we have chosen to label fragments of proteins with an active β-galactosidase moiety by the approaches described above. That is, we genetically fuse a protein which is ordinarily located in the cytoplasm (β-galactosidase) to one whose cellular location is elsewhere. By determining the location of the hybrid β-galactosidase molecule, we can obtain information on the gene components involved in protein transport.

As an example of the approach and the results it yields, we will describe studies on the bacteriophage λ receptor protein, which is located in the outer membrane of *E. coli*. The λ receptor is coded for by the *lamB* gene, which is part of an operon controlled by the sugar maltose (Fig. 7) (Schwartz 1967; Hofnung 1974). The *lamB* product also acts as a component of the transport system for maltodextrins (Szmelcman et al. 1976). We have isolated a number of strains in which bacteriophage Mu-1 DNA is inserted at different positions within the *lamB* gene. From these, using the Casadaban technique, we have isolated both operon fusions and gene fusions which generate hybrid proteins (Silhavy et al. 1977) (Fig. 7).

Strains carrying operon fusions, in which an intact *lacZ* gene is placed under the control of the promoter for the *lamB* gene, still show a cytoplasmic location for the β-galactosidase activity. Thus it appears that the transcriptional apparatus is not sufficient to determine the ultimate locations of gene products. However, one of the hybrid proteins generated by fusions between *lacZ* and *lamB* is located, in part, in the outer membrane. When a substantial portion of the amino-terminal sequence of the λ receptor protein is attached to β-galactosidase (Fig. 7, I), such a result is obtained. When only a very small portion is attached (Fig. 7, II), the β-galactosidase activity is found entirely in the cytoplasm. These preliminary results indicate that this approach to the mechanism of protein localization should allow us to define the region of the *lamB* gene involved in the process. This can be done by characterization of a series of fusions of this type.

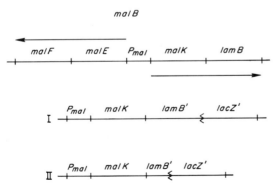

Figure 7 The *malB* region and protein fusions of *lacZ* and *lamB*. In protein fusion I, approximately 15,000 daltons of the amino-terminal sequence of the *lamB* gene product has been added to β-galactosidase. In protein fusion II, very little of the *lamB* sequence is added.

An unexpected finding in the study of certain *lacZ-lamB* fusions may allow us to define more exactly the important *lamB* components. The production of these hybrid proteins is controlled by the *mal* regulatory elements. When maltose is present in the growth media, the synthesis of the hybrid β-galactosidase is induced. Concomitant with this induction is a rapid and severe inhibition of bacterial growth. Cells do not divide effectively and some cell lysis is observed. Thus, although fusion strains producing the outer membrane hybrid protein grow normally on various minimal media, they are growth-inhibited if maltose is present. Prolonged growth in maltose-containing media results in selection for mutants which no longer make the hybrid protein. We suspect that the growth inhibition is due to the incorporation of the hybrid protein into the outer membrane or some aspect of its transport to that location. Therefore, we predict that certain of the mutants which are resistant to the growth-inhibitory effects of maltose should be altered in the transport process. The fusion strains may then allow a direct selection of mutants altering this process.

Finally, the construction of strains which produce hybrid proteins between β-galactosidase and membrane proteins may provide a handle on purifying certain membrane proteins. Heretofore the detection and purification of cytoplasmic membrane proteins involved in transport have been extremely difficult. For instance, the lactose permease (M protein) has been detected and partially purified, but the lack of an appropriate in vitro assay system and the hydrophobic nature of membrane proteins have not allowed further purification.

The existence of β-galactosidase–membrane protein hybrids, such as that involving the *malF* gene product (Silhavy et al. 1976), permits purification of whatever fragment of the membrane protein exists in the hybrid. The use of antibody to β-galactosidase, or simply separation of proteins according to molecular weight,[3] can allow rapid purification of hybrid proteins. The protein is assayed by its β-galactosidase activity. In addition to providing a portion of the membrane protein for analysis, such a purified hybrid protein may be used to elicit antibody to that portion. In turn, this antibody preparation may be used to detect and possibly purify the membrane protein itself from a wild-type strain. Experiments using this approach with a *malF-lacZ* protein fusion are presently under way (H. Shuman, unpubl.).

SUMMARY

We have reviewed some of the methods available for constructing genetic fusions with the *lac* operon of *E. coli*. The properties of these fusions

---

[3]The monomer of β-galactosidase has such a high molecular weight (approximately 116,000 daltons [Fowler and Zabin 1977]) that it is one of the few *E. coli* proteins seen in this size range. Thus, hybrid proteins are of the same or even higher molecular weight.

have opened up new approaches to several problems of gene regulation. In particular, the study of control of regulatory genes and of genes for stable RNA synthesis has been greatly facilitated by such fusions. In addition, the use of fusion techniques to isolate strains which produce hybrid proteins has generated a novel approach to certain biological processes. These techniques permit β-galactosidase activity to be used as a tag or marker for examining the synthesis, localization, and behavior of other bacterial proteins.

ACKNOWLEDGMENTS

This work was supported by grants to J. B. from the National Institutes of Health, the National Science Foundation, and the American Cancer Society. The authors are presented in alphabetical order by affiliation.

REFERENCES

Accolla, R. S. and F. Celada. 1976. Antibody-mediated activation of a deletion-mutant β-galactosidase defective in the α region. *FEBS Lett.* **67**:299.

Adhya, S. L. and J. A. Shapiro. 1969. The galactose operon of *E. coli* K-12. I. Structural and pleiotropic mutations of the operon. *Genetics* **62**:231.

Beckwith, J. R. 1970. *Lac*: The genetic system. In *The lactose operon* (ed. J. R. Beckwith and D. Zipser), p. 5. Cold Spring Harbor Laboratory, Cold Spring Harbor, New York.

Beckwith, J. R., E. R. Signer, and W. Epstein. 1967. Transposition of the *lac* region of *E. coli*. *Cold Spring Harbor Symp. Quant. Biol.* **31**:393.

Berman, M. 1977. Transfer RNA gene fusions and the study of stable RNA regulation. Ph.D. thesis, Harvard University, Cambridge, Massachusetts.

Bukhari, A. I., J. A. Shapiro, and S. L. Adhya, eds. 1977. *DNA insertion elements, plasmids, and episomes*. Cold Spring Harbor Laboratory, Cold Spring Harbor, New York.

Casadaban, M. 1976a. Transposition and fusion of the *lac* genes to selected promoters in *Escherichia coli* using bacteriophage lambda and Mu. *J. Mol. Biol.* **104**:541.

——. 1976b. Regulation of the regulatory gene for the arabinose pathway, *araC*. *J. Mol. Biol.* **104**:557.

Cohen, G. and F. Jacob. 1959. Sur la répression de la synthèse des enzymes intervenant dans la formation de tryptophane chez *E. coli*. *C.R. Acad. Sci* **248**:3490.

Cuzin, F. and F. Jacob. 1964. Délétions chromosomiques et intégration d'un épisome sexual F-*lac*+ chez *Escherichia coli* K12. *C.R. Acad. Sci.* **258**:1350.

Eckhardt, T. 1977. Use of *argA-lac* fusions to generate lambda *argA-lac* bacteriophages and to determine the direction of *argA* transcription in *Escherichia coli*. *J. Bacteriol.* **132**:60.

Englesberg, E., J. Irr, J. Power, and N. Lee. 1965. Positive control of enzyme synthesis by gene *C* in the L-arabinose system. *J. Bacteriol.* **90**:946.

Englesberg, E., R. Anderson, R. Weinberg, N. Lee, D. Hoffee, G. H. Henhauer, and H. Boyer. 1962. L-arabinose-sensitive–L-ribulose-5-phosphate-4-epimerase-deficient mutants of *E. coli. J. Bacteriol.* **84**:137.

Epp, C. and M. L. Pearson. 1976. Association of bacteriophage lambda *N* gene protein with *E. coli* RNA polymerase. In *RNA polymerase* (ed. R. Losick and M. Chamberlin), p. 683. Cold Spring Harbor Laboratory, Cold Spring Harbor, New York.

Errington, L., R. E. Glass, R. S. Hayward, and J. G. Scaife. 1974. Structure and orientation of an RNA polymerase operon in *Escherichia coli. Nature* **249**:519.

Fowler, A. V. and I. Zabin. 1977. The amino-acid sequence of β-galactosidase of *Escherichia coli. Proc. Natl. Acad. Sci.* **74**:1507.

Franklin, N. C. 1974. Altered reading of genetic signals fused to the *N* operon of bacteriophage λ: Genetic evidence for modification of polymerase by the protein product of the *N* gene. *J. Mol. Biol.* **89**:33.

Gronenborn, B. 1976. Overproduction of the phage λ repressor under control of the *lac* promoter of *Escherichia coli. Mol. Gen. Genet.* **148**:243.

Guarente, L. and J. Beckwith. 1978. A mutant RNA polymerase of *E. coli* which terminates transcription in strains making defective rho factor. *Proc. Natl. Acad. Sci.* **75**:294.

Guarente, L., D. H. Mitchell, and J. Beckwith. 1977. Transcription termination at the end of the *trp* operon of *E. coli. J. Mol. Biol.* **112**:423.

Heidecker, G. and B. Müller-Hill. 1977. Synthetic multifunctional proteins: Isolation of covalently linked tryptophan synthetase α-subunit–*lac*-repressor–β-galactosidase chimeras. *Mol. Gen. Genet.* **155**:301.

Hofnung, M. 1974. Divergent operons and the genetic structure of the maltose B region in *Escherichia coli* K12. *Genetics* **76**:169.

Hopkins, J. D. 1974. A new class of promoter mutations in the lactose operon of *Escherichia Coli. J. Mol. Biol.* **87**:715.

Ino, I., P. Hartman, Z. Hartman, and J. Yourno. 1975. Deletions fusing the *hisG* and *hisD* genes in *Salmonella typhimurium. J. Bacteriol.* **123**:1254.

Jackson, E. and C. Yanofsky. 1974. Localization of two functions of the phosphoribosyl anthranilate transferase of *E. coli* to distinct regions of the polypeptide chain. *J. Bacteriol.* **117**:502.

Jacob, F., A. Ullmann, and J. Monod. 1965. Délétions fusionnant l'opéron lactose et un opéron purine chez *E. coli. J. Mol. Biol.* **13**:704.

Kania, J. and B. Müller-Hill. 1977. Construction, isolation and implications of repressor-galactosidase:β-galactosidase hybrid molecules. *Eur. J. Biochem.* **79**:381.

Kelker, N. and T. Eckhardt. 1977. Regulation of *argA* expression in *Escherichia coli* K-12. Cell-free synthesis of β-galactosidase under *argA* control. *J. Bacteriol.* **132**:67.

Kessler, D. and E. Englesberg. 1969. Arabinose-leucine deletion mutants of *E. coli* B/r. *J. Bacteriol.* **98**:1159.

Ketner, G. and A. Campbell. 1974. A deletion mutation placing the galactokinase gene of *E. coli* under control of the biotin promoter. *Proc. Natl. Acad. Sci.* **71**:2698.

Miller, J. H., W. S. Reznikoff, A. E. Silverstone, K. Ippen, E. R. Signer, and J. R. Beckwith. 1970. Fusions of the *lac* and *trp* regions of the *E. coli* chromosome. *J. Bacteriol.* **104**:1273.

Mitchell, D. H., W. S. Reznikoff, and J. Beckwith. 1975. Genetic fusions defining *trp* and *lac* regulatory elements. *J. Mol. Biol.* **93**:331.

———. 1976. Genetic fusions that help define a transcription termination region in *E. coli. J. Mol. Biol.* **101**:441.

Müller-Hill, B. and J. Kania. 1974. *Lac* repressor can be fused to β-galactosidase. *Nature* **249**:561.

Müller-Hill, B., B. Gronenborn, J. Kania, M. Schlotmann and K. Beyreuther. 1977. Similarities between lac repressor and lambda repressor. In *Nucleic acid-protein recognition* (ed. H. Vogel), p. 219. Academic Press, New York.

Müller-Hill, B., G. Heidecker, and J. Kania. 1976. Repressor-galactosidase chimeras. In *Proceedings of the Third John Innes Symposium: Structure-function relationships of proteins* (ed. R. Markham and R. W. Horne), p. 167. Elsevier/North-Holland, Amsterdam.

Nomura, M. and F. Engbaek. 1972. Expression of ribosomal protein genes as analyzed by bacteriophage Mu-induced mutations. *Proc. Natl. Acad. Sci.* **69**:1526.

Nomura, M., A. Tissières, and P. Lengyel, eds. 1974. *Ribosomes.* Cold Spring Harbor Laboratory, Cold Spring Harbor, New York.

Reznikoff, W. and J. R. Beckwith. 1969. Genetic evidence that the operator locus is distinct from the Z gene in the *lac* operon of *E. coli. J. Mol. Biol.* **43**:215.

Reznikoff, W. and K. Thornton. 1972. Isolating tryptophan regulatory mutants in *E. coli* by using a *trp-lac* fusion strain. *J. Bacteriol.* **109**:526.

Reznikoff, W., J. H. Miller, J. G. Scaife, and J. R. Beckwith. 1969. A mechanism for repressor action. *J. Mol. Biol.* **43**:201.

Schwartz, M. 1967. Sur l'existence chez *Escherichia coli* K12 d'une régulation commune à la biosynthèse des récepteurs du bactériophage λ et au métabolisme du maltose. *Ann. Inst. Pasteur* (Paris) **113**:685.

Silvahy, T. J., M. J. Casadaban, H. A. Shuman, and J. R. Beckwith. 1976. Conversion of β-galactosidase to a membrane-bound state by gene fusion. *Proc. Natl. Acad. Sci.* **73**:3423.

Silhavy, T. J., H. A. Shuman, J. Beckwith, and M. Schwartz. 1977. The use of gene fusions to study outer membrane protein localization in *Escherichia coli. Proc. Natl. Acad. Sci.* **74**:5411.

Smith, J. D. 1973. Genetic and structural analysis of transfer RNA. *Br. Med. Bull.* **29**:220.

Szmelcman, S., M. Schwartz, T. J. Silhavy, and W. Boos. 1976. A comparison of transport kinetics in wild-type and λ-resistant mutants with the dissociation constants of the maltose-binding protein as measured by fluorescence quenching. *Eur. J. Biochem.* **65**:13.

Taylor, A. L. 1963. Bacteriophage-induced mutations in *Escherichia coli. Proc. Natl. Acad. Sci.* **50**:1043.

Yourno, J., T. Kohno, and J. Roth. 1970. Enzyme evolution: Generation of a bifunctional enzyme by fusion of adjacent genes. *Nature* **228**:820.

Zabin, I., A. V. Fowler, and J. R. Beckwith. 1978. Position of the mutation in beta-galactosidase ochre mutant U118. *J. Bacteriol.* **133**:437.

Zubay, G., D. E. Morse, W. Schrenk, and J. Miller. 1972. Detection and isolation of the repressor protein for the tryptophan operon of *E. coli. Proc. Natl. Acad. Sci.* **69**:1100.

Regulation of Gene Expression in the Tryptophan Operon of *Escherichia coli*

Terry Platt
Department of Molecular Biophysics and Biochemistry
Yale University
New Haven, Connecticut 06510

INTRODUCTION

The classic model of Jacob and Monod (1961) for induction and repression of operon expression provided a conceptual framework for integrating observations on cellular metabolism with a mechanism of regulation at the molecular level. In recent years, direct physical evidence has confirmed the essential predictions of their hypothesis for the lactose operon, as summarized elsewhere in this volume. In general, their ideas have been exceptionally valuable when applied to other systems as well. However, regulation of the *lac* gene cluster has proved more intricate than originally envisioned, and regulatory features have been discovered which cannot be accommodated in the simple repressor-operator model of regulation. The tryptophan (*trp*) operon of *Escherichia coli* also possesses regulatory features of several types in addition to repressor-operator interaction, and the purpose of this review is to summarize current knowledge of the molecular aspects of structure and regulation within the *trp* operon.

The tryptophan operon consists of five contiguous structural genes (which code for enzymes participating in the biosynthetic pathway from chorismic acid to tryptophan) and the associated control elements (see Fig. 1). The five genes are transcribed as a single polycistronic messenger RNA approximately 7000 nucleotides long. Initiation of transcription is controlled by the interaction of the tryptophan repressor (the protein product of *trpR*) with its target site on the DNA, the operator (*trpO*). Repressor binding at *trpO* competes with RNA polymerase binding at the adjacent promoter site, *trpP* (Squires et al. 1975). Transcription of the messenger RNA is initiated within the promoter-operator region 162 nucleotides before the first structural gene (*trpE*), and this point defines the beginning of the "leader region," which is the transcribed segment of DNA between *trpO* and *trpE* (Bronson et al. 1973; Squires et al. 1976; Lee et al. 1978). The leader region contains an "attenuator" site (*trp a*)

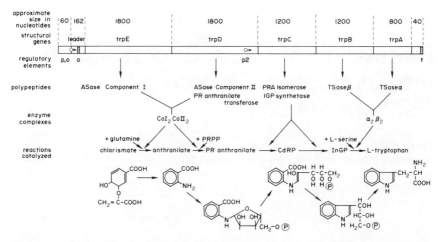

Figure 1 Genes of the tryptophan operon of *E. coli*, their polypeptide products, and reactions catalyzed by polypeptides or polypeptide complexes. Regulatory elements are the primary promoter (*trpP*), the operator (*trpO*), the attenuator (*trp a*), the secondary internal promoter (*trpP2*), and the terminator (*trp t*). Sites of mRNA initiation are given by ○→, sites of termination by ▨. CoI and CoII signify components I and II, respectively, of the anthranilate synthetase complex; PR-anthranilate is *N*-5′-phosphoribosyl-anthranilate; CdRP is 1-(*o*-carboxy-phenylamino)-1-deoxyribulose-5-phosphate; InGP is indole-3-glycerol phosphate; and PRPP is 5-phosphoribosyl-1-phyrophosphate. The convention has been adopted to use uppercase letters for structural genes and lowercase letters for regulating elements. (Adapted from Yanofsky 1971.)

approximately 140 nucleotides from the 5′ end of the mRNA, which causes partial termination of transcription and thus regulates the fraction of initiated RNA polymerase molecules that actually transcribe the structural genes of the operon (Bertrand et al. 1975; Pannekoek et al. 1975; Morse and Morse 1976). At the end of the operon, termination of transcription occurs within a few hundred nucleotides beyond the end of *trpA*, the last structural gene of the operon (Rose and Yanofsky 1971; A. M. Wu and T. Platt, in prep.). Figure 2 shows the location on the *E. coli* genetic map of some additional unlinked genes whose products are involved in regulating or responding to the intracellular levels of tryptophan. These include, in addition to the repressor gene (*trpR*), the genes for the tryptophanyl-tRNA synthetase (*trpS*), tRNA^{Trp} (*trpT*), and transcription termination factor (rho).

Many factors thus contribute to the level of *trp* operon expression in the cell, including (1) feedback inhibition of enzyme activity, (2) repression, (3) attenuation of transcription, (4) metabolic regulation (growth-rate dependence of RNA and protein synthesis), (5) internal initiation of transcription, and possibly (6) the rate of mRNA degradation. There is as

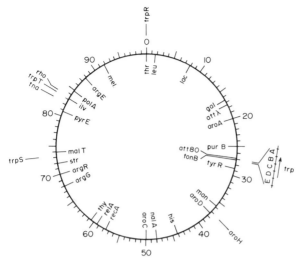

Figure 2 Genetic map of *E. coli*, indicating positions for some of the genes involved in *trp* operon expression or a response to tryptophan. In addition to the *trp* operon (*trpEDCBA*), these include the *trp* repressor (*trpR*), the 3-deoxy-D-arabinoheptulosonic acid-7-phosphate (DAHP) synthetase (*aroH*), the tryptophanyl tRNA synthetase (*trpS*), the tryptophanyl tRNA (*trpT*), tryptophanase (*tna*), and transcription termination factor rho (*rho*).

yet no evidence that termination of transcription at the end of the operon has any effect on the levels of gene products produced.

FEEDBACK INHIBITION AND ALLOSTERIC REGULATION

A classic mechanism for regulating the activity of a pathway is end-product inhibition (of an early enzyme in the pathway), as shown for the *trp* operon by Cohen and Jacob (1959). The first enzyme complex unique to tryptophan biosynthesis is the anthranilate synthetase aggregate, a tetrameric molecule consisting of two subunits of component I and two of component II, the polypeptide products of *trpE* and *trpD*, respectively (Ito and Yanofsky 1966). This enzyme complex functions both to produce anthranilate on one subunit (from chorismate and glutamine) and to consume it on the other (by conversion to phosphoribosyl-anthranilate), as shown in Figure 1. Both of these activities are feedback-inhibited by L-tryptophan, the ultimate end product of the pathway (Ito and Yanofsky 1969). The binding site for tryptophan is on the component-I subunit, and tryptophan can inhibit the synthetase activity of component I completely (the K_i for tryptophan inhibition is 1×10^{-6} M); in contrast, the maximum observable inhibition by tryptophan of the phosphoribosyl-anthranilate transferase activity of component II is only 70% (Ito and Yanofsky 1969). Since component II uncomplexed with component I is not susceptible to tryptophan inhibition, the component-II moiety of the aggregate must become sensitive to tryptophan-stimulated changes in the conformation of component I.

Tryptophan binding and inhibition of the anthranilate synthetase reaction are competitive with chorismate on component I (Baker and Crawford 1966; Henderson and Zalkin 1971). Yet they do not appear to share the same binding site: the K_i for tryptophan inhibition can be altered by a single-site mutation in *trpE* without affecting the K_m (5×10^{-6} M) for chorismate (Somerville and Yanofsky 1965; Pabst et al. 1973). The anthranilate synthetase reaction requires the hydrolysis of glutamine (if glutamine is the amino donor, as it is under most physiological conditions), but binding and hydrolysis of glutamine take place on the component-II subunit. Glutamine binding can occur in the absence of chorismate (Pabst et al. 1973), but glutamine hydrolysis by the anthranilate aggregate is greatly stimulated by the binding of chorismate and is inhibited by tryptophan (Somerville and Elford 1967; Pabst and Somerville 1971). Since double reciprocal plots of kinetic data indicate a pattern of competitive interaction between glutamine and tryptophan, and since their binding sites are on opposite subunits, glutamine too must participate in the regulatory properties of the aggregate.

It is thus apparent that recognition of the different substrates on their respective subunit binding sites can be communicated, presumably by allosteric conformational changes, to the opposite subunits. Pabst et al. (1973) have presented a model, shown in Figure 3, which is consistent with the known binding and kinetic data for tryptophan, chorismate, and glutamine interaction with the enzyme complex. Although the molecular details are not yet known and the overall picture of ligand interactions and conformational changes in vivo is far more complex, the model may be regarded as a description of one aspect of anthranilate aggregate function and provides a useful framework for predictions and future experiments.

REPRESSION AND THE INITIATION OF TRANSCRIPTION

Expression of the tryptophan operon is subject to negative control mediated by a regulatory gene, *trpR*, unlinked to the tryptophan operon (Cohen and Jacob 1959; see Fig. 2). This gene codes for a *trans*-dominant activity that reduces expression of the operon in the presence of excess tryptophan. Constitutive mutations which result in elevated levels of enzyme synthesis have been isolated both in *trpR* (Cohen and Jacob 1959; Morse and Yanofsky 1969a; Gardner et al. 1974) and in the operator, *trp o* (Hiraga 1969); those in the operator site are *cis*-dominant, indicating

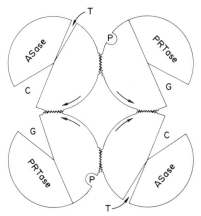

Figure 3 Model for regulation of the anthranilate aggregate. The model shows the four subunits of the anthranilate aggregate interconnected by gear teeth, which represent the bonding domains constituting the mechanism of communication between the subunits. The areas labeled C, T, G, and P are, respectively, the chorismate-binding site, the tryptophan-binding site, the site of glutamine hydrolysis, and the phosphoribosyl-transferase active site. Anthranilate synthesis probably takes place at or near the site of the chorismate binding. The outer segments of each subunit are supposed to be stationary, while the inner segments are capable of movement in the directions indicated by the arrows. The model is shown in the activated conformation. The chorismate site is open and the tryptophan site is closed. At the same time, the glutamine site is open, and the phosphoribosyl-transferase site is exposed and functioning. When tryptophan binds, the T site is enlarged. This results in a conformational change indicated by the arrows which close the chorismate site. Each conformational change is communicated to all other subunits through the gear teeth. The result is that the sites of glutamine hydrolysis on the phosphoribosyl-transferase subunits are closed, and the phosphoribosyl-transferase-active site is partially buried. This signal is also communicated to the opposite anthranilate synthetase subunit where the tryptophan site is partially opened and the chorismate site partially closed, encouraging the binding of a second molecule of tryptophan, and thus exhibiting cooperativity. (Adapted from Pabst et al. 1973.)

that *trpO* is the target site in the DNA for the *trpR* product, the repressor. When a cell is deprived of functional repressor, *trp*-specific enzyme synthesis is induced about 70-fold above the basal or "repressed" level. Some *trpR* constitutive mutations are suppressed by amber suppressors, indicating that the gene product is a protein (Morse and Yanofsky 1969a).

The repressor has been partially purified and studies in vitro confirm that the active form of repressor is a protein (the aporepressor) of about 58,000 daltons (Zubay et al. 1972) complexed with its corepressor, L-tryptophan (Squires et al. 1973; McGeoch et al. 1973). It is not known whether the repressor consists of more than one polypeptide chain. The active repressor complex binds to the *trp* operator with a dissociation constant of about 2×10^{-10} M in 0.12 M salt at 37°C, and the half-time for this dissociation is less than 2 minutes (Rose and Yanofsky 1974). In vivo, when the cytoplasmic levels of free tryptophan drop to a low level (the K_m of tryptophan for the aporepressor is $1-2 \times 10^{-5}$ M [Rose et al. 1973]), the repressor dissociates from the operator, permitting transcription to proceed at an elevated level. Some tryptophan analogs, such as 4-, 5-, and 6-methyltryptophan, can also activate aporepressor (Mosteller and Yanofsky 1971; Cohen and Jacob 1959), whereas others such as indole-3-propionic acid and indole-acrylic acid are competitive inhibitors that prevent tryptophan binding and thereby effectively inactivate the repressor (Doolittle and Yanofsky 1968; Rose et al. 1973; Squires et al. 1975). As is the case with many regulatory proteins, there are only 20–30 molecules of repressor per cell (Zubay et al. 1972; Rose and Yanofsky 1974). For this reason, purification and further characterization of the repressor have been difficult.

The *trp* promoter (*trpP*), the site of initiation of transcription by RNA polymerase, is located shortly before the structural genes of the operon (Bronson et al. 1973), as is the operator. In vitro, when repressor (aporepressor + tryptophan) is added to a minimal transcription system consisting of a *trp* DNA template, RNA polymerase, and nucleoside triphosphates in an appropriate buffer, transcription of *trp* mRNA is specifically inhibited. This effect is dependent on the presence of both tryptophan and aporepressor (Rose et al. 1973; McGeoch et al 1973). Moreover, it has been shown in vitro that, in a functional sense, the promoter and operator sites overlap one another: when repressor is prebound to the operator, it prevents the initiation of *trp*-specific transcription, and conversely, prebound RNA polymerase cannot be prevented from transcribing the operon by the subsequent addition of repressor (Squires et al. 1975). Interactions in this region appear to be confined to competition between the *trp* repressor and RNA polymerase for their respective (overlapping) binding sites on the DNA. Contrary to early suggestions, a direct involvement in the repressor-mediated regulation of transcription by either tRNA^{Trp} or by the tryptophanyl-tRNA synthetase has now been ruled out by experiments performed in vivo (Mosteller and Yanofsky 1971) and in vitro (Squires et al. 1973).

The entire nucleotide sequence of the *trp* promoter-operator region is now known (Bennett et al. 1976, 1977, 1978b) and is shown in Figure 4. Squires et al. (1976) identified the 5' terminus of the mRNA as pppAAG . . ., thus localizing the point of transcription initiation on the DNA. When an initiation complex between RNA polymerase and the DNA is formed in the absence of one or more triphosphates, elongation does not occur, but the bound polymerase is capable of protecting the region from position -19 to $+18$ from digestion by DNase, where the $+1$ position is defined as the first transcribed nucleotide (Bennett et al. 1976;

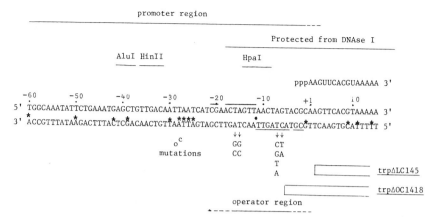

Figure 4 The promoter-operator region of the tryptophan operon. The sequence shown is from *E. coli* (asterisks indicate the positions which differ in *S. typhimurium*) and probably is sufficient for full promoter function. The region protected by RNA polymerase from DNase-I digestion is indicated, and protection from restriction endonuclease cleavage extends to the *Hpa*I, *Hin*II, and *Alu*I sites as well (see text). The start point of *trp* mRNA occurs at position +1. Repressor also protects the *Hpa*I site, and the five *trpO^c* mutations bracket this region, which possesses an axis of symmetry (shown by bars). Of the two deletions, *trpΔLD145* is *trpO^+* and *trpΔOC1419* is *trpO^-* (both retain *trpO* activity). Both promoter and operator must extend leftward beyond position −17 or so. (Data adapted from Bertrand et al. 1976; Bennett et al. 1976, 1977, 1978a,b); Brown et al. 1978; Bennett and Yanofsky 1978).

Brown et al. 1978) (see Fig. 4). Bennett et al. (1976) showed that polymerase bound to this region prevented cleavage by the restriction endonuclease *Hpa*I at a site (−9 to −14) in the DNA, and that repressor, if bound independently, also protected this same site from cleavage. This confirms directly that the promoter and operator sites overlap one another, as previously indicated by the results of Squires et al. (1975).

Bennett and Yanofsky (1978) have defined the extent of the operator more accurately by analyzing deletion mutants with endpoints in the operator region and by identifying the base-pair changes in operator-constitutive point mutations. The deletion *trpΔLD145* removes all of the sequence to the right of the +1 position and trtains full operator activity; a second deletion, *trpΔOC1418*, removes all of the sequence to the right of the −5 position and is operator-negative (Bertrand et al. 1976; Bennett et al. 1976; Bennett and Yanofsky 1978) (see Fig. 4). Thus the functional right-hand endpoint of the *trp* operator must lie between −5 and +1, and the features conveying specificity cannot extend significantly into the transcribed leader region. The early (left-hand) portion of the *trp* regulatory region is lacking in the transducing phage *λtrp*ED46, which only carries *trp* operon sequences from approximately −17 rightward through *trpD*. Although λ*trp*ED46 does carry the *Hpa*I site (at −9 to −14), the *trp* repressor is unable to bind and protect this site from cleavage, in contrast to the normal situation (Bennett et al. 1976). Thus, sequence information important for binding must occur within the portion of *trp* DNA not carried on λ*trp*ED46. The required sequences probably do not extend as far left as the *Hin*II site (−32 to −37) in the regulatory region, since bound *trp* repressor cannot protect this site from endonuclease cleavage (Bennett and Yanofsky 1978). Overall, these data imply that the functional sequences of the *trp* operator are located between −37 and +1 in the regulatory region, including at least the portion between −17 and −5 as indicated in Figure 4 (Bennett and Yanofsky 1978).

A closer look at the DNA sequence across the operator region shows that it possesses striking twofold symmetry (in 18 of the 20 base pairs between −21 and −2), centered around the *Hpa*I cleavage site (Bennett et al. 1976). Bennett and Yanofsky (1978) analyzed nine independently isolated operator-constitutive (*trpO*^{c}) mutations and found five different base-pair changes occurring at positions −6, −7, −15, and −16 (Fig. 4). One of the mutations at −7 is symmetrically equivalent to the one at −16, both being A:T to C:G transversions (Bennett and Yanofsky 1978). These two mutations exhibit nearly the same levels of *trp* operon expression, in contrast to that given by the other observed base alteration at −7 (A:T to T:A) (Bennett and Yanofsky 1978). It is probably not accidental that the two clusters of *trpO*^{c} mutations are separated by about one turn of the DNA helix, but it is surprising that no mutations between −7 and −15 have been identified. Possibly conservation of this region is required for maximum promoter function, as suggested by Bennett et al. (1978a).

The entire sequence from position −2 to −24 in *Salmonella typhimurium* is identical to that in *E. coli* (Bennett et al. 1978a), which explains the ability of *S. typhimurium* repressor to regulate the *E. coli* operon normally, and vice versa (Somerville 1966; Manson and Yanofsky 1976). Manson and Yanofsky (1976) have shown that such interspecific repression in heterologous hybrids exists as well between *E. coli* and *Shigella dysenteriae, Klebsiella aerogenes, Serratia marcescens*, and *Proteus mirabilis*. It therefore seems likely that the *trp* operator is highly conserved throughout the enterobacteria. One possible explanation for the lack of divergence is that there may be other constraints on repressor-operator interaction. For example, in *E. coli*, the *aroH* locus[1] is also under the control of *trpR* (Brown 1968; Camakaris and Pittard 1971) (see Fig. 2). Thus the repressor must interact with at least two operators.

The DNA sequences involved in interaction with RNA polymerase

[1]The *aroH* product is one of the three DAHP synthetases that catalyze the first step in aromatic amino acid biosynthesis (Brown 1968).

appear to extend over a region somewhat broader than the operator. In addition to the 37 base pairs protected by RNA polymerase from DNase-I digestion (Bennett et al. 1976), polymerase also protects a *Hin*II site from −32 to −37 and an *Alu*I site from −38 to −41 from cleavage by the respective restriction endonuclease (Jones and Reznikoff 1977; Brown et al. 1978) (see Fig. 4).

Transcription of the leader region can be observed in vitro using certain fragments obtained by restriction endonuclease digestion. In particular, a fragment bounded by the *Hha*I cut at −78 can promote *trp* transcription, whereas an *Alu*I fragment that ends at −39 cannot (Brown et al. 1978). Thus, sequences to the left of −78 are not necessary for promoter function, whereas some region (or perhaps just more DNA) to the left of the *Alu*I site at −39 is required (Fig. 4). Analogous studies by Bennett et al. (1978a) with this region from *S. typhimurium*, which is very similar to the *E. coli* sequence, suggest that promoter function is contained within the 59 base pairs preceding the mRNA initiation site. Although the "promoter region" may be considered to include the DNA sequences protected by RNA polymerase from nuclease attack, strict sequence conservation within this region is clearly not required for function. The five different *trpO^c* mutations (Fig. 4) have no significant effect on *trp* promoter activity, although they are within the region protected from DNase I and bracket the *Hpa*I cleavage site mentioned above (Bennett and Yanofsky 1978). Likewise, the deletions *trpΔLD145* and *trpΔOC1418*, which end at +1 and −5, respectively (Fig. 4), exhibit less than a twofold reduction of operon expression, suggesting that base specificity beyond −5 is not crucial for promoter activity (Bennett et al. 1976; Bertrand et al. 1976; Bennett and Yanofsky 1978).

A detailed comparison of the *E. coli* sequence in this regulatory region with the same region of *S. typhimurium* shows that the sequence differences (which average about one in six) appear confined to certain regions of the DNA (Bennett et al. 1977, 1978a). On the basis of these differences and an analysis of other promoter regions, Bennett et al. (1978a) suggest that (1) there are sequence-specific polymerase contacts in the −38 to −31 region (which is highly conserved), (2) there are weak interactions in the AT-rich "bridge" from −30 to −25, (3) there is tight binding in the −20 to −5 region preceding the mRNA start point, and (4) a specific sequence is not required in the −5 to +18 region. These results are consistent with observations in other systems that a critical region for RNA polymerase function occurs approximately 35 nucleotides prior to the site of mRNA initiation as well as in the region immediately preceding the point of transcription initiation (see discussion in Gilbert 1976; Reznikoff and Abelson, this volume). Further studies on the *trp* promoters of other enterobacteria may be expected to yield insights into promoter and operator relationships which cannot be obtained by comparisons between unrelated systems, where differing functional and regulatory requirements may dominate the primary structure and obscure common features.

Promoter regions may occur elsewhere than at the beginning of operons. Bauerle and Margolin (1967) reported the discovery in *S. typhimurium* of an internal promoter in the wild-type *trp* operon, which they called *p2* (here *trpP2*; see Fig. 1); the same feature was subsequently found in *E. coli* by Morse and Yanofsky (1968). In *E. coli*, this low-level promoter results in nonrepressible synthesis of the *trpC*, *trpB*, and *trpA* gene products at about 3% of the derepressed levels; initiations at *trpP2* appear to be responsible for about 80% of the *trpC*, *trpB*, and *trpA* polypeptides present in repressed cells (see Table 1). Jackson and Yanofsky (1972a) subsequently mapped this promoter late within the *trpD* structural gene, but operator-proximal to at least two *trpD* point mutations. Recent evidence indicates that *trpP2* must occur within 200 nucleotides of the beginning of the following gene, *trpC* (G. E. Christie and T. Platt, unpubl.), but its functional significance in the operon is unknown.

Internal promoters have also been observed as the result of mutational events in the *trp* operons of *S. typhimurium* (Wuesthoff and Bauerle 1970) and *E. coli* (McPartland and Somerville 1974). One constitutive promoter in *trpE* isolated by Morse and Yanofsky (1969b) is unusual because its low reversion rate (2×10^{-8}) is not affected by various mutagens, and reversion restores only partial activity to *trpE*. It has not been determined whether this promoter represents an insertion of a foreign promoter into *trpE* or is the fortuitous result of a small deletion or other unusual alteration in the DNA.

There are numerous other sites in the *trp* operon where new constitutive promoters can arise by mutation (McPartland and Somerville 1974), and two high-efficiency promoters of this type have been analyzed

Table 1 The internal promoter *P2* of the *E. coli trp* operon

Strain	trpR	trpP2	PRATase (trpD)	TSase β_2 (trpB)
Wild type	+	+	0.031	0.6
Wild type	−	+	2.3 (74)	12.5 (21)
trpΔED53	+	−	0	0.15
trpΔED53	−	−	0	11.0 (73)

The numbers are specific activities in units/mg in extracts of cells grown in the presence of excess tryptophan; the numbers in parentheses are derepression ratios. All strains had a normal primary promoter. Deletion of the internal promoter, *trpP2* in strain (*trpΔED53*) indicates that it is responsible for about 0.45 units/mg of β_2 activity, or 3% of the derepressed level, and that normally promoted synthesis of *trpD* and *trpB* proteins is increased 70–75-fold upon derepression. (Data adapted from Jackson and Yanofsky 1972a.)

in detail (McPartland and Somerville 1976). Under repressed conditions, both yield 15-fold higher levels of *trpC*, *trpB*, and *trpA* gene products than the wild type, and reversion analysis indicates that they are probably single base changes. Precise mapping for one of these, *trp-3B*, was not possible—it is most likely a noncritical missense mutation within *trpD*, though insertion of a foreign promoter into the *trpD-trpC* intercistronic region has not been excluded. The other mutation, *trpD11*, creates a UAA nonsense codon located, by deletion mapping, between the *P2* promoter and the *trpD-trpC* junction. Introduction of an ochre suppressor into this strain restores phosphoribosyl-anthranilate transferase activity (see Fig. 1), but suppression does not reduce the high levels of distal enzyme synthesis promoted by *trpD11*. At this same site, UAG and UGA, but not AGA, also exhibit high promoter activity. Classes of pseudo wild-type revertants (i.e., possessing *trpD* activity) from each of the four codons are found which also retain promoter activity (Hausler and Somerville 1977). Altogether, 16 codon changes from the wild-type CAA (glutamine) codon at this site have been characterized, and 10 of these have high-level promoter activity (R. L. Somerville, pers. comm.). It is not known whether the high-efficiency initiation of transcription brought about by these mutations is dependent on *trpP2* function. However, in this general region of DNA, a number of different sequences can clearly function as promoters and single base changes can have dramatic effects on their efficiencies.

THE LEADER SEQUENCE AND ATTENUATION

In 1973, Bronson et al. established the existence of a significant length of mRNA preceding the first known structural gene in the tryptophan operon messenger RNA. The transcribed segment of 162 nucleotides preceding the initiation codon of *trpE* was called the "leader sequence" (see Fig. 5) and exhibited some remarkable features that now explain earlier puzzling observations on the regulation of *trp* expression. Jackson and Yanofsky (1973) had observed that two particular internal *trp* deletions resulted in a *cis*-dominant increase in the expression of distal genes in the operon; since one endpoint of both deletions was between *trpE* and the *trp* operator, they postulated a regulatory function for this region of the operon. Subsequent studies (Bertrand et al. 1975) demonstrated that this leader region contained a site or sites responsible for partial termination of transcription of *trp* mRNA, thus explaining why deletion of this locus resulted in increased distal gene expression.

Kasai (1974) observed that the histidine operon in *S. typhimurium* had a similar transcription barrier, which he called the "attenuator," between the promoter and the first gene (*hisG*) that, when deleted, permitted RNA polymerase to transcribe the operon with enhanced frequency.

```
                            leader polypeptide (hypothetical)

                    MET-LYS-ALA-ILE-PHE-VAL-LEU-LYS-GLY-TRP-TRP-ARG-THR-SER
pppAAGUUCACGUAAAAAGGGUAUCGACA AUG AAA GCA AUU UUC GUA CUG AAA GGU UGG UGG CGC ACU UCC UGAAACGGGCAGUGUA
           ─────────────────────
                ribosome protection

                                                                       trpE protein
                                                       MET-GLN-THR-GLN-LYS-PRO
UUCACCAUGCGUAAAGCAAUCAGAUACCCAGCCCGCCUAAUGAGCGGGCUUUUUUUUGAACAAAAUUAGAGAAUAACA AUG CAA ACA CAA AAA CCG
                                                                   ─────────────────────
                                                                   ribosome protection
```

Figure 5 The 5′-terminal region of tryptophan operon mRNA. The 162 transcribed nucleotides preceding *trpE* are called leader mRNA and serve no known function. An early ribosome-binding site may initiate synthesis of a small peptide as shown, and the tandem tryptophan codons may play a role in regulation at the attenuator. This sequence is considerably larger than that preceding the first structural gene in the *lac* and *gal* operons (Maizels 1974; Musso et al. 1974; and this volume). (Data from Squires et al. 1976; Platt et al. 1976; Lee and Yanofsky 1977; Lee et al. 1978.)

Studies with a DNA-dependent protein-synthesizing system in vitro supported Kasai's genetic observations (Artz and Broach 1975) and provided evidence for an independent positive control system for this operon as well, involved ppGpp (Stephens et al. 1975). The attenuator in the *his* operon of *S. typhimurium* is similar to the partial transcriptional barrier in the *trp* operon of *E. coli* in that (1) it acts as a transcription termination site, (2) it is located between the promoter and the first structural gene, (3) deletion of the attenuator enhances expression of the operon, and (4) one or more protein factors may interact to regulate transcription termination at the site.

In *E. coli*, the internal *trp* deletion strain *trp*Δ*LD102* yields distal enzyme levels eight- to tenfold above wild type (Jackson and Yanofsky 1973; Bertrand et al. 1976), but regulation by the *trp* repressor is normal in this strain (Table 2). Thus the operator is still functionally intact, and since it is the basal (repressed) levels of enzyme that are proportionally higher in the deletion strains, the regulatory site in the leader region must be functioning independently of repressor-operator interaction (Yanofsky 1976b). Experiments performed in *trpR* strains therefore permit attenuation effects to be separated from repressor effects.

In *trpR trp+* cells, the rate of synthesis of *trp* mRNA from the leader region is eight to ten times greater than the rate of distal (*trpBA*) mRNA synthesis, an effect probably not due to an altered rate of messenger degradation (Betrand et al. 1975; Pannekoek et al. 1975; Bertrand et al. 1976; Bertrand and Yanofsky 1976). Bertrand et al. (1976) detected a major, discrete species of mRNA corresponding to the first 140-nucleotide pairs of the leader region. This species is present in large molar excess over distal mRNA, which suggests that partial termination of transcription is occurring about 20 base pairs before *trpE*. The

Table 2 Attenuation is independent of repression

Strain	$trpR^+$	$trpR^-$
$trp\Delta ED53$ (*trp* a^+)	0.17	11.8 (69)
$trp\Delta LD102$ (*trp* a^-)	1.32	100 (76)

The numbers are tryptophan-synthetase-β_2-specific activities in units/mg, in extracts of cells grown in the presence of excess tryptophan; derepression ratios are in parentheses. Both strains delete the *trpP2* (see Table 1), though neither deletes *trpP* or *trpO*. Deletion of the attenuator by $trp\Delta LD102$ increases repressed and derepressed enzyme levels by eight to tenfold without significantly affecting the derepression ratio. (Data from Yanofsky 1976a.)

efficiency of this termination event, however, depends on the level of tryptophan present. Starvation for tryptophan "relieves" attenuation and permits most RNA polymerase molecules to read through the attenuation signal (Bertrand and Yanofsky 1976; Morse and Morse 1976).

Recent observations on the suppression of polarity support the notion that attenuation is mediated by transcription termination. In the polarity-supressing strain *suA*, the *E. coli* transcription termination factor rho, first characterized by Roberts (1969), has been shown to be altered (Ratner 1976). Several suppressors of mutational polarity isolated by Korn and Yanofsky (1976a) relieve *trp* attenuation and also elevate the synthesis of distal gene products in the wild-type operon (Table 3) without

Table 3 Attenuation is affected by *rho*, *trpT*, *trpX*, and *trpS* mutations in *trpR* strains

Strain (*trpR* derivative)	Enzyme levels (normalized)	
	wild type (*trp* a^+)	$trp\Delta LD102$ (*trp* a^-)
Wild type	1.0	7.1
rho102	2.8	7.0
$trpT_{ts}$	7.1	—
trpX	4.5	6.7
trpS9969	2.7	7.5

All strains were *trpR* (derepressed) and grown in the presence of excess tryptophan; $trp\Delta LD102$ deletes the attenuator. Enzyme levels were measured on anthranilate synthetase for the $trpT_{ts}$ strain, and tryptophan synthetase for the *rho102*, *trpX*, and *trpS9969* strains. (Data adapted from Korn and Yanofsky 1976a; Yanofsky 1976b; Yanofsky and Soll 1977.)

affecting the rates of *trp* mRNA degradation. An altered rho protein has been identified in some of these polarity-suppressing strains (Korn and Yanofsky 1976b), and the lesion in rho is presumed to result in less efficient termination than usual at the attenuator site. However, not all polarity suppressors with an altered rho protein have an effect upon *trp* attenuation. Among suppressors of this class are *suA*, *rho103*, *rho104*, and *rho201* (Korn and Yanofsky 1976b; Guarente et al. 1977; Guarente and Beckwith 1978).

Several important observations on the nature of attenuation have been described by Morse and Morse (1976). First, their data indicate that in vivo this tryptophan-mediated arrest of transcription within the leader sequence is resistant to rifampicin (which has its effect on the initiation of transcription) but sensitive to streptolidigin (which affects the process of elongation). Second, if initiation of *trp* mRNA is halted by the addition of rifampicin, and immediately afterward the cells are starved for tryptophan, pulse-labeling of the mRNA demonstrates an increase in *trp* operon expression. These points indicate that attenuation must occur after RNA polymerase initiates transcription of *trp* mRNA and that it has its effect during the elongation process. Furthermore, the effect is specific to tryptophan, since neither starvation for other amino acids (histidine, arginine, cysteine, or isoleucine) nor the addition of chloramphenicol relieves attenuation of *trp* transcription. The increase in *trp* expression upon tryptophan starvation is also specific to the trytophan operon, since total mRNA synthesis (and, for example, *lac* operon mRNA synthesis) actually decreases under these conditions. Regulation at this early site is coordinate across the operon. Deletion of any of the *trp* operon genes does not affect attenuation, suggesting that none of the structural gene products are directly involved (Morse and Morse 1976).

Finally, experiments comparing the response to tryptophan starvation in a $relA^+$ strain to that in a $relA^-$ strain suggest that some ribosomal component or product may be involved (Morse and Morse 1976) (see Table 4). The $relA^-$ strain has an altered ribosomal factor that is deficient in ppGpp synthesis in response to starvation conditions (Haseltine et al. 1972), and it is apparent that relief of attenuation is weak in this strain. It has been reported that ppGpp stimulates *trp* expression in vitro (Yang et al. 1974), but a direct effect by ppGpp in vivo is excluded by the fact that starvation for other amino acids, which leads to an accumulation of ppGpp, does not affect attenuation (Morse and Morse 1976). These results imply that the *relA* gene product is necessary but not sufficient for normal relief of attenuation—starvation for tryptophan is also required. Although ppGpp may play a general role in the regulation of amino acid biosynthetic operons (Stephens et al. 1975), lesions in *relA* also exert ubiquitous effects upon cellular metabolism and an indirect effect may well account for the lack of an attenuation response to tryptophan starvation in a $relA^-$ strain.

Table 4 Relaxed vs stringent response

	trpR argA relA⁺		*trpR argA relA⁻*	
	trpA	total	*trpA*	total
+ trp + arg	103 /	290,000	100 /	220,000
+ trp − arg	58 /	35,000	78 /	230,000
+ IA + arg	706 /	110,000	180 /	250,000

The genetically derepressed arginine auxotrophs were pulse-labeled in the presence or absence of tryptophan, arginine, and indoleacrylic acid (IA) as indicated. Tryptophan starvation is induced by IA, an efficient competitive inhibitor of tRNA synthetase (as well as repressor). The numbers are cpm 10 μg of RNA for *trpA*-specific mRNA compared to total RNA. The "stringent" reduction of total RNA syntheses is seen in the *relA⁺* strain. This response is "relaxed" in the *relA⁻* strain, yet levels of *trpA* mRNA are far below those in the *relA⁺* strain during tryptophan starvation. Thus, the *relA* product seems to be required for maximum expression of *trp*. (Data adapted from Morse and Morse 1976.)

Several lines of evidence suggest that a major factor which influences the extent of attenuation is the intracellular concentration of tryptophan, probably mediated by the level of charged tRNA^{Trp} in the cell (Bertrand and Yanofsky 1976; Morse and Morse 1976; Yanofsky and Soll 1977). In *trpR* strains grown in the presence of tryptophan, the introduction of certain mutations affecting tRNA^{Trp} and its charging elevates expression in the wild-type operon, but not in *trpΔLD102* (in which the attenuator is deleted). The effect of *trpT*, *trpS*, and *trpX* mutations is as shown in Table 3. The response to these mutations is similar to that elicited by tryptophan starvation and is consistent with an overall scheme in which charged tRNA^{Trp} acts in concert with one or more additional factors to promote termination at *trp a*. However, alternate possibilities are by no means ruled out, and some of the limitations of this simplified model will become apparent later.

The *trpT* mutation isolated by Yanofsky and Soll (1977) is a temperature-sensitive lesion on the tRNA^{Trp} gene (*trpT*$_{ts}$), which even at permissive temperatures does not allow a normal level of termination at the attenuator. The restoration of termination upon starvation for isoleucine, which inhibits protein synthesis, is attributed to the accumulation of charged tRNA species under these conditions (presumably including the tRNA$^{Trp}_{ts}$, thought to be otherwise mostly uncharged).

The presence of a mutation in *trpS* (the tRNA synthetase gene) relieves attenuation by nearly threefold in a *trp a⁺* strain but does not increase expression in *trpΔLD102* (Table 3). The mutant tryptophanyl-tRNA synthetase resulting from *trpS9969* has a 100-fold weaker affinity for tryptophan than the wild-type enzyme (Squires et al. 1973), and the intracellular levels of charged tRNA^{Trp} will thus be much lower than normal. However, when charging of tRNA^{Trp} is forced by altering the metabolic state of the cell (in this case, by valine inhibition of protein synthesis in the presence of tryptophan), distal *trp* mRNA is reduced to *trpS$^+$* levels, indicating that the attenuation response has been restored to normal (Yanofsky and Soll, 1977). A similar correlation between the extent of tRNA^{Trp} aminoacylation and the level of *trp* operon expression has been observed by Morse and Morse (1976) in studies employing the synthetase mutation *trpS10330* and the analogs 6-methyltryptophan and 7-azatryptophan.

The structure of the tRNA^{Trp} is also crucial for the attenuation response. The *trpX* mutation (identified as one of the lesions in a double mutation, *psu2*, originally detected by Korn and Yanofsky [1976a]) has a significant effect in relieving attenuation (Table 3) and results in an altered tRNA^{Trp}, although it does not map within the structural gene *trpT* (Yanofsky and Soll 1977). It appears likely that *trpX* leads to a defect in modification of the adenine adjacent to the anticodon sequence of the tRNA (S. Eisenberg et al., pers. comm.). This is consistent with earlier observations which suggested that a fully modified cognate tRNA might be necessary for normal regulation, since starvation of *E. coli* for iron leads to a similar defect in modification in several tRNA species (Rosenberg and Gefter 1969) and also causes elevated *trp* operon expression (McCray and Herrmann 1976). In a *trpT* merodiploid that synthesizes higher levels of tRNA^{Trp}, the presence of *trpX* has less effect than it does in the haploid strain. Moreover, the effect of *trpX* is negated when *trpT sup9^2* (Hirsch 1971) is introduced into a *trpX* strain, i.e., attenuation functions normally (Yanofsky and Soll 1977). The explanation for this effect is not clear. One simple possibility which has not been excluded is that *trpT sup9* suppresses a possible UGA nonsense mutation in *trpX*. Alternatively, significant differences in the tertiary structure of the *trpT sup9* species (see Hirsch 1971) may permit it to function in regulation at the attenuator, despite the presence of *trpX*.

Yanofsky and Soll (1977) have also observed an effect on attenuation upon introduction of the suppressor tRNA resulting from *trpT sup7*, which reads the termination codon UAG instead of the tryptophan codon UGG (Soll 1974) and is mischarged with glutamine as well as tryptophan in a 9:1 ratio (Celis et al. 1976; Knowlton and Yarus 1976). When a *trpT$^+$/F'14 trpT sup7* heterozygote is starved for tryptophan, there is only a twofold increase in synthesis of distal *trp* mRNA; in contrast, distal *trp* mRNA in the control strain, *trpT$^+$/F'14 trpT$^+$*, is increased by six- to sevenfold, as expected by the relief of attenuation. This suggests strongly that the *glutamine*-charged tRNA^{Trp} *sup7* is almost as effective as *tryp-*

---

[2]The *sup9* mutation results in a UGA suppressor.

tophan-charged wild-type tRNA^{Trp} in preventing relief of attenuation. Since the *sup7* species has a 50-fold weaker affinity for tryptophanyl-tRNA synthetase than does the wild-type tRNA^{Trp} (Yarus et al. 1977), it seems unlikely that the synthetase itself is interacting directly with tRNA^{Trp} to mediate the response at the attenuator.

However, the mechanism that regulates the level of transcription termination at the attenuator must include some sort of interactions (though not necessarily direct ones) involving the *trpS* and *trpT* products. Whether the primary regulatory function is the promotion of read-through by the uncharged species of tRNA^{Trp} or the stimulation of termination by the charged species is still an open question. The situation may be even more complex, in fact, and may depend on the intracellular ratio of the two species as well as on the absolute concentrations, as suggested by Yanofsky and Soll (1977).

Many of the properties of the attenuator inferred from observations made in vivo have been confirmed in vitro. In a purified system, consisting of RNA polymerase, a DNA template carrying the *trp* operon, nucleoside triphosphates, and buffer, transcription is unable to proceed at a significant level beyond nucleotide 141–142 (Lee et al. 1976; Lee and Yanofsky 1977) (see Fig. 5). In this case, termination is clearly very efficient, even in the complete absence of accessory components, although previous results (Rose et al. 1973; Pannekoek et al. 1974) suggest that at least a small fraction of polymerase molecules can traverse the entire leader region and continue into the structural genes. *Trp* operon transcription in a coupled system does yield structural gene mRNA (Zalkin et al. 1974), but the S30 extract employed in these studies may contain cellular components which allow transcription initiated at the *trp* promoter to proceed beyond the termination site in the leader region. The partial purification of a protein factor that appears to be a positive effector for read-through at the attenuator has been reported (Pannekoek et al. 1975; Pouwels and van Rotterdam 1975), but detailed characterization of this factor has not yet been carried out.

The product of *trp* leader region transcription in vitro is an RNA molecule about 140 nucleotides long, which terminates with a very U-rich oligonucleotide sequence, carrying a 3'-OH. The exact site of termination is not unique, as two major T_1 oligonucleotides, CU_7-OH and CU_8-OH, are found (Lee et al. 1976). Bertrand et al. (1977) have shown more recently that transcripts produced in vivo when cells are grown in the presence of excess tryptophan (i.e., under conditions where the levels of charged *trp*-tRNA^{Trp} are high and termination at the attenuator is most efficient) are very similar to those synthesized in vitro and have terminal oligonucleotide sequences of the general form $C(U)_n$-OH, where $n = 3$ to 7 (Fig. 6). These sequences are strikingly similar to the 3' termini of other small RNA molecules, such as the U_6A-OH of lambda 4S and 6S RNA, the CU_5-OH of $\phi80$ M_3 RNA, the U_6A-OH of *E. coli* band IV RNA, and the U_6G-OH of 5S rRNA precursor

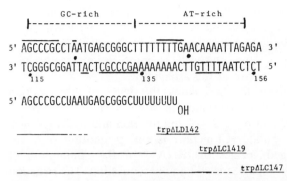

Figure 6 The attenuator region of the tryptophan operon. The sequence of *trp* mRNA terminated at the attenuator site is shown; the 3' end within the run of uridine residues is actually somewhat heterogeneous both in vivo and in vitro. The GC-rich and AT-rich regions are indicated, as is the dyad symmetry (heavy bars with dots at the center). Nucleotide position is relative to the mRNA initation site at +1 (see also Figs. 4 and 5). The approximate position of the deletion endpoints is shown, and only that of *trpΔLC1419* is known precisely. As discussed in the text, the attributes of attenuator function are present in *trpΔLC147*, partially evident in *trpΔLC1419*, and lacking in *trpΔLD142*. (Data and figure adapted from Bertrand et al. 1977.)

(Lebowitz et al. 1971; Pieczenik et al. 1972; Ikemura and Dahlberg 1973; Sogin et al. 1976). Although it is almost impossible to eliminate completely the involvement of nuclease degradation in the production of such termini in vivo, the facts that these oligonucleotides are discrete and that they correspond to those seen in vitro suggest that degradation and/or processing are unlikely possibilities.

Several properties are characteristic of wild-type attenuator function in vivo, including (1) the production of terminated transcripts, (2) the regulation of termination by tRNA^{Trp}, and (3) the rho-dependence of this termination. Bertrand et al. (1977) have analyzed several deletion mutants with endpoints in the vicinity of the termination region (see Fig. 6) which permits these functions to be localized more precisely. The latest deletion endpoint in the leader region is located between positions 145 and 152. Transcription both in vivo and in vitro for a template carrying this deletion (*trpΔLC147*) yields normal 3' ends, indicating normal attenuation. The site of rho action also appears to be intact, and the response to tryptophan starvation is normal. In contrast, the deletion *trpΔLD142*, which ends between positions 119 and 125, clearly inactivates the attenuator—there is no termination of transcription in vivo or in vitro, nor do altered rho factors influence read-through transcription to the distal genes.

The endpoint of *trpΔLC1419* in the leader region is at position 137, in the midst of the tract of AT base pairs that contains the wild-type termination site; this deletion removes nearly all of the AT-rich sequence block. Bertrand et al. (1977) found that, in *trpΔLC1419* strains, synthesis of *trpB* protein and mRNA (used as a measure of distal transcription) is elevated about threefold; this partial increase suggests that attenuator function is reduced but not completely eliminated. Moreover, the 3' oligonucleotides CU_4-OH and CU_4G-OH have been isolated from *trpΔLC1419* mRNA labeled in vivo, indicating significant termination of transcription directly at the deletion endpoint. This residual termination in vivo is suppressed by tryptophan starvation, but the involvement of rho factor has not been observed. Studies with this DNA template in vitro, by contrast, lead to a slightly different conclusion: transcription in the purified system does not terminate, nor is there any evidence of any 3'-OH ends corresponding to sequences in this region; moreover, no sign of attenuator function is restored even with the addition of rho protein (Bertrand et al. 1977).

On the basis of this deletion analysis, Bertrand et al. (1977) concluded that sequences critical for transcription termination, rho action, and response to tRNA^{Trp} occur between positions 119 and 152. A shorter sequence between 119 and 137 may be sufficient to signal partial termination. It is reasonable to propose that rho and perhaps tRNA^{Trp} interact with RNA polymerase and/or the nascent RNA chain in the immediate vicinity of the termination site itself. Rosenberg et al. (1976) noted that, although the lambda 6S and 4S transcripts have extensive homology in their 3' termini, there is little additional homology in the DNA sequences beyond the ends of these transcripts. This suggests that the DNA region which specifies termination is largely in the transcribed region preceding the termination site. In the case of *trpΔLC1419*, however, some portion of the AT-rich sequences removed by the deletion appears to be essential for complete function.

Gilbert (1976) has suggested that the GC-rich region that precedes many termination sites by about 10 base pairs may enhance termination. Advancement of the polymerase might be hindered either as a result of difficulty in initially unwinding the DNA helix in these regions or by increased stability of the nascent RNA-DNA hybrid in GC-rich sequences. The finding that C-rich ribopolymers are especially good substrates for the RNA-dependent ATPase reaction catalyzed by rho also raises the possibility that rho may preferentially interact with RNA transcribed from the GC-rich sequences which precede termination sites (Lowery and Richardson 1977).

The primary structure of the attenuator region has several remarkable features shared by other terminator regions (see review by Adhya and Gottesman 1978). Attenuation of transcription occurs (1) downstream from a region rich in GC base pairs, (2) within a run of uridine residues in an AT-rich region of the DNA, and (3) just beyond a region of dyad symmetry in the DNA (see Fig. 6). In the symmetric region, the self-complementary bases of the RNA transcript could form a fairly stable stem-end-loop structure. Lee and Yanofsky (1977) have presented evidence that, under conditions favoring base-pairing in vitro, certain regions of leader mRNA are less susceptible to nuclease attack. Two mutually exclusive secondary structures are compatible with the data, and Lee and Yanofsky (1977) suggest that one of these structures may favor termination, while the other favors read-through. In their model, the equilibrium between these two structures is shifted by translation of the leader mRNA, an event predicted by the identification of a ribosome-binding site near the 5' terminus of *trp* mRNA (Platt et al. 1976) (see Fig. 5 and next section). Because of the two tryptophan codons at positions 10 and 11 of the putative translation product, termination of transcription at the attenuator is linked to translation of this region via the intracellular levels of charged tyrptophanyl tRNA. This model requires only translation itself, and not the product of translation. However, the short polypeptide resulting from translation could also possess a role essential to regulatory interactions at the attenuator. At present, no experimental results exist which can distinguish between these and numerous other possibilities.

The possible importance of stem-and-loop formation in termination regions is discussed by Rosenberg et al. (1978) and Adhya and Gottesman (1978). Support for the role of RNA secondary structure in termination function at the *trp* attenuator is provided by a comparison of the *E. coli* sequence with that of *S. typhimurium* (Lee and Yanofsky and 1977; Lee et al. 1978). The predicted stability of the secondary structures correlates with the efficiency of termination in vitro in each case. Moreover, the incorporation in vitro of ITP instead of GTP increases read-through at the attenuators of both *E. coli* and *S. typhimurium* to nearly 100% (Lee and Yanofsky 1977). The use of ITP weakens base-pairing interactions by substituting two hydrogen bonds for the three found in a normal GC base pair. Both RNA-RNA and RNA-DNA interactions will be affected, and it is not known which of these is more critical for attenuation.

Preliminary evidence from sucrose gradient analysis of *trp* transcription reactions performed in vitro indicates that, although mRNA synthesis halts at the *trp* attenuator in the absence of rho factor, the mRNA is not released from the termination complex (F. Lee and C. Yanofsky, pers. comm.; R. S. Fuller and T. Platt, unpubl.). The addition of rho releases leader mRNA from the fast-sedimenting termination complex (R. S. Fuller and T. Platt, unpubl.), suggesting that rho is acting as a release factor under these conditions rather than causing cessation of transcription. When rho factor is present during a transcription reaction with limiting RNA polymerase, the yield of leader mRNA is increased three-fold (R. S. Fuller and T. Platt, unpubl.). Howard et al. (1977) have seen a similar increase in the yield of the lambda 4S *oop* RNA in vitro upon the addition of rho, and they ascribe this effect to a rho-mediated release of stalled polymerase molecules that permits each molecule to transcribe more frequently. Further experiments along these lines are expected to clarify the role of rho factor in attenuation.

METABOLIC REGULATION

Observations by Rose and Yanofsky (1972) have indicated that in cultures of *trpR* strains growing on different carbon sources the rates of synthesis of *trp* mRNA and *trp* operon polypeptides vary directly with the cell growth rate. This phenomenon was called "metabolic regulation" and has been interpreted as a control of operon expression at the level of transcription initiations—at low growth rates, initiation by RNA polymerase is less frequent. This may function as a general mechanism to prevent runaway expression of particular operons. The involvement of the attenuator in this phenomenon has been apparently ruled out by comparing the specific activities of tryptophan synthetase in four *trpR* strains, two with and two without the attenuator, grown on different growth-rate-limiting carbon sources (Table 5). Since strains lacking the attenuator are still subject to metabolic regulation, although their enzyme levels are several times as great as in *trp a*$^+$ controls, these results demonstrate that metabolic regulation seems to be independent of attenuation. P. H. Pouwels (pers. comm.) also finds that enzyme levels are not affected in a strain without the attenuator, with respect to one with the attenuator.

However, on the basis of hybridization competition measurements of *trp* mRNA obtained from cells growing in different media, Pouwels and

Table 5   Metabolic regulation and attenuation

Carbon source	Generation time (min)	Relative amount of *trp* mRNA per genome	Specific-activity ratios	
			trpΔLD102/trpΔED24	*trpΔLE1413/trp*$^+$
Glucose	66–80	1.0	8.1	12
Glycerol	100–144	0.52	8.3	10
Proline	180–600	0.14	14	11

All strains are *trpR* derivatives and were grown at 37°C with shaking on the carbon sources indicated. Generation times and tryptophan synthetase (TSase)-β_2-specific activities were determined. Ratios of specific activities for a strain without the attenuator (*trpΔLD102* or *trpΔLE1413*) and a strain with it (*trpΔED24* or *trp*$^+$) are presented. Since the ratios are similar in all cases, the *trp a*$^-$ strains must respond to the different carbon sources just as the *trp a*$^+$ strains do. (Data adapted from Yanofsky 1976a.)

Pannekoek (1976) concluded that the levels of transcription do vary. Because of the differences in mRNA levels in the two strains ($trp\ a^+$ and $trp\ a^-$), these authors postulate that metabolic regulation does, therefore, involve interactions at the attenuator. This response is possibly regulated by a positive control factor (Pouwels and van Rotterdam 1975) and in a different fashion than the $tRNA^{Trp}$-mediated effects on attenuation (P. H. Pouwels, pers. comm.). Further experimentation is necessary to clarify these effects, and at present the actual mechanism linking cellular growth rate to the level of transcription of the trp structural genes remains unknown.

MESSENGER DEGRADATION

The effects of repression and attenuation on the levels of trp messenger RNA synthesis were discussed above. However, the steady-state level of trp mRNA and thus of trp enzymes is dependent not only on the rate of synthesis of trp message, but also on its stability. Transcription time for the 7000-nucleotide-long trp mRNA is about 4 minutes at 30°C (Rose et al. 1970; Forchhammer et al. 1972) or slightly longer at high cell densities (Schlessinger et al. 1977). Early studies on decay of trp operon mRNA established that degradation occurs in the 5'-to-3' direction (Morikawa and Imamoto 1969; Morse et al. 1969). Moreover, the disappearance of trp mRNA is exponential and decay is initiated randomly after the initiation of transcription (Mosteller et al. 1971). Numerous models for messenger turnover are possible, and several of the simpler ones are outlined in Figure 7.

Measurements of trp mRNA decay rates vary somewhat under different conditions but generally indicate that decay occurs more slowly in the 3'-distal gene segments, from a half-life of 60–100 seconds for $trpE$ to between 100 and 240 seconds for $trpA$ (Morikawa and Imamoto 1969; Rose et al. 1970; Forchhammer et al. 1972; Imamoto and Schlessinger 1974). More recently, Schlessinger et al. (1977) reported that (1) at the time transcription terminates, 30–40% of total $trpA$ sequences are in full-size trp mRNA, (2) a relative lag of up to 5 minutes occurs before bulk decay of most $trpA$-specific sequences, and (3) discrete species of size CBA, BA, and A are seen as transient intermediates, with CBA appearing and disappearing more rapidly than BA, which in turn appears more rapidly than A.

These observations rule out the simple models of uniform exonucleolytic degradation in the 5'-to-3' direction and random fragmentation at many sites (Fig. 7, models 1 and 4). In an effort to distinguish between two alternative mechanisms, Schlessinger et al. (1977) carried out extensive studies on trp mRNA labeled in the 3' region; labeling was done after shutdown of mRNA initiation by the addition of rifampicin plus

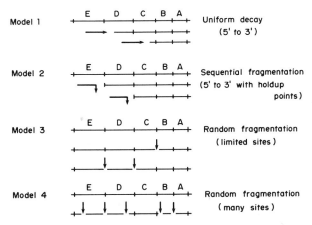

Figure 7 Models for the decay of individual mRNA chains. In model 1, exonucleolytic degradation proceeds continuously and uniformly from the 5' end of the mRNA to the 3' end. Model 2 differs from model 1 only by the postulated delays in exonucleolytic decay, which may occur near intercistronic junctions. Model 3 proposes that a few "special" sites (as shown here, the intercistronic regions) are involved and each is subject from the time of its synthesis to random cleavage that initiates further decay. With model 4, every segment of an mRNA is exposed to endonucleolytic attack from the moment of its synthesis (this can produce apparent 5'-to-3' degradation because the 5' end is synthesized first and therefore begins to decay first). The evidence discussed in the text suggests that model 3 is the most consistent with observations on the degradation of *trp* operon mRNA. (Adapted from Schlessinger et al. 1977.)

tryptophan. One hypothesis, referred to as "sequential fragmentation" (model 2), suggests that during normal 5'-to-3' degradation there are delay points at specific sites within the operon. An alternative scheme, "random fragmentation" (model 3), has been proposed for the *lac* (Blundell and Kennell 1974) and *gal* (Achord and Kennell 1974) operons, in which each intercistronic region (or special sites nearby) is subject to random cleavage from the time of its synthesis. This alternative was ruled out in the case of the *trp* operon by analysis of the size distribution of end-labeled mRNA, and the fact remains that the half-lives of mRNA fragments required to fit a random fragmentation model are two to three times longer than any previously measured times (Schlessinger et al. 1977).

Overall, the best fit for the existing data is the model for sequential fragmentation, and this hypothesis is supported by additional evidence. First, differential variation of decay rates of *trp* genes with temperature should be a sensitive indication of independent inactivation sites. Yet there is no difference in the response for the *ED* and *BA* segments, even though they must have different decay rates at 30°C (Wice and Kennell 1974). Since initial events in 5'-proximal segments will set limits on the decay rate of subsequent segments, this result is consistent with sequential fragmentation. Second, when internal deletions are introduced in the *trp* operon, the 3'-distal *BA* mRNA decays faster as it is brought closer to the 5' end, whereas the decay of 5'-proximal regions remains the same (Forchhammer et al. 1972). The remaining data of Forchhammer et al. (1972) can also be accommodated in a sequential-fragmentation model. These observations are contrary to the prediction of the simple random-fragmentation model, in which rate is dependent on primary structure rather than on distance from the 5' end. Further tests to confirm or disprove the model of sequential fragmentation must await in vitro studies that demonstrate the specific action of relevant nucleases on *trp* operon mRNA (or mRNA from another polycistronic operon). And of course, it is not known how the sites postulated to function as holdup points become exposed as targets for degradation. In this model, specific base sequences may function independently of translation or may be coupled somehow to the translational machinery. An intriguing possibility is that degradation may "pause" at each intercistronic junction until the last ribosome initiates there. However, in the *trp* operon, any model for processing at the intercistronic boundaries must take into account the fact that these junctions may be very small—for example, only two untranslated nucleotides separate *trpB* from *trpA* (Platt and Yanofsky 1975).

RIBOSOME-BINDING SITES AND INTERCISTRONIC REGIONS

Bronson et al. (1973) obtained the first bacterial mRNA sequence corresponding to a known protein sequence, the amino-terminal region of the *trpE* gene product. Since then, nucleotide sequences corresponding to the initiator regions of three of the five structural genes in the operon have been determined (Platt and Yanofsky 1975; T. Platt, unpubl.); in addition, a previously unknown site in the leader region has been identified (Platt et al. 1976). These sequences are compared with other bacterial initiator regions in Table 6.

A promising hypothesis proposed by Shine and Dalgarno (1974, 1975) for explaining the specificity of ribosome recognition of initiator sequences in mRNA suggests that a sequence near the 3' end of 16S ribosomal RNA (3'OH-AUUCCUCCAC-5') is involved in hydrogen-bonded base-pairing with a more-or-less complementary polypurine sequence in mRNA three to four codons 5' to the AUG (or rarely, GUG) initiation codon. The thermodynamic stability of this interaction would depend on the precise sequence occurring in the mRNA, and this variable may partly explain the differential affinity of the ribosome for different initiator

Table 6 Gene initiator regions of *E. coli*

Region	Sequence	References
trp leader	CAC GUA AAA AGG GUA UCG ACA AUG AAA GCA AUU UUC GUG	Bertrand et al. (1975), Platt et al. (1976)
trpE	GAA CAA AAU UAG AGA AUA ACA AUG ACA CAA CAA AAA CCG	Bronson et al. (1973), Platt et al. (1976)
trpC	CUG GCG GCA CGA GGG UAA AUG AUG CAA ACC GUU UUA GCG	G. E. Christie and T. Platt (unpubl.)
trpA	GAA AGC ACG AGG GGA AAU CUG AUG GAA CGC UAC GAA UCU	Platt and Yanofsky (1975)
lacZ	AAU UUC ACA CAG GAA ACA GCU AUG ACC AUG AUU ACG GAU	Maizels (1974)
lacI	AGU CAA UUC AGG GUG GUG AAU GUG AAA CCA GUA ACG	Steege (1977)
araB	UUU UUU GGA UGG AGU GAA ACG AUG GCG AUU GCA AUU	Lee and Carbon (1977)
galE	AUA AGC CUA AUG GAG CGA AUU AUG AGA GUU CUG GUU ACC	Musso et al. (1974)
galT	TAT CCC CAT TAA GGA ACG ACC ATG ACG CAA TTT AAT CCC	Grindley (1978)

The known ribosome-binding regions in the *trp* operon are compared with those of other *E. coli* genes, aligned relative to the initiating AUG codon. The underlined nucleotides are those which can potentially base-pair with the 3' end of 16S ribosomal RNA according to the model of Shine and Dalgarno (1974, 1975). A thorough discussion of the significant common features of these sequences is found in Steitz (1978).

regions.[3] Potential complementarity between the 3' end of 16S RNA and the *trp* operon initiator regions is rather weak, comprising only 3 or 4 base pairs. It seems likely, therefore, that additional factors are probably important in the ribosomal selection of these initiator regions.

Ribosome-binding experiments in vitro with operator-proximal *trp* mRNA yielded the protected sequence for the *trpE* initiator region predicted by Bronson et al. (1973). Unexpectedly, a second region was also protected, centered about an AUG codon near the 5' end of the leader sequence and approximately 140 nucleotides prior to the *trpE* initiation codon (Platt et al. 1976). Binding to this site was independent of the presence of the *trpE* initiation sequence, and recently Sommer et al. (1978) have shown that when the *trp* leader region is fused genetically to *lacI*, translation can actually initiate at this site in vivo. The amino-terminal sequence of the fusion protein produced corresponds to the first seven amino acids predicted for an initiation event directed by the *trp* leader ribosome-binding site. The nucleotide sequence of the wild-type leader region predicts the synthesis of a leader polypeptide only 14 amino acids long (Lee et al. 1978) (see Fig. 5), and its possible role in attenuation has been mentioned above.

For the *trpC* initiator region, the precise nucleotide sequence is not yet known, but an interesting situation is created by the internal deletion *trpΔLD102*. The operator-proximal endpoint of this deletion is at nucleotide 25 in the leader region (Bronson et al. 1973) and the distal endpoint is beyond all known markers in *trpD* (Jackson and Yanofsky 1972b, 1973). The *trpC* structural gene cannot be affected, since the *trpC* protein possesses a wild-type amino-terminal sequence (T. Platt et al., unpubl.). A purified *trp* mRNA fragment carrying the sequences from the *trpΔLD102* endpoint through *trpC* does not bind ribosomes in vitro. However, if "trimming" of the RNA with ribonuclease is omitted during the hybridization steps of the mRNA purification procedure so that the short leader portion remains attached to the *trpC* sequences, then ribosome binding is observed (T. Platt, unpubl.). We have now shown that the deletion creates a new "hybrid" initiator region for *trpC*, which possesses a 5' portion from the *trp* leader ribosome-binding site and a 3' portion (including the AUG codon) from the *trpC* site (G. E. Christie and T. Platt, unpubl.). Apparently, the leader nucleotides preceding the deletion (which include a potential polypurine sequence for ribosome recognition) supply sufficient additional specificity for ribosomes to bind and initiate translation of *trpC*. Moreover, the efficiency of initiation with the hybrid site is approximately the same as the wild type, since a strain

[3]The mRNA:rRNA complexes predicted by the hypothesis of Shine and Dalgarno (1974, 1975) have been verified for the A-protein initiator region of bacteriophage R17 RNA (Steitz and Jakes 1975) and for a λ P_R RNA ribosome-binding site encoding the amino terminus of the λ *cro* protein (Steitz and Steege 1977).

carrying *trpΔLD102* (which deletes the attenuator) overproduces *trpC* protein to the same level as *trpB* and *trpA* (Jackson and Yanofsky 1973). Although the extent of similarity between the wild-type *trpC* initiator sequence and the *trp* leader is not known, it is not unlikely that proximal and distal elements (in sequence or structure) which determine ribosome-binding recognition and specificity may be independent of one another.[4]

The *trpA* initiator sequence is particularly unusual because it provided an early example of overlapping genes in bacteria. Not only does the ribosome-protected region include the end of the preceding gene, *trpB*, but also the *trpB* translation termination codon (UGA) actually overlaps the *trpA* initiation codon: UGAUG (Platt and Yanofsky 1975). One significant implication of this finding is that the RNA sequences in this region are multifunctional, coding simultaneously for the ribosome-recognition function, termination and initiation of translation, and for the amino acid sequences of both the carboxy terminus of *trpB* protein and the amino terminus of *trpA* protein.[5]

The question of initiation of translation by ribosomes is further complicated in the case of the *trpBA* intercistronic region, which consists of only two untranslated nucleotides. This raises a fundamental question about the mechanism of translation of a polycistronic operon: What is the origin of ribosomes translating the distal genes? One may consider three major possibilities: (1) the same ribosome traverses the entire operon; (2) new ribosomes initiate at each cistron; (3) ribosomes continue into distal genes at less than 100% efficiency, for which new initiations compensate.

In the case of the *trp* operon, Zalkin et al. (1974) have shown that ribosomes translating in vitro cannot traverse the entire *trp* operon if kasugamycin, an inhibitor of translational initiation, is present. Their data do not exclude the possibility that some ribosomes may continue on into subsequent genes, but if they do, it must be at less than 60–70% efficiency. We also know that new ribosomes are capable of initiating internally, since translation of *trpA* mRNA can occur even when *trpB* mRNA is not being translated (Morse et al. 1970). Sufficient information for ribosome binding in vitro is contained within the 220-nucleotide sequence of the *trpB-trpA* fragment spanning the initiator region (Platt and Yanofsky 1975).

One might ask, however, If *trpB* mRNA *is* being translated, what

[4]Backman and Ptashne (1978) have constructed a similar, functional hybrid site in vitro between the 5' region of the *lacZ* initiator and the AUG and the 3' portion of the λ*CI* initiator.

[5]Further evidence that nucleic acid sequences may be far more information-dense than imagined is illustrated by the complete nucleotide sequence of the bacteriophage φX174, in which there is not only a similar overlap between termination and initiation codons, but also the remarkable occurrence of two entire genes within other genes (for a summary, see Sanger et al. 1977). In each of these cases two unrelated polypeptides are translated from the same nucleotide sequence in two different reading frames.

happens to the ribosome upon release of the completed *trpB* polypeptide? If ribosomes dissociate from the mRNA upon termination of translation of *trpB*, and if they are closely packed on the mRNA during translation, it is not clear how the *trpA* initiator region can become accessible to free 30S ribosomal subunits. Instead, perhaps termination of *trpB* does not result in complete release of the ribosome from the mRNA chain, but only in dissociation of the 50S subunit, leaving mRNA complexed to the 30S subunit. Realignment of the 30S subunit from its termination configuration (with the UGA codon in the "A" site) to an initiation configuration (with AUG in the "P" site) would only involve a shift of a few nucleotides along the mRNA, and this might easily occur via base-pairing of the 16S RNA with the polypurine sequence or the ribosome-binding site, as proposed by Shine and Dalgarno (1974). In this way the 30S-mRNA complex (remaining from chain termination) could associate directly with fMet-tRNA$_F^{Met}$ and a new 50S particle and immediately initiate translation of *trpA*. In essence, the cell would bypass some of the "normal" steps in termination and initiation (perhaps including a requirement for initiation factors) in order to translate polycistronic messenger RNA more efficiently. Martin and Webster (1975) have in fact found a transient 46S complex during chain termination in vitro with bacteriophage f2 RNA, which they believe is composed of the RNA template and the 30S ribosomal subunit. A model involving partial ribosome dissociation is not inconsistent with the results of Zalkin et al (1974), since kasugamycin inhibition of initiation is thought to involve interaction with the 3′ end of 16S ribosomal RNA (Helser et al. 1971); hence, release of the 50S subunit alone could readily expose the 30S subunit to kasugamycin inhibition.

Although the situation with *trpB* and *trpA* may not be a common one, it is clear that simple mutations in or near the small intercistronic region could easily fuse *trpB* with *trpA*. The *trpD* and *trpC* proteins in *E. coli*, which each possess two separate enzymatic functions in single polypeptide chains (see Fig. 1), might have arisen by deletion or alteration of previously existing intercistronic regions. Gene fusions of various types have been suggested by Bonner et al. (1965) as being an important mechanism in the evolution of new proteins.

TERMINATION

Evidence from various systems suggests that partial termination of transcription is an important element in the regulation of gene expression and can provide a crucial modulating effect on the levels of RNA elongated from initiations at promoter sites (for review, see Adhya et al. 1976; Roberts 1976; Adhya and Gottesman 1978). In these cases, regulation results in detectable effects on the expression of distal genes in an operon. At the ends of gene clusters, however, mutations altering the efficiency of transcription termination are not expected to change the normal functioning of those genes. To study termination in the *trp* operon, Guarente et al. (1977) have selected deletions in a strain with the *lac* operon transposed to a site near the *trp* operon such that *lac* operon expression is fused to the *trp* controlling elements. Presumably, some of these deletions alter or eliminate a termination signal at the end of the *trp* operon. Mitchell et al. (1976) have shown that some deletions which express the *lac* genes still retain an intact *trpA* structural gene. Therefore the *trp* terminator (*trp t*) must lie beyond the end of *trpA*.

Several years ago Rose and Yanofsky (1971) estimated that *trp* mRNA contained no more than 300 nucleotides beyond *trpA*, based on extrapolations from kinetic measurements of *trp* mRNA labeled in vivo. Recent experiments (A. M. Wu and T. Platt, in prep.) have provided more detailed information about the termination region. A 3' fragment of *trp* mRNA approximately 150 nucleotides long can be isolated from cells labeled in vivo by hybridization to a transducing phage DNA that carries only the distal portion of *trpA* and bacterial DNA through the *tonB* locus (see Fig. 2). About 120 nucleotides of the RNA sequence of this fragment can be assigned to the end of *trpA* by correlation with the amino acid sequence of the protein product. Sequence analysis of the DNA corresponding to this region confirms the alignment of RNA and protein sequence and extends the total sequence information nearly 60 nucleotides beyond the end of *trpA* (Fig. 8). An oligonucleotide with a 3'-hydroxyl can be isolated from a T_1 ribonuclease digest of the mRNA by chromatography on a dihydroxyboryl-aminoethyl cellulose column. The tentative sequence of this oligonucleotide is CAUUUU-OH, and the large T_1 product that would be found if transcription continued 14 nucleotides farther has not been detected (A. M. Wu and T. Platt, in prep.; see Fig. 8). The simplest interpretation of these data is that transcription of the tryptophan operon structural genes in *E. coli* is

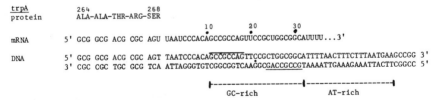

Figure 8 The termination region of the tryptophan operon. Transcription of the *trp* operon halts about 35 nucleotides beyond *trpA*, for which the carboxy-terminal protein sequence is shown. Termination of mRNA synthesis occurs at or near the run of uridine residues as indicated. The skewed distribution of GA and AT base pairs is remarkable, but of unknown significance. The dyad symmetry (heavy bars with a dot at the center) is also striking and common to other terminator regions. (Data from A. M. Wu and T. Platt, in prep.)

terminated about 35 nucleotides beyond the end of *trpA*. The absence of distal oligonucleotide sequences suggests that this termination is at least 90% efficient in vivo.

This region of DNA is strikingly similar to the *trp* attenuator region (see Figs. 6 and 8). Termination of transcription occurs (1) distal to a region rich in GC base pairs, (2) within a run of uridine residues in an AT-rich region of the DNA, and (3) just beyond a region of dyad symmetry in the DNA (Fig. 8). In the symmetric region, the RNA transcript potentially can form a stable stem-and-loop structure, with 7 GC base pairs out of the 8 in the stem; this structure is even more stable than that in the leader mRNA, as shown in Figure 9.

Still unexplained is the identification by Hardman et al. (1975) of a mutationally altered *trpA* protein some 50–70 amino acids longer than normal, which was thought to be due to a simple frameshift mutation late in *trpA* and would require the transcription of more than 150 nucleotides beyond *trpA*. Their alternate explanation that this could be due to an insertion of foreign DNA now seems more likely, since there are nonsense codons in the other reading frames of late *trpA* sequence that would preclude the translation required for the mutationally altered protein (A. M. Wu and T. Platt, unpubl.).

An alternative possibility to efficient termination shortly beyond *trpA* that cannot easily be excluded is the processing of a longer transcript down to the observed size with concomitant degradation of the distal portion. However, in a strain carrying the polarity suppressor mutation *rho201* (formerly *tsu1*), *trpR*-controlled read-through into the *lac* genes 1800 nucleotides away is quite efficient in vivo (Guarente et al.

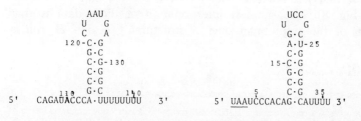

(a)   Attenuator site   (b)   Terminator site

Figure 9 The 3'-terminal regions of the tryptophan operon mRNA. Possible secondary structures for *trp* mRNA terminated (*a*) at the attenuator and (*b*) at the end of the operon. It is not known whether these structures simply reflect the dyad symmetry present in the DNA sequence or whether they are required for direct interactions with rho or RNA polymerase or other regulatory molecules acting at these sites. A discussion of the significance of such stem-and-loop structures has been presented by Lee and Yanofsky (1977) and Rosenberg et al. (1978). (Data from Lee and Yanofsky 1977; A. M. Wu and T. Platt, in prep.)

1977). When *rho201* is transferred into a wild-type background, a much longer and more complex transcript is obtained by hybridization than is obtained from the control strain (A. M. Wu et al., unpubl.). This suggests that termination in vivo at *trp t* is a rho-dependent event, and that if RNA processing does occur, it is defective in the *rho201* strain.

The response of *trp t* to a particular altered rho factor is a feature shared with the attenuator, although *rho201*, which suppresses termination at *trp t* very efficiently, has no detectable effect at the *trp* attenuator (Guarente et al. 1977). Another response probably occurring at *trp t* is seen with a mutation to rifampicin resistance in RNA polymerase which is capable of compensating for the defect in *rho201* to terminate efficiently in the region between *trp* and *lac*, apparently by creating a "rho-independent" polymerase (Guarente et al. 1977; Guarante and Beckwith 1978).

The most striking common features of both major transcription termination regions in the *trp* operon are the long GC-rich regions followed by long AT-rich regions and the dyad symmetry preceding the T-rich sequence where the mRNA presumably terminates (Fig. 8). It is not known whether the dyad symmetry is necessary for protein recognition of the DNA sequence or for a stem-and-loop structure in the RNA transcript. A stable structure in the RNA could facilitate release of the completed RNA molecule from the DNA template to which it has been base-paired, or it could interact directly with polymerase and termination factors. Changes that reduce the dyad symmetry (even though increasing the GC content of the region) have been shown to weaken termination at the bacteriophage λ termination site T_L (Rosenberg et al. 1978). This is also consistent with the differences between the attenuator regions of *E. coli* and *S. typhimurium* (Lee and Yanofsky 1977), as discussed earlier. Other portions of the sequence in the vicinity of termination are important as well. In the *trp* attenuator region, the distal portion of the T-rich sequence must contribute to the termination function, since deletion of the last four T residues elicits higher levels of read-through in vivo and eliminates termination in vitro (Bertrand et al. 1978). The isolation of additional point and deletion mutations in both the attenuator and terminator regions is expected to shed more light on the processes involved in termination at these sites.

A complete analysis of termination mechanisms must consider at least three of the elements involved: (1) cessation of mRNA synthesis, (2) release of completed mRNA from the template, and (3) release of RNA polymerase from the DNA or DNA-RNA complex. Some evidence suggests that rho factor may act at the third level (Howard et al. 1977). However, Rosenberg et al. (1978) and others have shown that RNA polymerase can pause at certain sites in vitro and that point mutations in a normal termination region can affect the extent of this pausing in the complete absence of rho factor. Thus, although the presence of rho factor may increase the specificity or efficiency of termination at some sites, RNA polymerase alone is also capable of terminating transcription. Finally, in several cases the use of modified nucleotides in vitro has been shown to affect termination efficiency. Use of ITP rather than GTP virtually eliminates termination at *trp a* (Lee and Yanofsky 1977). Similar effects are seen with transcription in vitro on bacteriophage T7 and T3 DNA, and the opposite effect (to strengthen termination) is seen if BrCTP is used (Neff and Chamberlin 1978). These effects are consistent with the expectation that RNA:RNA or RNA:DNA base-pairing is important for the termination event.

It is clear that termination of transcription is a subtle and intricate process that can easily provide sensitive regulation of gene expression and integrate it with cellular metabolism when necessary. It may often occur with less than 100% efficiency, and it responds to alterations in (1) the nucleotide sequence being transcribed, (2) the RNA polymerase, (3) the termination and antitermination factors, and even (4) the nature of the ribonucleotides incorporated. As additional termination regions are sequenced and characterized, the detailed interactions occurring at these sites will undoubtedly become more clear.

SUMMARY AND CONCLUSIONS

The tryptophan gene cluster in *E. coli* is one of the best-characterized biosynthetic operons in bacteria and is therefore extremely well suited for detailed studies of the mechanisms regulating operon expression in prokaryotes. Moreover, the final level of expression is subject to control by integrative feedback mechanisms at many different levels. End-product inhibition modulates the enzyme activity level leading into the tryptophan biosynthetic pathway. At the translational level, the synthesis of a small polypeptide from the leader sequence may link *trp*-tRNA^{Trp} concentration to the production of structural gene mRNA. Alternatively, the response to the level of tRNA^{Trp} may involve other effector molecules with early termination of transcription at the attenuator. Attenuation, an important feature governing the level of transcription, is independent of regulation at the level of transcription initiation, in which RNA polymerase and repressor compete for the promoter/operator site on the DNA near the mRNA start point. Together, repression and attenuation probably control transcription of the *trp* operon over a wider range than is possible with either one alone. Some details of these and other aspects of *trp* regulation have been described in this paper, yet numerous questions still remain to be answered at the molecular level.

The specific recognition features necessary for repression and RNA-polymerase binding are only beginning to be analyzed and understood. Even though the primary features of the leader region and the attenuator are now fairly clear, the function of the 140 nucleotides which precede the termination region is still obscure, as is the function of the early ribosome-binding site. It is tempting to predict that a polypeptide is synthesized from this region which would be involved in regulation at the attenuator, but none has yet been found. Other molecules, including tryptophanyl tRNA and tRNA synthetase, have been implicated in attenuator regulation, but the detailed interactions of these species with other protein factors (or nonprotein cofactors) to terminate or antiterminate transcription are not known. Likewise, the significance of the *relA* locus and ppGpp in the starvation response and the mechanism of "metabolic regulation" linking *trp* operon expression to cellular growth rate are still obscure.

The low-level internal promoter, *trpP2*, while providing a promising system for the study of initiation of transcription, has itself no clear purpose in tryptophan biosynthesis. Models both for messenger processing and degradation and for the relationship of polarity suppression to rho factor and transcription termination can be readily tested in the *trp* operon; definitive answers in this area are not yet available, but future experiments should provide more detailed information. Significant contributions to our knowledge of how polycistronic operons are translated by the ribosome and of the function of intercistronic regions are also likely to result from further studies in the *trp* system.

In conclusion, it seems reasonable to predict that, although a great deal is known about the molecular details governing expression of the tryptophan operon of *E. coli*, there is yet much more to be discovered, and we may look to the future with great anticipation.

ACKNOWLEDGMENTS

The thorough and valuable comments of my colleagues during the preparation of this manuscript are gratefully acknowledged, in particular those of Deborah Steege, Nigel Grindley, and Laurence Korn. In addition, I especially thank Charles Yanofsky for his patient sharing of tryptophan operon lore with me and for his generous and enthusiastic support for my own work in this area.

REFERENCES

Achord, D. and D. Kennell. (1974). Metabolism of messenger RNA from the *gal* operon of *Escherichia coli*. *J. Mol. Biol.* **90**:581.

Adhya, S. and M. Gottesman. 1978. Control of transcription termination. *Annu. Rev. Biochem.* (in press).

Adhya, S., M. Gottesman, B. de Crombrugghe, and D. Court. 1976. Transcription termination regulates gene expression. In *RNA polymerase* (ed. R. Losick and

M. Chamberlin), p. 719. Cold Spring Harbor Laboratory, Cold Spring Harbor, New York.

Artz, S. W. and J. R. Broach. 1975. Histidine regulation in *Salmonella typhimurium*: An activator-attenuator model of gene regulation. *Proc. Natl. Acad. Sci.* **72**:3453.

Backman, K. and M. Ptashne. 1978. Maximizing gene expression on a plasmid using recombination *in vitro. Cell* **13**:65.

Baker, T. J. and I. P. Crawford. 1966. Anthranilate synthetase partial purification and some kinetic studies on the enzyme from *Escherichia coli. J. Biol. Chem.* **241**:5577.

Bauerle, R. H. and P. Margolin. 1967. Evidence for two sites for initiation of gene expression in the tryptophan operon of *Salmonella typhimurium. J. Mol. Biol.* **26**:423.

Bennett, G. N. and C. Yanofsky. 1978. Sequence analysis of operator constitutive mutants of the tryptophan operon of *Escherichia coli. J. Mol. Biol.* **121**:179.

Bennett, G. N., K. D. Brown, and C. Yanofsky. 1977. Nucleotide sequence of the promoter-operator region of the tryptophan operon for *E. coli* and *S. typhimurium. Fed. Proc.* **36**:878 (Abstr.).

————. 1978a. Nucleotide sequence of the promoter-operator region of the tryptophan operon of *Salmonella typhimurium. J. Mol. Biol.* (in press).

Bennett, G. N., M. E. Schweingruber, K. D. Brown, C. Squires, and C. Yanofsky. 1976. Nucleotide sequence of region preceding *trp* mRNA initiation site and its role in promoter and operator function. *Proc. Natl. Acad. Sci.* **73**:2351.

————. 1978b. Nucleotide sequence of the promoter-operator region of the tryptophan operon of *Escherichia coli. J. Mol. Biol.* **121**:113.

Bertrand, K. and C. Yanofsky. 1976. Regulation of transcription termination in the leader region of the tryptophan operon of *Escherichia coli* involves tryptophan or its metabolic product. *J. Mol. Biol.* **103**:339.

Bertrand, K., C. Squires, and C. Yanofsky. 1976. Transcription termination *in vivo* in the leader region of the tryptophan operon of *Escherichia coli. J. Mol. Biol.* **103**:319.

Bertrand, K., L. J. Korn, F. Lee, and C. Yanofsky. 1977. The attenuator of the tryptophan operon of *Escherichia coli*. Heterogeneous 3'-OH termini *in vivo* and deletion mapping of functions. *J. Mol. Biol.* **117**:229.

Bertrand, K., L. Korn, F. Lee, T. Platt, C. L. Squires, C. Squires, and C. Yanofsky. 1975. New features of the regulation of the tryptophan operon. *Science* **189**:22.

Blundell, M. and D. Kennell. 1974. Evidence for endonucleolytic attack in decay of *lac* messenger RNA in *Escherichia coli. J. Mol. Biol.* **83**:143.

Bonner, D. M., J. A. DeMoss, and S. E. Mills. 1965. The evolution of an enzyme. In *Evolving genes and proteins* (ed. V. Bryson and H. J. Vogel), p. 305. Academic Press, New York.

Bronson, M. J., C. Squires, and C. Yanofsky. 1973. Nucleotide sequences from tryptophan messenger RNA of *Escherichia coli*: The sequence corresponding to the amino-terminal region of the first polypeptide specified by the operon. *Proc. Natl. Acad. Sci.* **70**:2335.

Brown, K. D. 1968. Regulation of aromatic amino acid biosynthesis in *Escherichia coli* K12. *Genetics* **60**:31.

Brown, K. D., G. N. Bennett, M. E. Schweingruber, and C. yanofsky. 1978. Functional analysis of restriction fragments from the promoter-operator region of the tryptophan operon of *Escherichia coli* and *Salmonella typhimurium. J. Mol. Biol.* (in press).

Camakaris, J. and J. Pittard. 1971. Repression of 3-deoxy-D-arabinoheptulosonic acid-7-phosphate synthetase (*trp*) and enzymes of the tryptophan pathway in *Escherichia coli* K12. *J. Bacteriol.* **107**:406.

Celis, J. E., C. Coulondre, and J. H. Miller. 1976. Suppressor su^+7 inserts tryptophan in addition to glutamine. *J. Mol. Biol.* **104**:729.

Cohen, G. N. and F. Jacob. 1959. Sur la répression de la synthèse des enzymes intervenant dans la formation du tryptophan chez *E. coli. C. R. Acad. Sci.* **248**:3490.

Doolittle, W. F. and C. Yanofsky. 1968. Mutants of *Escherichia coli* with an altered tryptophanyl-transfer ribonucleic acid synthetase. *J. Bacteriol.* **95**:1283.

Forchhammer, J., E. N. Jackson, and C. Yanofsky. 1972. Different half-lives of messenger RNA corresponding to different segments of the tryptophan operon of *Escherichia coli. J. Mol. Biol.* **71**:687.

Gardner, J. F., O. H. Smith, W. W. Fredricks, and M. A. McKinney. 1974. Secondary-site attachment of coliphage lambda near the *thr* operon. *J. Mol. Biol.* **90**:613.

Gilbert, W. 1976. Starting and stopping sequences for the RNA polymerase. In *RNA polymerase* (ed. R. Losick and M. Chamberlin), p. 193. Cold Spring Harbor Laboratory, Cold Spring Harbor, New York.

Grindley, N. 1978. IS*1* insertion generates duplication of a nine base pair sequence at its target site. *Cell* **13**:419.

Guarente, L. P. and J. Beckwith. 1978. Mutant RNA polymerase of *Escherichia coli* terminates transcription in strains making defective rho factor. *Proc. Natl. Acad. Sci. U.S.A.* **75**:294.

Guarente, L. P., D. H. Mitchell, and J. Beckwith. 1977. Transcription termination at the end of the tryptophan operon of *E. coli. J. Mol. Biol.* **112**:423.

Hardman, J. K., H. Berger, and M. Goodman. 1975. Tryptophan operon read-through: Isolation and characterization of an abnormally long tryptophan synthetase α subunit from a frame-shift mutant of *E. coli. J. Biol. Chem.* **250**:4634.

Haseltine, W. A., R. Block, W. Gilbert, and K. Weber. 1972. MSI and MSII made on ribosome in idling step of protein synthesis. *Nature* **238**:381.

Hausler, B. and R. L. Somerville. 1977. On the degeneracy of promoter structure. *Fed. Proc.* **36**:783 (Abstr.).

Helser, T. L., J. E. Davies, and J. E. Dahlberg. 1971. Change in methylation of 16S ribosomal RNA associated with mutation to kasugamycin resistance in *Escherichia coli. Nat. New Biol.* **233**:12.

Henderson, E. J. and H. Zalkin. 1971. On the composition of anthranilate synthetase-anthranilate 5-phosphoribosylpyrophosphate phosphoribosyltransferase from *Salmonella typhimurium. J. Biol. Chem.* **246**:6891.

Hiraga, S. 1969. Operator mutants of the tryptophan operon in *Escherichia coli. J. Mol. Biol.* **39**:159.

Hirsch, D. 1971. Tryptophan transfer RNA as the UGA suppressor. *J. Mol. Biol.* **58**:439.

Howard, B. H., B. de Crombrugghe, and M. Rosenberg. 1977. Transcription *in vitro* of bacteriophage lamba 4S RNA: Studies on termination and rho protein. *Nucleic Acids Res.* **4**:827.

Ikemura, T. and J. E. Dahlberg. 1973. Small ribonucleic acids of *Escherichia coli*. *J. Biol. Chem.* **248**:5024.

Imamoto, F. and D. Schlessinger. 1974. Bearing of some recent results on the mechanisms of polarity and messenger RNA stability. *Mol. Gen. Genet.* **135**:29.

Ito, J. and C. Yanofsky. 1966. The nature of the anthranilic acid synthetase complex of *Escherichia coli*. *J. Biol. Chem.* **241**:4112.

———. 1969. Anthranilate synthetase, an enzyme specified by the tryptophan operon of *Escherichia coli*: comparative studies on the complex and the subunits. *J. Bacteriol.* **97**:734.

Jackson, E. N. and C. Yanofsky. 1972a. Internal promoter of the tryptophan operon of *Escherichia coli* is located in a structural gene. *J. Mol. Biol.* **69**:307.

———. 1972b. Internal deletions in the tryptophan operon of *Escherichia coli*. *J. Mol. Biol.* **71**:149.

———. 1973. The region between the operator and first structural gene of the tryptophan operon of *Escherichia coli* may have a regulatory function. *J. Mol. Biol.* **76**:89.

Jacob, F. and J. Monod. 1961. Genetic regulatory mechanisms in the synthesis of proteins. *J. Mol. Biol.* **3**:318.

Jones, B. B. and W. S. Reznikoff. 1977. Tryptophan-transducing bacteriophages: *In vitro* studies with restriction endonucleases *Hind*II + III and *Escherichia coli* ribonucleic acid polymerase. *J. Bacteriol.* **132**:270.

Kasai, T. 1974. Regulation of the expression of the histidine operon in *Salmonella typhimurium*. *Nature* **249**:523.

Knowlton, R. G. and M. Yarus. 1976. Amino acid accepting specificity of *su7*[+] tRNA. *Fed. Proc.* **35**:1735.

Korn, L. J. and C. Yanofsky. 1976a. Polarity suppressors increase expression of the wild-type tryptophan operon of *Escherichia coli*. *J. Mol. Biol.* **103**:395.

———. 1976b. Polarity suppressors defective in transcription termination at the attenuator of the tryptophan operon of *Escherichia coli* have altered rho factor. *J. Mol. Biol.* **106**:231.

Lebowitz, P., S. M. Weissman, and C. M. Radding. 1971. Nucleotide sequence of a ribonucleic acid transcribed *in vitro* from λ phage DNA. *J. Biol. Chem.* **246**:5120.

Lee, F. and C. Yanofsky. 1977. Transcription termination at the *trp* operon attenuators of *E. coli* and *S. typhimurium*: RNA secondary structure and regulation of termination. *Proc. Natl. Acad. Sci.* **74**:4365.

Lee, F., K. Bertrand, G. Bennett, and C. Yanofsky. 1978. Comparison of the nucleotide sequences of the initial transcribed regions of the tryptophan operons of *Escherichia coli* and *Salmonella typhimurium*. *J. Mol. Biol.* **121**:193.

Lee, F., C. L. Squires, C. Squires, and C. Yanofsky. 1976. Termination of transcription *in vitro* in the *Escherichia coli* tryptophan operon leader region. *J. Mol. Biol.* **103**:383.

Lee, N. and J. Carbon. 1977. Nucleotide sequence of the 5' end of *araBAD* operon messenger RNA in *Escherichia coli* B/r. *Proc. Natl. Acad. Sci.* **74**:49.

Lowery, C. and J. P. Richardson. Characterization of the nucleotide triphosphate phosphohydrolase (ATPase) activity of RNA synthesis termination factor ρ. II. Influence of synthetic RNA homopolymers and random copolymers on the reaction. *J. Biol. Chem.* **252**:1381.

Maizels, N. 1974. *E. coli* lactose operon ribosome binding site. *Nature* **249**:647.

Manson, M. D. and C. Yanofsky. 1976. Tryptophan operon regulation in interspecific hybrids of enteric bacteria. *J. Bacteriol.* **126**:679.

Martin, J. and R. Webster. 1975. The *in vitro* translation of a terminating signal by a single *Escherichia coli* ribosome. *J. Biol. Chem.* **250**:8132.

McCray, J. W., Jr. and K. M. Herrmann. 1976. Derepression of certain aromatic amino acid biosynthetic enzymes of *Escherichia coli* K-12 by growth in Fe-deficient medium. *J. Bacteriol.* **125**:608.

McGeoch, D., J. McGeoch, and D. Morse. 1973. Synthesis of tryptophan operon RNA in a cell-free system. *Nat. New Biol.* **245**:137.

McPartland, A. and R. L. Somerville. 1974. Isolation and properties of new high efficiency promoters. *Genetics* **77**:s43.

————. 1976. Isolation and characterization of mutation creating high-efficiency transcription initiation signals within the *trp* operon of *Escherichia coli*. *J. Bacteriol.* **128**:557.

Mitchell, D. H., W. L. Reznikoff, and J. Beckwith. 1976. Genetic fusions that help define transcription termination region in *Escherichia coli*. *J. Mol. Biol.* **101**:441.

Morikawa, N. and F. Imamoto. 1969. On the degradation of messenger RNA for the tryptophan operon in *Escherichia coli*. *Nature* **223**:37.

Morse, D. E. and A. N. C. Morse. 1976. Dual-control of the tryptophan operon is mediated by both tryptophanyl-tRNA synthetase and the repressor. *J. Mol. Biol.* **103**:209.

Morse, D. E. and C. Yanofsky. 1968. The internal low-efficiency promoter of the tryptophan operon of *Escherichia coli*. *J. Mol. Biol.* **38**:447.

————. 1969a. Amber mutants of the *trpR* regulatory gene. *J. Mol. Biol.* **44**:185.

————. 1969b. A transcription-initiating mutation within a structural gene of the tryptophan operon. *J. Mol. Biol.* **41**:317.

Morse, D. E., R. D. Mosteller, and C. Yanofsky. 1970. Dynamics of synthesis, translation, and degradation of *trp* operon messenger RNA in *E. coli*. *Cold Spring Harbor Symp. Quant. Biol.* **34**:725.

Morse, D. E., R. Mosteller, R. F. Baker, and C. Yanofsky. 1969. Direction of *in vivo* degradation of tryptophan messenger RNA—A correction. *Nature* **233**:40.

Mosteller, R. D. and C. Yanofsky. 1971. Evidence that tryptophanyl transfer ribonucleic acid is not the corepressor of the tryptophan operon of *Escherichia coli*. *J. Bacteriol.* **105**:268.

Mosteller, R. D., J. K. Rose, and C. Yanofsky. 1971. Transcription initiation and degradation of *trp* mRNA. *Cold Spring Harbor Symp. Quant. Biol.* **35**:461.

Musso, R. E., B. de Crombrugghe, I. Pastan, J. Sklar, P. Yot, and S. Weissman. 1974. The 5'-terminal nucleotide sequence of galactose messenger ribonucleic acid of *Escherichia coli*. *Proc. Natl. Acad. Sci.* **71**:494.

Neff, N. F. and M. J. Chamberlin. 1978. Termination of transcription of *Escherichia coli* RNA polymerase *in vitro* is affected by ribonucleoside triphosphate base analogs. *J. Biol. Chem.* **253**:2455.

Pabst, M. J. and R. L. Somerville. 1971. A comparison of hydroxylamine and

N-methylhydroxylamine as probes for the mechanism of action of the anthranilate synthetase of *Escherichia coli*. *J. Biol. Chem.* **246**:7214.

Pabst, M. J., J. C. Kuhn, and R. L. Somerville. 1973. Feedback regulation in the anthranilate aggregate from wild type and mutant strains of *Escherichia coli*. *J. Biol. Chem.* **248**:901.

Pannekoek, H., W. J. Brammar, and P. H. Pouwels. 1975. Punctuation of transcription *in vitro* of the tryptophan operon of *Escherichia coli*. A novel type of control of transcription. *Mol. Gen. Genet.* **136**:199.

Pannekoek, H., B. Perbal, and P. H. Pouwels. 1974. The specificity of transcription *in vitro* of the tryptophan operon of *Escherichia coli*. II. The effect of rho factor. *Mol. Gen. Genet.* **132**:291.

Pieczenik, G., B. G. Barrell, and M. L. Gefter. 1972. Bacteriophage ϕ80-induced low molecular weight RNA. *Arch. Biochem. Biophys.* **152**:152.

Platt, T. and C. Yanofsky. 1975. An intercistronic region and ribosome-binding site in bacterial messenger RNA. *Proc. Natl. Acad. Sci.* **72**:2399.

Platt, T., C. Squires, and C. Yanofsky. 1976. Ribosomal-protected regions in the leader-*trpE* sequence of *E. coli* tryptophan operon mRNA. *J. Mol. Biol.* **103**:411.

Pouwels, P. H. and H. Pannekoek. 1976. A transcriptional barrier in the regulatory region of the tryptophan operon of *Escherichia coli*: Its role in the regulation of repressor-independent RNA synthesis. *Mol. Gen. Genet.* **149**:255.

Pouwels, P. H. and J. van Rotterdam. 1975. *In vitro* synthesis of enzymes of the tryptophan operon of *Escherichia coli*: Evidence for positive control of transcription. *Mol. Gen. Genet.* **136**:215.

Ratner, D. 1976. Evidence that mutations in the *suA* polarity suppressing gene directly affect termination factor rho. *Nature* **259**:151.

Roberts, J. 1969. Termination factor for RNA synthesis. *Nature* **224**:1168.

———. 1976. Transcription termination and its control in *E. coli*. In *RNA polymerase* (ed. R. Losick and M. Chamberlin), p. 247. Cold Spring Harbor Laboratory, Cold Spring Harbor, New York.

Rose, J. K. and C. Yanofsky. 1971. Transcription of the operator proximal and distal ends of the tryptophan operon: Evidence that *trpE* and *trpA* are the delimiting structural genes. *J. Bacteriol.* **108**:615.

———. 1972. Metabolic regulation of the tryptophan operon of *Escherichia coli*: Repressor-independent regulation of transcription initiation frequency. *J. Mol. Biol.* **69**:103.

———. 1974. Interaction of the operator of the tryptophan operon with repressor. *Proc. Natl. Acad. Sci.* **71**:3134.

Rose, J. K., R. D. Mosteller, and C. Yanofsky. 1970. Tryptophan messenger ribonucleic acid elongation rates and steady-state levels of tryptophan operon enzymes under various growth conditions. *J. Mol. Biol.* **51**:541.

Rose, J. K., C. L. Squires, C. Yanofsky, H.-L. Yang, and G. Zubay. 1973. Regulation of *in vitro* transcription of the tryptophan operon by purified RNA polymerase in the presence of partially purified repressor and tryptophan. *Nat. New Biol.* **245**:133.

Rosenberg, A. H. and M. L. Gefter. 1969. An iron-dependent modification of several transfer RNA species in *Escherichia coli*. *J. Mol. Biol.* **46**:581.

Rosenberg, M., B. de Crombrugghe, and R. Musso. 1976. Determination of nucleotide sequences beyond the sites of transcriptional termination. *Proc. Natl. Acad. Sci.* **73:** 717.

Rosenberg, M., D. Court, D. L. Wulff, H. Shimatake, and C. Brady. 1978. The relation between function and DNA sequence in an intercistronic regulatory region in phage λ. *Nature* **272:** 414.

Sanger, F., G. M. Air, B. G. Barrell, N. L. Brown, A. R. Coulson, J. C. Fiddes, C. A. Hutchinson III, P. M. Slocombe, and M. Smith. 1977. Nucleotide sequence of bacteriophage φX174 DNA. *Nature* **265:** 687.

Schlessinger, D., K. A. Jacobs, R. S. Gupta, Y. Kano, and F. Imamoto. 1977. Decay of individual *Escherichia coli* *trp* mRNA molecules is sequentially ordered. *J. Mol. Biol.* **110:** 421.

Shine, J. and L. Dalgarno. 1974. The 3'-terminal sequence of *Escherichia coli* 16S ribosomal RNA: Complementarity to nonsense triplets and ribosome binding sites. *Proc. Natl. Acad. Sci.* **71:** 1342.

———. 1975. Determinant of cistron specificity in bacterial ribosomes. *Nature* **254:** 34.

Sogin, M. L., N. R. Pace, M. Rosenberg, and S. M. Weissman. 1976. Nucleotide sequence of a 5S ribosomal RNA precursor from *Bacillus subtilis*. *J. Biol. Chem.* **251:** 3480.

Soll, L. 1974. Mutational alterations of tryptophan-specific transfer RNA that generate translation suppressors of the UAA, UAG, and UGA nonsense codons. *J. Mol. Biol.* **86:** 233.

Somerville, R. L. 1966. Tryptophan operon of *Escherichia coli* regulatory behavior in *Salmonella typhimurium* cytoplasm. *Science* **154:** 1585.

Somerville, R. L. and R. Elford. 1967. Hydroxamate formation by anthranilate synthetase of *Escherichia coli* K12. *Biochem. Biophys. Res. Commun.* **28:** 437.

Somerville, R. L. and C. Yanofsky. 1965. Studies on the regulation of tryptophan biosynthesis in *Escherichia coli*. *J. Mol. Biol.* **11:** 747.

Sommer, H., A. Schmitz, U. Schmeissner, and J. H. Miller. 1978. Genetic studies of the *lac* repressor. VI. The B116 repressor: An altered *lac* repressor containing amino acids specified by both the *trp* and *lacI* leader regions. *J. Mol. Biol.* (in press).

Squires, C., F. Lee, K. Bertrand, C. L. Squires, M. J. Bronson, and C. Yanofsky. 1976. Nucleotide sequence of the 5' end of tryptophan messenger RNA of *E. coli*. *J. Mol. Biol.* **103:** 351.

Squires, C. L., F. D. Lee, and C. Yanofsky. 1975. Interaction of the *trp* repressor and RNA polymerase with the *trp* operon. *J. Mol. Biol.* **92:** 93.

Squires, C. L., J. K. Rose, C. Yanofsky, H.-L. Yang, and G. Zubay. 1973. Tryptophanyl-tRNA and tryptophanyl-tRNA synthetase are not required for *in vitro* repression of the tryptophan operon. *Nat. New Biol.* **245:** 131.

Steege, D. A. 1977. 5'-Terminal nucleotide sequence of *Escherichia coli* lactose repressor mRNA: Features of translational initiation and reinitiation sites. *Proc. Natl. Acad. Sci.* **74:** 4163.

Steitz, J. A. 1978. Genetic signals and nucleotide sequences in messenger RNA. In *Biological regulation and control* (ed. R. Goldberger). Plenum Press, New York. (in press.)

Steitz, J. A. and K. Jakes. 1975. How ribosomes select initiator regions in mRNA: Base pair formation between the 3' terminus of 16S rRNA and the mRNA during initiation of protein synthesis in *E. Coli. Proc. Natl. Acad. Sci.* **72:**4734.

Steitz, J. A. and D. A. Steege. 1977. Characterization of two mRNA · rRNA complexes implicated in the initiation of protein biosynthesis. *J. Mol. Biol.* **114:**545.

Stephens, J. C., S. W. Artz, and B. N. Ames. 1975. Guanosine 5'-diphosphate 3'-diphosphate (ppGpp): Positive effector for histidine operon transcription and general signal for amino acid deficiency. *Proc. Natl. Acad. Sci.* **72:**4389.

Wice, M. and D. Kennell. 1974. Decay of messenger RNA from the tryptophan operon of *Escherichia coli* as a function of growth temperature. *J. Mol. Biol.* **84:**649.

Wuesthoff, G. and R. H. Bauerle. 1970. Mutations creating internal promoter elements in the tryptophan operon of *Salmonella Typhimurium. J. Mol. Biol.* **49:**171.

Yang, H. L., G. Zubay, E. Urm, G. Reiness, and M. Cashel. 1974. Effects of guanosine tetraphosphate, guanosine pentaphosphate, and β-γ methylenyl-guanosine pentaphosphate on gene expression of *Escherichia coli in vitro. Proc. Natl. Acad. Sci.* **71:**63.

Yanofsky, C. 1971. Tryptophan biosynthesis in *Escherichia coli. J. Am. Med. Assn.* **218:**1026.

———. 1976a. Control sites in the tryptophan operon. *Alfred Benson Symposium IX: Control of ribosome synthesis* (ed. N.C. Kjeldgaard and O. Maaløe), p. 149. Munksgaard, Copenhagen.

———. 1976b. Regulation of transcription initiation and termination in the control of expression of the tryptophan operon of *E. coli. ICN-UCLA Symp. Mol. Cell. Biol.* **5:**75.

Yanofsky, C. and L. Soll. 1977. Mutations affecting tRNA[trp] and its charging and their effect on regulation of transcription termination at the attenuator of the tryptophan operon. *J. Mol. Biol.* **113:**663.

Yarus, M., R. Knowlton, and L. Soll. 1977. Aminoacylation of the ambivalent su^+7 amber suppressor tRNA. In *Columbia Symposium on Nucleic Acid-Protein Recognition* (ed. H. J. Vogel), p. 391. Academic Press, New York.

Zalkin, H., C. Yanofsky, and C. L. Squires. 1974. Regulated *in vitro* synthesis of *Escherichia coli* tryptophan operon messenger ribonucleic acid and enzymes. *J. Biol. Chem.* **249:**465.

Zubay, G., D. E. Morse, W. J. Schrenk, and J. H. M. Miller. 1972. Detection and isolation of the repressor protein for the tryptophan operon of *Escherichia coli. Proc. Natl. Acad. Sci.* **69:**1100.

Cyclic AMP, the Cyclic AMP Receptor Protein, and Their Dual Control of the Galactose Operon

Benoit de Crombrugghe and Ira Pastan
Laboratory of Molecular Biology
National Cancer Institute
Bethesda, Maryland 20014

INTRODUCTION

In this paper we summarize the experimental evidence which led to the demonstration of the role of cyclic AMP and its receptor protein (CRP) in the activation of gene transcription in bacteria. We also examine the function of this protein in the control of the galactose operon of *Escherichia coli*. Regulation of this operon is more complex than that of the *lac* operon: two interspersed promoters which respond to different regulatory mechanisms control the expression of the *gal* genes. The activity of one *gal* promoter is stimulated and the activity of the other *gal* promoter is inhibited by cyclic AMP and CRP.

CYCLIC AMP AND CATABOLITE REPRESSION

When *E. coli* find both glucose and lactose in their environment, they metabolize glucose and repress the utilization of lactose. This phenomenon has been called "catabolite or glucose repression of lactose utilization," and it results in the inhibition of the synthesis of the enzymes for lactose metabolism (Monod 1947; Magasanik 1962). This repression by glucose is not unique for the lactose metabolizing enzymes and has been observed for the enzymes which degrade a number of other carbohydrates (Epps and Gale 1942; Magasanik 1962; Koch et al. 1964). One intracellular compound which varies when the composition of the medium changes is the cyclic nucleotide adenosine-3',5'-monophosphate (cyclic AMP). Sutherland and his colleagues, who had first discovered cyclic AMP in animal cells, found that when *E. coli* were growing in a glucose-containing medium they had low levels of cyclic AMP and that withdrawal of glucose from the medium produced a rapid increase in cyclic AMP (Makman and Sutherland 1965).

The finding of low cyclic AMP levels in cells growing in glucose, coupled with the observation that glucose repressed the synthesis of β-galactosidase and a number of other enzymes, prompted the hypothesis that the repression of catabolic enzyme synthesis by glucose might be mediated by a decrease in the intracellular levels of cyclic AMP. To test this idea, Perlman and Pastan added cyclic AMP to *E. coli* growing in glucose medium and found that the cyclic nucleotide could overcome the glucose repression of β-galactosidase synthesis (Perlman and Pastan 1968). Subsequently, it was found that cyclic AMP controlled the synthesis of other inducible enzymes which were subject to catabolite repression (de Crombrugghe et al. 1969) and also regulated the synthesis of the flagellum of *E. coli* (Yokota and Gots 1970). Later it was shown that cyclic AMP could influence the life cycle of some bacteriophages, such as λ and P22, by favoring their lysogenic pathway over their lytic pathway (Hong et al. 1971; Grodzicker et al. 1972).

A good correlation was found between the intracellular levels of cyclic AMP in *E. coli* and the ability of these cells to synthesize β-galactosidase (Epstein et al. 1975). The carbohydrates which produce the most severe repression in enzyme synthesis, such as glucose-6-phosphate and glucose, also cause the most pronounced reduction in cyclic AMP concentration. If glycerol and glucosamine are the carbon sources, the cells synthesize much more β-galactosidase and have higher cyclic AMP levels.

Several investigators have studied the mechanism by which glucose lowers the intracellular concentrations of cyclic AMP. The lowering of cyclic AMP in the cells is not the result of a more rapid degradation of the cyclic nucleotide, since the decrease occurs even in cells with no detectable phosphodiesterase activity (Nielsen et al. 1973). Peterkofksy and Gazdar (1973) measured the rate of synthesis of cyclic AMP in growing cells and showed that glucose reduced the synthesis of cyclic AMP and did not affect release of cyclic AMP into the medium. Indeed, the rate of release of cyclic AMP into the medium varies proportionally with the intracellular concentration of the nucleotide (Epstein et al. 1975). Extensive metabolism of glucose is not required to inhibit cyclic AMP synthesis, since α-methylglucoside is as effective as glucose in inhibiting cyclic AMP synthesis (α-methylglucoside is transported into the cells by the phosphotransferase system as α-methylglucoside-6-P and is not metabolized further). Studies with several mutants of the phosphotransferase carbohydrate transport system (PTS) indicate that the ability of glucose or α-methylglucoside to inhibit adenylate cyclase activity is mediated by one or more components of the PTS system (Pastan and Perlman 1969; Peterkofsky and Gazdar 1975), probably by a phosphorylation-dephosphorylation mechanism of either adenylate cyclase itself (Peterkofsky and Gazdar 1975) or of a membrane component interacting with adenylate cyclase (Saier and Feucht 1975).

CRP MEDIATES THE EFFECTS OF CYCLIC AMP

Two types of experiments were critical for our understanding of the role of cyclic AMP in controlling the synthesis of a number of inducible enzymes. First, two classes of mutants were isolated which were unable to ferment lactose and many other carbohydrates. One such mutant (Cya⁻) has a defective adenylate cyclase enzyme and is unable to convert ATP to cyclic AMP (Perlman and Pastan 1969). This mutant grows very poorly even in rich medium, suggesting an important role of cyclic AMP for normal growth of the cells. Addition of cyclic AMP to the cells restores their ability to ferment lactose and other sugars and to synthesize β-galactosidase and other inducible catabolic enzymes (Perlman and Pastan 1969; Miller et al. 1971). The second class of mutants (Crp⁻) obtained were unable to synthesize β-galactosidase and other inducible enzymes even when cyclic AMP was added to the cells (Emmer et al. 1970; Schwartz and Beckwith 1970). The isolation of this second class of mutants suggested that another factor in *E. coli* might be responsible for the action of cyclic AMP on enzyme synthesis. A protein which binds cyclic AMP was indeed found in extracts of wild-type cells (Emmer et al. 1970). (The protein is called CRP for cyclic AMP receptor protein, or CAP for catabolite activator protein [Zubay et al. 1970], or CGA for catabolite gene activator protein [Riggs et al. 1971].) The cyclic AMP binding protein was absent or greatly reduced in the second class of mutants (Emmer et al. 1970; Zubay et al. 1970).

The development of DNA-dependent cell-free systems for the synthesis of β-galactosidase (Chambers and Zubay 1969) and other enzymes and for the synthesis of *lac* and *gal* mRNA (de Crombrugghe et al. 1971a,b; Nissley et al. 1971) greatly aided in elucidating the mechanism of action of cyclic AMP. It was first shown that the synthesis of β-galactosidase was stimulated 20-fold by cyclic AMP in a crude *E. coli* extract (S30) supplemented with DNA from the transducing phage ϕ80d*lac* DNA (Chambers and Zubay 1969). If the S30 extract was made from cells which were defective in the CRP protein, cyclic AMP was unable to stimulate β-galactosidase synthesis (Emmer et al. 1970; Zubay et al. 1970). However, the addition of an extract from wild-type cells or of a purified preparation of CRP restored the cyclic-AMP-dependent synthesis of β-galactosidase in this *lac* DNA-directed cell-free system. This experiment suggested that the action of cyclic AMP on catabolic enzyme synthesis was mediated by CRP.

After the purification of CRP had been achieved, it was shown that CRP and cyclic AMP were essential for initiation of *lac* mRNA synthesis in a completely defined cell-free system (de Crombrugghe et al. 1971a; Eron and Block 1971). Hence, no other factors are involved which could possibly mediate the action of CRP. In the same system, the *lac* repressor was shown to prevent *lac* mRNA synthesis, and this block was overcome by adding inducers of the *lac* operon. CRP thus mediates directly the action of cyclic AMP on *lac* mRNA synthesis at the *lac* promoter. In several other inducible bacterial operons, a similar role for CRP and cyclic AMP as a positive factor in gene regulation was demonstrated (Parks et al. 1971; Nissley et al. 1971; Wetekam et al. 1971; Greenblatt and Schlief 1971; Wilcox et al. 1974; Lee et al. 1974).

CRP AND THE REGULATION OF THE *gal* OPERON

The *gal* operon of *E. coli* consists of three contiguous genes, *E*, *T*, and *K*, specifying three enzymes which participate in the metabolism of galactose: UDP-galactose 4-epimerase, galactose 1-phosphate uridyltransferase, and galactokinase. The size of each cistron is approximately 1100 base pairs (Wilson and Hogness 1968). *Gal* mRNA synthesis proceeds from *E* through *K* (Michaelis and Starlinger 1967; Adhya and Shapiro 1968) and the synthesis of the three *gal* enzymes is induced by D-galactose or D-fucose (Buttin 1963a).

Negative control of the operon is exerted by the *gal* repressor protein, the product of the *galR* gene which is unlinked to the *gal* operon (Buttin 1963b). Most mutations in *galR* result in the constitutive synthesis of the *gal* enzymes, i.e., the enzymes are synthesized without inducer. Other *gal*-linked mutations are also constitutive but are *cis*-dominant: they are mutations in the *gal* operator (Buttin 1963b; Adhya and Echols 1966). The *gal* repressor protein has been purified from strains which either were made lysogenic with a λ*galR* transducing phage (Parks et al. 1971) or harbor a plasmid in which the *galR* gene had been introduced by in vitro recombination (R. DiLauro, pers. comm.). The *gal* repressor binds specifically to *gal* DNA (Parks et al. 1971) and represses the synthesis of *gal* mRNA in a defined in vitro system (Nakanishi et al. 1973). The repressor is active with a λp*gal* DNA template containing a normal *gal* operator, but not with *gal* operator constitutive (O^c) templates.

CONTROL BY CRP AND CYCLIC AMP

In Vivo Studies

That CRP and cyclic AMP are important for *gal* enzyme synthesis was first suggested by the finding that cyclic AMP could overcome the repression by glucose of galactokinase synthesis (de Crombrugghe et al. 1969). Furthermore, in Cya$^-$ or Crp$^-$ mutants, the induced levels of galactokinase and of *gal* mRNA were found to be much reduced (Miller et al. 1971). The inducers, D-galactose or D-fucose, had little effect on *gal* expression in these mutant strains. Although high concentrations of inducer were used in these experiments, it is probable that the uptake of inducer was limited either by glucose itself (Adhya and Echols 1966) or as a result of the absence of cyclic AMP or functional CRP in the cells (S. Gottesman and S. Adhya, pers. comm.). It was noted, however, that both Cya⁻ and Crp⁻ mutants, which are unable to ferment lactose, arabinose, and maltose, were capable of utilizing galactose as their sole carbon source (Perlman and Pastan 1969).

Recently, S. Adhya performed induction experiments using growth conditions different from those previously used. He found that the synthesis of galactokinase in *cya* or *crp* strains was inducible by D-fucose or D-galactose. Furthermore, the induced level was only moderately reduced in comparison to the fully induced enzyme levels in Cya⁺ or Crp⁺ cells (S. Adhya, in prep.). Consistent with this observation, mutations in the *gal* repressor gene or in the *gal* operator locus resulted in a high level of constitutive *gal* expression whether or not cyclic AMP or CRP were present in the cells (Rothman-Denes et al. 1973; S. Adhya, in prep.).

In Vitro Studies

In contrast to the in vivo results, the in vitro results showed a very striking stimulatory effect of CRP and cyclic AMP on *gal* expression. First in a cell-free DNA-dependent system for protein synthesis, cyclic AMP stimulated galactokinase synthesis five- to tenfold (Parks et al. 1971; Wetekam et al. 1971). The synthesis of *gal* mRNA was also studied in vitro in a completely defined system consisting of DNA from a transducing phage λp*gal*, *E. coli* RNA polymerase, CRP, cyclic AMP, buffers, and nucleoside triphosphates (Nissley et al. 1971). *Gal* mRNA synthesis was measured by hybridization to the separated strands of λp*gal* DNA after a prehybridization to λ DNA. In this defined transcription system, the synthesis of *gal* mRNA was completely dependent on CRP and cyclic AMP and required an intact *gal* promoter. No stimulation of *gal* mRNA transcription was found with the DNA of a *gal* promoter mutant (Pastan and Adhya 1976; P. Nissley, unpubl.). Thus an obvious discrepancy existed between the in vivo observations, which indicated little or no dependency on cyclic AMP, and the in vitro results, which demonstrated an almost absolute requirement for CRP and cyclic AMP. One solution to this enigma was that the operon might be controlled by two promoters, one dependent on cyclic AMP and CRP and the other independent of these factors.

Based on studies with *capR*⁻ mutants that have elevated *gal* enzyme levels in vivo, it has also been proposed that other types of elements regulate *gal* operon expression (Hua and Markovitz 1972; Mackie and Wilson 1972). This mode of regulation has not as yet been demonstrated in vitro. *capR*⁻ mutants have a complex phenotype including hyper-mucoidicity, higher ultraviolet (UV) sensitivity, and defective cell division; these mutants are also able to suppress some missense mutations (Gottesman and Zipser 1978; J. Schrenk, pers. comm.) and degrade nonsense polypeptide fragments more slowly than normal cells (Shineberg and Zipser 1973).

Nucleotide Sequence of the *gal* Regulatory Region

To understand in more detail the molecular basis of the regulation of the galactose operon, the nucleotide sequence of the segment of DNA involved in the control of this operon was determined. The nucleotide sequence of the initial 5′-terminal 70 bases of *gal* mRNA was first established by conventional RNA sequencing techniques (Musso et al. 1974). The 5′-terminal *gal* mRNA was obtained from a CRP- and cyclic-AMP-stimulated, kinetically controlled, in vitro transcription reaction using as template λp*gal* DNA. The RNA was first hybridized to λ DNA and subsequently to the *l* strand of λp*gal*8 DNA. To obtain the nucleotide sequence preceding the start point of transcription, a restriction map of the DNA region surrounding the regulatory region of *gal* was first established (Fig. 1) (Sklar et al. 1977; Musso et al. 1977b). Restriction sites recognized by *Hin*f and by *Hha* were located about 60 and 90 bases, respectively, preceding the point at which mRNA transcription began. The DNA sequence of the 93 residues preceding the initiation site was determined (Musso et al. 1977b; Sklar et al. 1977) both by sequencing the RNA transcripts of the restriction fragments and by direct DNA sequence analysis of the fragments by the method of Maxam and Gilbert (1977). Figure 2 shows the DNA sequence of a segment covering the 93 base pairs preceding the start site for cyclic AMP–CRP-dependent *gal* mRNA and 46 base pairs corresponding to the initial 5′ terminus of *gal* mRNA: +1 corresponds to the first nucleotide present in *gal* mRNA when cyclic AMP and CRP are used to promote *gal* transcription.

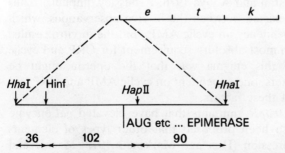

Figure 1   Relevant restriction sites in the regulatory segment preceding the structural genes of the galactose operon.

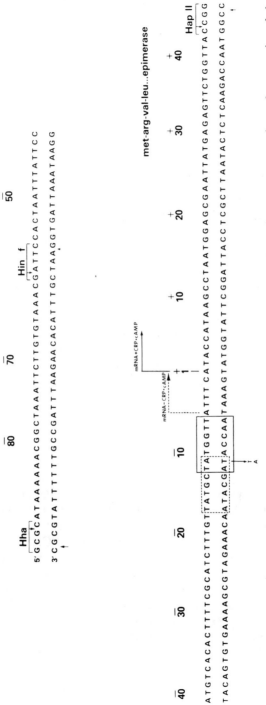

Figure 2 DNA sequence of the operator-promoter region of the galactose operon. The +1 corresponds to the start site of the CRP–cyclic-AMP-dependent mRNA. The two Pribnow heptamers preceding each start site are boxed.

The Two Promoters of the *gal* Operon

When the same restriction fragments containing the *gal* regulatory region were transcribed in vitro, it became clear that transcription initiated from two different start points, depending on the presence or absence of cyclic AMP and CRP (Musso et al. 1977a). For these experiments, the transcription reactions were conducted at low nucleoside-triphosphate concentrations, using conditions which cause the enzyme RNA polymerase to pause early after initiation (see also Maizels 1973). In the presence of CRP and cyclic AMP, the majority of the *gal* transcripts pause at several points within the first 9 bases of the 5′ end of the CRP- and cyclic-AMP-dependent *gal* mRNA (Fig. 2, +1 to +9) (Musso et al. 1974). These short transcripts were fractionated by polyacrylamide gel electrophoresis, and their RNA sequence determined. In the absence of CRP and cyclic AMP, transcription from the above start point was completely inhibited and instead was initiated 5 bases upstream from it and paused within a different 6-base sequence (Fig. 2, −5 to +1). Hence, in the absence of CRP and cyclic AMP, RNA polymerase initiates transcription at a site, S2, that is about half a turn in the DNA helix preceding S1, the CRP- and cyclic-AMP-dependent start site. CRP and cyclic AMP are not only required for transcription from S1, but they also abolish transcription from S2. Under our experimental conditions, the efficiency of initiation of transcription at S2 is about two to five times better than at S1 (R. DiLauro and B. de Crombrugghe, in prep.). Glycerol, which had been shown previously to stimulate *gal* transcription in the absence of CRP and cyclic AMP (Nakanishi et al. 1974), enhances transcription at S2 but not at S1 (Musso et al. 1977a).

It should be noted that transcription from each of the start sites is not limited to short transcripts. When the same fragment used for the above experiments was transcribed at high nucleoside-triphosphate concentrations, both in the presence and absence of CRP and cyclic AMP, long transcripts were synthesized. These were isolated and analyzed by RNA sequencing methods. The fingerprints of the two were identical except for the 5′-triphosphate-containing oligonucleotide which was 5 bases longer when the transcript came from a reaction without CRP and cyclic AMP (Musso et al. 1977a). It was interesting to note that even at a high nucleoside-triphosphate concentration a considerable proportion of the transcripts from S2 continued to pause within the sequence of 6–7 bases following S2. For the same conditions of high nucleoside-triphosphate concentrations, all CRP- and cyclic-AMP-dependent S1 transcripts are of large size (R. DiLauro and B. de Crombrugghe, in prep.). Thus the stuttering of transcription from S2 is not just a result of the low nucleoside-triphosphate concentrations but may represent an additional regulatory mechanism.

In many prokaryotic promoters, a sequence of 7 bases related to the sequence TATPuATG precedes the start point of transcription by a distance of 5 to 6 base pairs (Pribnow 1975; Schaller et al. 1975). This sequence is believed to play a role in the formation of a stable complex between RNA polymerase and promoters. Such stable complex formation appears to involve the melting of a small number of base pairs and is a prerequisite for correct initiation of transcription (Chamberlin 1974). A similar heptamer precedes both the S1 (TATGGTT) and S2 (TATGCTA) start sites. These heptamers are boxed in Figure 2.

The existence of two promoters in *gal* is further illustrated by a *gal* promoter mutation (Musso et al. 1977a). In vivo cells which harbor this *gal* promoter mutation are unable to ferment galactose. However, if cyclic AMP or CRP is eliminated by mutation as in Cya⁻ or Crp⁻ mutants, *gal* expression is increased. In vitro, with this mutant, transcription from S2 is unaltered but no transcription from S1 takes place. CRP and cyclic AMP still prevent transcription from S2 but are unable to activate transcription from S1. Thus, both in vivo transcription and in vitro transcription take place only in the absence of CRP and cyclic AMP. With CRP and cyclic AMP, transcription from S2 is blocked and transcription from S1 is abolished by the promoter mutation.

Interestingly, the base change caused by the mutation (an inversion of A/T to T/A) affects the second base of the heptamer sequence preceding S1 (see Fig. 2). Many promoters have an A residue in this position of their heptamer sequence. In *gal* the single base change completely abolishes the activity of the CRP- and cyclic-AMP-dependent promoter. The same base change also alters the seventh base of the heptamer preceding S2. In many promoters this seventh residue in the heptamer is highly variable. This base change does not affect initiation from S2 in vitro.

The differential regulation by CRP of transcription at two start sites (S1 and S2), the existence of a mutation which abolishes transcription from one but not the other site, the presence of two separate heptamers preceding the two start sites, and the premature termination of one of the transcripts all indicate that two overlapping promoters control *gal* transcription.

The demonstration of two promoters for *gal* transcription provides a rationale for the apparent lack of cyclic AMP dependency for *gal* expression in vivo. As for in vitro transcription, in vivo transcription presumably starts at S1 in the presence of cyclic AMP and CRP, but starts at S2 when cyclic AMP or CRP is low or absent from the cells.

Since S1 and S2 are separated by 5 base pairs, the sites for promoter-polymerase interaction and thus for formation of open promoter complexes are interspersed. Isolation of additional mutations that affect initiation of transcription at one or the other promoter or at both promoters, as well as direct protection experiments against chemical modification of the DNA, will help identify the bases which are important for the interactions of each promoter with RNA polymerase. The observation of two overlapping promoters in *gal* is analogous to the existence in the ϕX174 genome of sequences coding for two different proteins interspersed within the same DNA segment. In *gal*, two overlapping promoter sequences control a same set of structural genes.

THE *gal* OPERATOR AND A MODEL FOR *gal* REPRESSION

Recent experiments by S. Adhya clearly indicate that the *gal* operon can be induced by galactose even when cyclic AMP or functional CRP is eliminated from the cells by mutations (*cya* or *crp*) (S. Adhya, in prep.). Thus, under conditions where S1 is inactive, the operon is still inducible. In vitro, the *gal* repressor blocks cyclic-AMP- and CRP-dependent transcription from S1 but has no effect on initiation of transcription from S2 (R. DiLauro and B. de Crombrugghe, in prep.). The repressor binds to *gal* DNA in the absence of CRP and cyclic AMP but does not prevent RNA polymerase from initiating transcription at S2. Hence, the in vitro results reproduce the in vivo regulation by the *gal* repressor when transcription starts from S1. In the absence of cyclic AMP or CRP, however, repression of *gal* transcription occurs in vivo but not, under our experimental conditions, in vitro. This could suggest that our defined in vitro system is lacking one or more elements responsible for the repression at S2 in vivo.

Two lines of evidence mark the location of the *gal* operator. Formation of a complex between *gal* repressor and *gal* DNA protects the *Hin*f site at -60 (see Fig. 2) from being restricted (R. DiLauro and B. de Crombrugghe, in prep.). Two *gal* operator constitutive mutants have also lost this cleavage site and DNA sequence analysis of these and other *gal* operator mutants indicate that the operator mutations are all clustered between -66 and -60 (R. DiLauro et al., in prep.). A more complete definition of the *gal* repressor binding site will be obtained by direct protection experiments against chemical modification of the DNA. Such experiments are in progress.

The location of the *gal* operator contrasts with the location of the operator in the *lac*, *trp*, and lambda operons. In these systems repressor binds close to the transcription initiation site and thereby directly prevents RNA polymerase from forming a stable initiation complex. The location of the *gal* operator suggests a different mechanism for repression. Our simplest model postulates that the *gal* repressor inhibits transcription from S1 by preventing the interaction between CRP and DNA and/or between CRP and RNA polymerase.

The repression of *gal* expression from S2 which occurs in vivo obviously requires a more complex mechanism. In our earlier experiments using λ*gal* DNA as template, it was found that cyclic AMP and

CRP stimulated *gal* mRNA synthesis five- to tenfold (Nissley et al. 1971). *Gal* mRNA was measured by DNA-RNA hybridization and the majority of the RNA molecules were of large size. Our more recent experiments indicate that initiation of *gal* transcription at S2 is in fact more efficient than at S1 (R. DiLauro and B. de Crombrugghe, in prep.). Hence the intense stuttering of RNA polymerase transcription at S2, even with elevated concentrations of nucleoside triphosphates, indicates a high rate of initiation coupled with a high rate of premature termination. Thus the low levels of hybridizable *gal* mRNA found in vitro in the absence of cyclic AMP and CRP were probably due to a defect in elongation and not of initiation. In vivo, as indicated earlier, a high inducible level of *gal* operon expression can be observed in the absence of cyclic AMP or CRP (S. Adhya, in prep.). Under these conditions, initiation of transcription probably occurs from S2. Repression of *gal* transcription from S2, as is observed in vivo, might therefore be mediated by a mechanism that would control the rate of premature termination.

THE CRP RECOGNITION SITE IN *gal* COULD BE DIFFERENT FROM THE *lac* CRP SITE

Two lines of evidence suggest that the DNA segment to the left of −60 in Figure 2 may contain at least part of the CRP recognition site. First, the *Hin*f site at −60 in Figure 2 is protected against restriction when a CRP-dependent transcription-initiation complex is formed, but no protection of this site occurs when a similar complex is formed at the second promoter without CRP (Musso et al. 1977b). Second, comparison of the *gal* sequence near this site with the CRP binding site in *lac* reveals several striking similarities. In *lac*, two types of experiments have identified the CRP binding site. By binding CRP to a small DNA fragment, J. Majors (1978) could protect from methylation by dimethylsulfate symmetrically located G residues at −55 and −57 on one strand and at −68 and −66 on the other strand (see Fig. 3). These residues are part of a sequence with twofold rotational symmetry, centered at −62/61. In addition, two of these residues, −57 and −66, symmetrically located within the symmetry element are the sites where all CRP site mutations occur (Dickson et al. 1977). These results strongly suggest that, in *lac*, CRP recognizes a symmetrical DNA sequence.

In *gal*, the DNA sequence in this region presents striking similarities with the *lac* sequence. The G-T-G (−68 to −66) and C-A-C (−39 to −55) residues which define the outside bases of the CRP symmetry in *lac* are also the outside segments of a similar symmetrical element in *gal* centered at −61/60. However, the size of this symmetrical element is slightly larger in *gal* than in *lac*. In addition, two sequences which are very similar in *gal* and *lac* overlap these symmetries (Fig. 3). Sequence AATTCTTGTG in *gal* resembles the sequence AATTAATGTG in *lac*; both sequences are

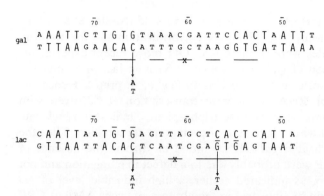

Figure 3 Comparison of the CRP binding site in *lac* and an analogous segment in *gal*. The base change in *gal*, indicated by the arrow, is the 126 mutation (R. DiLauro and B. de Crombrugghe, unpubl.). The base changes in *lac* correspond to class-1 promoter mutations sequenced by Dickson et al. (1977). The symmetrical sequences are underscored. Bars above bases in the *lac* sequence indicate sites of protection by CRP against methylation (Majors 1978).

exactly aligned with respect to the start point of transcription. On the other side of the symmetrical element, the *gal* sequence CACTAATT (−55 to −48) resembles the *lac* sequence CACTCATT (−57 to −50).

Although there are similarities, both in sequence and in symmetry, between the CRP binding site in *lac* and an analogous segment in *gal*, a change of the same G residue to A at −66, which lies within this similar and symmetrical sequence, produces a very different result on promoter activity in *lac* and *gal*. The change which alters the twofold rotational symmetry shown in Figure 3 results in a high level of constitutive expression of the *gal* operon in vivo. In vitro, with this mutant, transcription from S1 still exhibits complete CRP and cyclic-AMP dependency and transcription from S2 is not different from S2 transcription with wild-type DNA. In contrast, an identical G/C-to-A/T change at −66 in *lac*, which alters the same symmetrical sequence, results in a severe loss of promoter activity (Hopkins 1974). Although the CRP concentration dependencies of the *lac* promoter and the P1 *gal* promoter are identical (J. Majors, pers. comm.), it is conceivable that in *gal* CRP binds only to the right part (most proximal to the initiation site) of the symmetrical element. In fact, all *gal* operator constitutive mutants that we have studied map between −66 and −60 and show a normal pattern of in vitro transcription at both the S1 and S2 promoters (R. DiLauro and B. de Crombrugghe, in prep.). It is clear that the *gal* CRP recognition site will be better defined by the isolation of mutations in this site and also by performing chemical protection experiments similar to those conducted by J. Majors with *lac*.

Examination of the DNA sequence in the promoter of the arabinose operon, another CRP-dependent operon, fails to show similarities with the CRP binding site in *lac* or with the analogous segment in *gal* (R. Schleif, pers. comm.). This suggests that CRP is capable of activating gene transcription by interacting with a different set of sequences in different CRP-sensitive promoters.

STRUCTURE AND MECHANISM OF ACTION OF CRP

The original method for purifying CRP to homogeneity was developed by Anderson et al. (1971). This method was then slightly modified to allow the purification of larger amounts of material necessary for structural studies (Pastan et al. 1974). More recently, J. S. Krakow (pers. comm.) has developed a simpler method employing DNA chromatography that also gives quite good yields of CRP. Attempts to purify CRP by affinity chromatography of cyclic-AMP columns have been unsuccessful.

A number of physical properties of CRP are listed in Table 1. CRP is a dimer composed of two identical subunits of 22,500 daltons each. One striking feature is its isoelectric point, $pI = 9.12$. David Schlesinger (University of Indiana) and others have attempted to determine the amino acid sequence of CRP (pers. comm.). A summary of the current state of this work follows.

CRP is composed of two identical subunits of approximately 200

Table 1   Summary of physical properties of CRP

Parameter	Calculated value
Molecular weight of native protein[a]	44,600
Molecular weight of reduced alkylated subunits in 6 M guanidine hydrochloride[a]	22,300
Sedimentation coefficient, $S_{20,w}$, of native protein[b]	3.53
Partial specific volume, V^c	0.752 ml/g
Diffusion coefficient, $D_{20,w}$, of native protein[d]	7.7×10^{-7} cm^2/sec
Frictional coefficient, f/f_0, of native protein[e]	1.17
Isoelectric point, pI[f]	9.12
Percent α-helical structure[g]	31

Data from Anderson et al. (1971).
[a]Determined by sedimentation equilibrium studies.
[b]Determined by sedimentation velocity studies.
[c]Calculated from the amino acid composition.
[d]Calculated from combined sedimentation and molecular-weight data.
[e]Calculated from combined sedimentation and molecular-weight data, but uncorrected for hydration.
[f]Determined by isoelectric focusing.
[g]Determined by circular dichroic measurements.

residues (22,500 daltons) each. Digestion of CRP in the presence of cyclic AMP with subtilisin results in a resistant-core, alpha CRP which retains cyclic-AMP binding but which has lost the cyclic-AMP-dependent DNA-binding activity (Krakow and Pastan 1973). Alpha CRP is approximately 60% the size of CRP and has been shown by automated amino acid sequence analysis to be N terminal in CRP. Interestingly, the largest fragment (CNBr-1) of CRP produced by cleavage of CRP with cyanogen bromide (CNBr) is also N terminal in CRP and consists of about half the intact CRP molecule.

The N-terminal ten-amino-acid segment has been published (Pastan and Adhya 1976), but extended automated sequence analysis has been limited due to poor solubility of intact CRP or CNBr-1 in the coupling buffer during sequence analysis. Partial sequence of the N-terminal half of CRP is presently being obtained from purified peptides following maleoylation and tryptic digestion of the N-terminal CNBr peptide.

Most of the C-terminal half of CRP has been sequenced and peptide segment overlaps with CNBr and tryptic peptides have been obtained for 80% of the region.

A number of nucleotides other than cyclic AMP bind to CRP. These include cyclic tubericidin monophosphate (cyclic TuMP), cyclic GMP, cyclic IMP, and 8-Br-cyclic AMP (Anderson et al. 1972). However, despite their ability to bind to CRP, they differ in their ability to promote binding of CRP to DNA. Only cyclic AMP and cyclic TuMP are active for DNA binding. The latter are also the only two nucleotides to promote gene transcription (Anderson et al. 1972). This is due to the fact that only cyclic AMP and cyclic TuMP induce a conformational change in CRP. Apparently, this conformational change is necessary for DNA binding. A reflection of this conformational change is the proteolysis of CRP that occurs in the presence of cyclic AMP (Krakow and Pastan 1973). Under these conditions, a fragment of CRP designated αCRP is generated that retains its ability to bind to DNA at pH 6 but has lost its cAMP-dependent DNA-binding activity at pH 8. αCRP is derived from the amino-terminal portion of the native molecule (see above).

Other evidence that cyclic AMP induces a conformational change in CRP comes from the studies of Wu and coworkers using temperature-jump and fluorescent-labeling methods (Wu and Wu 1974; Wu et al. 1974). Cyclic AMP also induces cross-linking of sulfhydryls of CRP in the presence of 4,4'-dithriodipyridine (Eilen and Krakow 1977).

Specificity of binding to CRP-dependent promoters has been difficult to demonstrate. Indeed, no difference in binding of CRP to intact λ DNA or λlac DNA is found, although the effect of CRP on activation of the *lac* promoter is highly specific. Furthermore, CRP binds as well to single-stranded λlac DNA as to native λlac DNA (Riggs et al. 1971; Nissley et al. 1972). This inability to demonstrate binding specificity could be due to

(1) the high affinity of CRP for random DNA and only a slightly more elevated affinity for specific binding sites, or (2) a very fast dissociation rate of CRP from both its specific and nonspecific sites. Only by using small DNA fragments (~200 base pairs) could specificity of binding of CRP to the *lac* and *gal* promoter regions be detected (Majors 1975; Mitra et al. 1975; J. S. Krakow et al., unpubl.). CRP binds much more strongly to a fragment containing the *lac* or *gal* promoter region than to other similar-sized fragments. Binding to a fragment containing a point mutation in the *lac* promoter is greatly reduced (Majors 1975). Moreover, in *lac* the exact location of the CRP binding site and the bases which make contact with this protein have been identified (Reznikoff and Abelson, this volume).

The function of CRP is to stimulate the formation of an initiation complex for a certain class of promoters. The structure of this class of promoters is obviously more complex than that of promoters which can be activated without additional factors. In some of the latter promoters, sequence specificity of only a small segment of untranscribed DNA seems essential for promoter function. In an fd promoter, the segment which lies upstream of residue -15 can be interchanged with other unrelated segments without considerable loss of promoter function (Okamoto et al. 1977). It is thus possible that for some minimal promoters the only essential feature is a seven-nucleotide sequence similar to or closely related to that described by Pribnow (1975). A second class of CRP-independent promoters, such as the λP_R and λP_L and the *lacI* promoter, need additional specific interaction sites for activity, including some around -35. Indeed, mutations around this site either inactivate or greatly enhance the function of these promoters (Maurer et al. 1974; Maniatis et al. 1975a,b; J. Miller, pers. comm.).

A third class is represented by CRP-regulated promoters. They are characterized by the extent of the interactions needed to be activated. A stable initiation complex is not formed in the absence of CRP. The sequence information, and hence the structure of the DNA, is insufficient by itself to allow RNA polymerase to form an initiation complex. The additional information and interactions for such a complex are provided by CRP and the CRP binding site.

The base changes in a *lac* promoter mutant and its UV5 revertant illustrate this concept. The mutant has a defective CRP site (Dickson et al. 1977; Majors 1975) and is unable to initiate *lac* transcription. In the pseudorevertant, UV5, promoter activity is restored but becomes independent of cyclic AMP and CRP (Silverstone et al. 1970). Two base pairs in the Pribnow box are changed so that RNA polymerase is now capable of forming a stable initiation complex without the interactions provided by CRP (Gilbert 1976).

There are two general models for the action of CRP on transcription.

The first model implies that CRP activates the promoter and the second postulates activation of RNA polymerase. According to the first model, the binding of CRP results in destabilizing the DNA helix at a distance ("telestability") and so allows the formation of an initiation complex between RNA polymerase and DNA. One argument in favor of this model was based on the presence of two G/C-rich segments bracketing an A/T-rich sequence in the *lac* promoter (Dickson et al. 1975). Binding of CRP to its recognition site would destabilize these G/C-rich segments. Such structures are not found in *gal*, although transcription from S1 is as dependent on CRP and cyclic AMP as in *lac*. The second model proposes that protein-protein contacts between CRP bound to DNA and RNA polymerase are needed for the formation of an initiation complex (Gilbert 1976).

It is possible that in some CRP-sensitive promoters the CRP site itself has a low degree of structural specificity and that the formation of an initiation complex takes place because of the simultaneous interaction between CRP and RNA polymerase and between these proteins and the promoter. In *gal* the signal for the formation of a stable initiation complex and the subsequent activation of transcription at S1 rather than at S2 is the presence of CRP already on the DNA or the simultaneous interactions between CRP and RNA polymerase at the promoter. If RNA polymerase were interacting first with this region, it would bind preferentially to the second promoter (S2).

Another important question is, How is transcription from S2 in *gal* inhibited by CRP and cyclic AMP? One possible mechanism is that the interaction of CRP with its recognition site on the DNA could create different protein-protein contacts which would facilitate the formation of a preinitiation complex at S1 and inhibit this reaction at S2. Alternatively, CRP might also interact with a second site on the DNA to inhibit transcription from S2. Another possible explanation would imply inactivation of free RNA polymerase by CRP. The concentration of CRP which produces half-maximal stimulation of transcription at S1 coincides with that which causes 50% inhibition at S2, hence favoring the first mechanism (T. Taniguchi et al., in prep.).

In the arabinose system, two adjacent promoters, one for the *araBAD* operon and one for the *araC* gene, are oriented in opposite directions. Initiation of transcription at the *araBAD* promoter requires, in addition to CRP and cyclic AMP, the *araC* protein. The activity of the *araC* promoter is stimulated by, but not dependent on, CRP and cyclic AMP. The corresponding start sites for these promoters are about 150 base pairs apart. As in *gal*, activation of one promoter inhibits transcription of the other (Hirsh and Schleif 1977). Here also, the formation of a stable preinitiation complex at one promoter could by protein-protein interactions inhibit its formation at the other promoter.

WHY TWO *gal* PROMOTERS?

What is the physiological significance of the complex regulation of *gal* expression? The dual control of *gal* transcription may reflect the dual role of galactose in cellular metabolism. When present in the medium, galactose can serve as a general carbon source for cell metabolism. Figure 4 shows the pathway for conversion of galactose to glucose-6-P. In the course of reaction 2, UDP-galactose is generated. UDP-galactose is a direct precursor for cell-wall biosynthesis. Even in the absence of galactose, UDP-galactose is needed for this function and is generated from UDP-glucose by the enzyme UDP-galactose-epimerase. This enzyme is specified by the promoter proximal cistron of the galactose operon.

Transcription from both promoters appears to be inducible. Thus, when galactose is present, the cells should be capable of synthesizing *gal* enzymes at a high rate whether they contain cyclic AMP or not. Uptake of galactose could, however, be a limiting factor in the absence of cyclic AMP. In addition, if galactose becomes the principal carbon source, the intracellular levels of cyclic AMP will be elevated. The presence of high intracellular concentrations of both galactose and cyclic AMP will cause activation of transcription at S1.

What may be critical for the cell is to maintain a constant basal level of *gal* enzyme synthesis (particularly UDP-galactose-epimerase) in the absence of galactose regardless of the physiological fluctuations in the intracellular concentrations of cyclic AMP. The basal uninduced level of *gal* expression is certainly higher vis-à-vis the fully induced level than in the *lac* operon (comparison of the induction ratios for the synthesis of the *lac* and *gal* enzymes indicates a 1000-fold difference between the induced and uninduced states in *lac* and only a 10- to 15-fold difference in *gal*). Both promoters could contribute to this basal level, depending on the cyclic AMP concentrations in the cell. In the absence of galactose, this basal rate of *gal* expression probably satisfies the cellular requirements to ensure adequate synthesis of UDP-galactose for cell-wall biosynthesis. The presence of two *gal* promoters could thus be a mechanism to maintain a stable basal level of *gal* expression whatever the cellular

(1) galactose + ATP $\xrightarrow{\text{galactokinase}}$ galactose-1-P + ADP

(2) galactose-1-P + UDP glucose $\xrightleftharpoons{\text{transferase}}$ UDP-galactose + glucose-1-P

(3) UDP-galactose $\xrightleftharpoons{\text{epimerase}}$ UDP-glucose.

(4) UDP-glucose + pyrophosphate $\xrightleftharpoons{\text{UDPG pyrophosphorylase}}$ UTP + glucose-1-P

(5) glucose-1-P $\xrightleftharpoons{\text{phosphoglucomutase}}$ glucose-6-P

Figure 4 Pathway of galactose metabolism in *E. coli*.

concentrations of cyclic AMP when no galactose is found in the cell's environment. It would also allow the operon to function maximally as an inducible cyclic-AMP-regulated unit when galactose becomes the principal carbon source.

Studies of the *gal* system and other systems illustrate the diversity of regulation of each bacterial operon. One may expect that even more complex mechanisms will be found to operate in the control of individual genes or groups of genes in higher organisms.

ACKNOWLEDGMENTS

We thank R. DiLauro and S. Adhya for communication of results prior to publication. We also thank R. DiLauro, R. Musso, and S. Adhya for many helpful discussions, Ray Steinberg for his work with the figures, and Alana Muto for typing the manuscript.

REFERENCES

Adhya, S. and H. Echols. 1966. Glucose effect and the galactose enzymes of *Escherichia coli*. Correlation between glucose inhibition of induction and inducer transport. *J. Bacteriol.* **92**:601.

Adhya, S. and J. A. Shapiro. 1968. The galactose operon of *E. Coli* K12. I. Structural and pleiotropic mutations of the operon. *Genetics* **62**:231.

Anderson, W. B., R. L. Perlman, and I. Pastan. 1972. Effect of adenosine 3',5'-monophosphate analogues on the activity of the cyclic adenosine 3',5'-monophosphate receptor in *Escherichia coli*. *J. Biol. Chem.* **247**:2717.

Anderson, W. B., A. B. Schneider, M. Emmer, R. L. Perlman, and I. Pastan. 1971. Purification of and properties of the cyclic adenosine 3',5'-monophosphate receptor protein which mediates cyclic adenosine 3',5'-monophosphate-dependent gene transcription in *Escherichia coli*. *J. Biol. Chem.* **246**:5929.

Buttin, G. 1963a. Mécanismes régulateurs dans la biosynthèse des enzymes du métabolisme du galactose chez *Escherichia coli* K12. I. *J. Mol. Biol.* **7**:169.

———. 1963b. Mécanismes régulateurs dans la biosynthèse des enzymes du métabolisme du galactose chez *Escherichia coli* K12. II. *J. Mol. Biol.* **7**:183.

Chamberlin, M. J. 1974. The selectivity of transcription. *Annu. Rev. Biochem.* **43**:721.

Chambers, D. A. and G. Zubay. 1969. The stimulatory effect of cyclic adenosine 3'5'-monophosphate on DNA-directed synthesis of β-galactosidase in a cell-free system. *Proc. Natl. Acad. Sci.* **63**:118.

de Crombrugghe, B., R. L. Perlman, H. E. Varmus, and I. Pastan. 1969. Regulation of inducible enzyme synthesis in *Escherichia coli* by cyclic adenosine 3',5'-monophosphate. *J. Biol. Chem.* **244**:5828.

de Crombrugghe, B., B. Chen, W. Anderson, P. Nissley, M. Gottesman, and I. Pastan. 1971a. *Lac* DNA, RNA polymerase and cyclic AMP receptor protein, cyclic AMP, *lac* repressor and inducer are the essential elements for controlled *lac* transcription. *Nat. New Biol.* **231**:139.

de Crombrugghe, B., B. Chen, M. Gottesman, I. Pastan, H. E. Varmus, M. Emmer, and R. L. Perlman. 1971b. Regulation of the mRNA synthesis in a soluble cell-free system. *Nat. New. Biol.* **230**:37.

Dickson, R. C., J. Abelson, W. M. Barnes, and W. S. Reznikoff. 1975. Genetic regulation: The *lac* control region. *Science* **187**:27.

Dickson, R. C., J. Abelson, P. Johnson, W. S. Reznikoff, and W. M. Barnes. 1977. Nucleotide sequence changes produced by mutations in the *lac* promoter of *Escherichia coli. J. Mol. Biol.* **111**:65.

Eilen, E. and J. S. Krakow. 1977. Cyclic AMP-mediated intersubunit disulfide crosslinking of the cyclic AMP receptor protein of *Escherichia coli. J. Mol. Biol.* **114**:47.

Emmer, M., B. de Crombrugghe, I. Pastan, and R. Perlman. 1970. Cyclic AMP receptor protein of *E. coli*: Its role in the synthesis of inducible enzymes. *Proc. Natl. Acad. Sci.* **66**:480.

Epps, H. M. R. and E. F. Gale. 1942. The influence of the presence of glucose during growth on the enzyme activities of *Escherichia coli*: Comparison of the effect with that produced by fermentation acids. *J. Biochem.* **36**:619.

Epstein, W., L. B. Rothman-Denes, and J. Hesse. 1975. Adenosine 3':5' cyclic monophosphate as mediator of catabolite repression in *Escherichia coli. Proc. Natl. Acad. Sci.* **72**:2300.

Eron, L. and R. Block. 1971. Mechanism of initiation and repression of *in vitro* transcription of the *lac* operon of *Escherichia coli. Proc. Natl. Acad. Sci.* **68**:1828.

Gilbert, W. 1976. Starting and stopping sequences for the RNA polymerase. In *RNA polymerase* (ed. R. Losick and M. Chamberlin), p. 193. Cold Spring Harbor Laboratory, Cold Spring Harbor, New York.

Gottesman, S. and D. Zipser. 1978. Deg phenotype of *Escherichia coli lon* mutants. *J. Bacteriol.* **133**:844.

Greenblatt, J. and R. Schleif. 1971. Arabinose C protein: Regulation of the arabinose operon *in vitro. Nat. New Biol.* **233**:166.

Grodzicker, T., R. R. Arditti, and H. Eisen. 1972. Establishment of repression by lamboid phage in catabolite activator protein and adenylate cyclase mutants of *Escherichia coli. Proc. Natl. Acad. Sci.* **69**:366.

Hirsh, J. and R. Schleif. 1977. The *ara* C promoter: Transcription, mapping and interaction with the *ura BAD* promoter. *Cell* **11**:545.

Hong, J. S., G. R. Smith, and B. N. Ames. 1971. Adenosine 3':5' cyclic monophosphate concentration in the bacterial host regulates the viral decision between lysogeny and lysis. *Proc. Natl. Acad. Sci.* **68**:2258.

Hopkins, J. D. 1974. A new class of promoter mutations in the lactose operon of *Escherichia coli. J. Mol. Biol.* **87**:715.

Hua, S. and A. Markovitz. 1972. Multiple regulatory gene control of the galactose operon in *Escherichia coli* K12. *J. Bacteriol.* **110**:1089.

Koch, J. P., S.-L. Hayashi, and E. C. C. Lin. 1964. The control of dissimilation of glycerol and 1-D-glycerophosphate in *Escherichia coli. J. Biol. Chem.* **239**:3106.

Krakow, J. S. and I. Pastan. 1973. Cyclic adenosine monophosphate receptor: Loss of cAMP-dependent DNA binding activity after proteolysis in the presence of cyclic adenosine monophosphate. *Proc. Natl. Acad. Sci.* **70**:2529.

Lee, N., G. Wilcox, W. Gielono, J. Arnold, P. Cleary, and E. Englesberg. 1974. *In vitro* activation of transcription of *ara* BAD operon and *ara* C activator. *Proc. Natl. Acad. Sci.* **71**:634.

Mackie, G. and D. B. Wilson. 1972. Regulation of the *gal* operon of *Escherichia coli* by the *cap* R gene. *J. Biol. Chem.* **247**:2973.

Magasanik, B. 1962. Catabolite repression. *Cold Spring Harbor Symp. Quant. Biol.* **26**:249.

Maizels, N. 1973. The nucleotide sequence of the lactose messenger ribonucleic acid transcribed from the UV5 promoter mutant of *E. coli. Proc. Natl. Acad. Sci.* **70**:3585.

Majors, J. 1975. Specific binding of CAP factor to *lac* promoter DNA. *Nature* **256**:672.

―――. 1978. A symmetric binding site for CAP factor within the *E. Coli lac* promoter. *J. Biol. Chem.* (in press).

Makman, R. S. and E. Q. Sutherland. 1965. Adenosine 3',5'-phosphate in *Escherichia coli. J. Biol. Chem.* **240**:1309.

Maniatis, T., A. Jeffrey, and D. Kleid. 1975a. Nucleotide sequence of the rightward operator of phage λ. *Proc. Natl. Acad. Sci.* **72**:1184.

Maniatis, T., M. Ptashne, K. Backman, D. Kleid, S. Flashman, A. Jeffrey, and R. Maurer. 1975b. Recognition sequences of repressor and polymerase in the operators of bacteriophage lambda. *Cell* **5**:109.

Maurer, R., T. Maniatis, and M. Ptashne. 1974. Promoters are in the operons in phage lambda. *Nature* **249**:221.

Maxam, A. M. and W. Gilbert. 1977. A new method for sequencing DNA. *Proc. Natl. Acad. Sci.* **74**:560.

Michaelis, G. and P. Starlinger. 1967. Sequential appearance of the galactose enzymes in *E. coli. Mol. Gen. Genet.* **100**:210.

Miller, Z., H. E. Varmus, J. S. Parks, R. L. Perlman, and I. Pastan. 1971. Regulation of *gal* messenger ribonucleic acid synthesis in *Escherichia coli* by 3',5'-cyclic adenosine monophosphate. *J. Biol. Chem.* **246**:2898.

Mitra, S., G. Zubay, and A. Landy. 1975. Evidence for the preferential binding of the catabolite gene activator protein (CAP) to DNA containing the *lac* promoter. *Biochem. Biophys. Res. Commun.* **61**:857.

Monod, J. 1947. The phenomenon of enzymatic adaptation. *Growth* **11**:223.

Musso, R. E., R. DiLauro, S. Adhya, and B. de Crombrugghe. 1977a. Dual control for transcription of the galactose operon by cyclic AMP and its receptor protein at two interspersed promoters. *Cell* **12**:847.

Musso, R., R. DiLauro, M. Rosenberg, and B. de Crombrugghe. 1977b. Nucleotide sequence of the operator-promoter region of the galactose operon of *Escherichia coli. Proc. Natl. Acad. Sci.* **74**:106.

Musso, R. E., B. de Crombrugghe, I. Pastan, J. Sklar, P. Yot, and S. Weissman. 1974. The 5'-terminal nucleotide sequence of galactose messenger ribonucleic acid of *Escherichia coli. Proc. Natl. Acad. Sci.* **71**:4940.

Nakanishi, S., S. Adhya, M. E. Gottesman, and I. Pastan. 1973. *In vitro* repression of the transcription of *gal* operon by purified *gal* repressor. *Proc. Natl. Acad. Sci.* **70**:334.

―――. 1974. Activation of transcription at specific promoters by glycerol. *J. Biol. Chem.* **249**:4050.

Nielsen, L. D., D. Monard, and H. V. Rickenberg. 1973. Cyclic 3′,5′ adenosine monophosphate phosphodiesterase of *Escherichia coli. J. Bacteriol.* **116**: 857.

Nissley, S. P., W. B. Anderson, M. Gallo, I. Pastan, and R. L. Perlman. 1972. The binding of cyclic adenosine monophosphate receptor to deoxyribonucleic acid. *J. Biol. Chem.* **247**: 4265.

Nissley, S. P., W. B. Anderson, M. E. Gottesman, R. L. Perlman, and I. Pastan. 1971. *In vitro* transcription of the *gal* operon requires cyclic adenosine monophosphate and cyclic adenosine monophosphate receptor protein. *J. Biol. Chem.* **246**: 4671.

Okamoto, T., K. Sugimoto, H. Sugisaki, and M. Takanami. 1977. DNA regions essential for the function of a bacteriophage *fd* promoter. *Nucleic Acids Res.* **4**: 2213.

Parks, J. S., M. Gottesman, R. L. Perlman, and I. Pastan. 1971. Regulation of galactokinase synthesis by cyclic adenosine 3′,5′-monophosphate in cell-free extracts of *Escherichia coli. J. Biol. Chem.* **246**: 2419.

Pastan, I. and S. Adhya. 1976. Cyclic adenosine 5′-monophosphate in *Escherichia coli. Bact. Rev.* **40**: 527.

Pastan, I. and R. L. Perlman. 1969. Repression of β-galactosidase synthesis by glucose in phosphotransferase mutants of *Escherichia coli*: Repression in the absence of glucose phosphorylation. *J. Biol. Chem.* **244**: 5836.

Pastan, I., M. Gallo, and W. B. Anderson. 1974. The purification and analysis of mechanism of action of a cyclic AMP-receptor protein from *Escherichia coli. Methods Enzymol.* **38C**: 367.

Perlman, R. L. and I. Pastan. 1968. Cyclic 3′,5′-AMP: Stimulation of β-galactosidase and tryptophanase induction in *E. coli. Biochem. Biophys. Res. Commun.* **30**: 656.

―――. 1969. Pleiotropic deficiency of carbohydrate utilization in an adenyl cyclase deficient mutant of *Escherichia coli. Biochem. Biophys. Res. Commun.* **37**: 151.

Peterkofsky, A. and C. Gazdar. 1973. Measurements of rates of adenosine 3′:5′-cyclic monophosphate synthesis in intact *Escherichia coli* B. *Proc. Natl. Acad. Sci.* **70**: 2149.

―――. 1975. Interaction of enzyme I of the phosphoenolpyruvate:sugar phosphotransferase system with adenylate cyclase of *E. coli. Proc. Natl. Acad. Sci.* **72**: 2920.

Pribnow, D. 1975. Bacteriophage T7 early promoters: Nucleotide sequences of two RNA polymerase binding sites. *J. Mol. Biol.* **99**: 419.

Riggs, A. D., G. Reiness, and G. Zubay. 1971. Purification and DNA-binding properties of the catabolite gene activator protein. *Proc. Natl. Acad. Sci.* **68**: 1222.

Rothman-Denes, L. B., J. E. Hesse, and W. Epstein. 1973. Role of cyclic adenosine 3′,5′-monophosphate in the *in vivo* expression of the galactose operon of *Escherichia coli. J. Bacteriol.* **114**: 1040.

Saier, M. H. and B. U. Feucht. 1975. Coordinate regulation of adenylate cyclase and carbohydrate permeases by the phosphoenolpyruvate:sugar phosphotransferase system in *Salmonella typhimurium. J. Biol. Chem.* **250**: 7078.

Schaller, H., C. Gray, and K. Herrmann. 1975. Nucleotide sequence of an RNA polymerase binding site from the DNA of bacteriophage *fd. Proc. Natl. Acad. Sci.* **72**:737.

Schwartz, D. and J. R. Beckwith. 1970. Mutants missing a factor necessary for the expression of catabolite-sensitive operons in *E. coli.* In *The lactose operon* (ed. J. R. Beckwith and D. Zipser), p. 417. Cold Spring Harbor Laboratory, Cold Spring Harbor, New York.

Shineberg, B. and D. Zipser. 1973. The *lon* gene and degradation of β-galactosidase nonsense fragments. *J. Bacteriol.* **116**:1469.

Silverstone, A. E., R. R. Arditti, and B. Magasanik. 1970. Catabolite-insensitive revertants of *lac* promoter mutants. *Proc. Natl. Acad. Sci.* **68**:773.

Sklar, J., S. Weissman, R. Musso, R. DiLauro, and B. de Crombrugghe. 1977. Determination of the nucleotide sequence of part of the regulatory region for the galactose operon from *Escherichia coli. J. Biol. Chem.* **252**:3538.

Wetekam, W., K. Staack, and R. Ehring. 1971. DNA-dependent *in vitro* synthesis of enzymes of the galactose operon of *Escherichia coli. Mol. Gen. Genet.* **112**:14.

Wilcox, G., P. Meuris, P. Bass, and E. Englesberg. 1974. Regulation of the L-arabinose operon *in vitro. J. Biol. Chem.* **249**:2946.

Wilson, D. B. and D. S. Hogness. 1968. The enzymes of the galactose operon in *Escherichia coli.* IV. The frequencies of translation of the terminal cistrons in the operon. *J. Biol. Chem.* **244**:2143.

Wu, C. and F. Y. H. Wu. 1974. Conformational transitions of cyclic adenosine monophosphate receptor protein of *Escherichia coli.* A temperature-jump study. *Biochemistry* **13**:2573.

Wu, F. Y. H., K. Nath, and C. Wu. 1974. Conformational transitions of cyclic adenosine monophosphate receptor protein of *Escherichia coli.* A fluorescent probe study. *Biochemistry* **13**:2567.

Yokota, T. and J. S. Gots. 1970. Requirement of adenosine 3′,5′-cyclic monophosphate for flagella formation in *Escherichia coli* and *Salmonella typhimurium. J. Bacteriol.* **103**:513.

Zubay, G., D. Schwartz, and J. Beckwith. 1970. Mechanism of activation of catabolite-sensitive genes: A positive control system. *Proc. Natl. Acad. Sci.* **66**:104.

λ Repressor Function and Structure

Mark Ptashne
The Biological Laboratories
Harvard University
Cambridge, Massachusetts 02138

INTRODUCTION

In this paper I will summarize our understanding of the molecular basis of the following phenomena involving the function and synthesis of the bacteriophage λ repressor.

1. In its classical role, repressor turns off transcription of other phage genes at the promoters P_L and P_R, thereby maintaining the phage chromosome as prophage in a lysogenic bacterium. These phage genes are thus *heterogenously* regulated by repressor (Fig. 1).
2. In lysogens the repressor gene (*CI*) is *autogenously* regulated. Repressor activates *CI* transcription at low concentrations and represses it at high concentrations. The promoter for *CI* transcription in lysogens is called P_{RM} (*p*romoter for *r*epressor *m*aintenance) (Fig. 1).
3. Upon infection of nonlysogens (i.e., in the absence of repressor), repressor is synthesized in a mode different from that in lysogens. In this case, *CI* is transcribed under the direction of regulatory proteins encoded by phage genes *CII* and *CIII*. The promoter used is called P_{RE} (*p*romoter for *r*epressor *e*stablishment) (Fig. 1). In a cell destined to become a lysogen, this burst of repressor turns off transcription of *CII* and *CIII* and of other phage genes as it turns on transcription of *CI* from P_{RM}.
4. Phage λ sometimes grows lytically in nonlysogens. In this case, synthesis of a second repressor encoded by the *cro* (or *tof*) gene is required. The *cro* product represses early genes, including *cro*, by blocking transcription beginning at P_L and P_R. In addition, the *cro* protein represses transcription of *CI* originating at P_{RM}.
5. Treatment of lysogens with ultraviolet (UV) irradiation—or more generally with activated carcinogens—results in repressor inactivation and phage growth.

Evidence supporting the above assertions is found in various reviews of the physiology and genetics of λ growth (Echols and Green 1971; Ptashne 1971; Eisen and Ptashne 1971; Herskowitz 1973; Weisberg et al. 1977). Before examining the issues listed above, I will describe certain aspects of

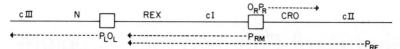

Figure 1 Schematic representation of transcriptional patterns in a portion of the λ genome. The arrows show the directions of transcription of genes *N, cro, CI, rex, CII,* and *CIII.* Genes *CI* and *rex* are transcribed either from the promoter P_{RM} in lysogens or from P_{RE} after phage infection of nonlysogens. The exact location of P_{RE} is unknown. $O_L P_L$ represents the leftward and $O_R P_R$ the rightward operator promoter.

the structure of the λ repressor and the λ operators. A more detailed review of some of the arguments set forth is contained in Ptashne et al. (1976).

THE λ REPRESSOR AND THE *CI* GENE

The repressor is an acidic protein whose monomer has a molecular weight of 26,228. These monomers are in concentration-dependent equilibrium with dimers ($K_D \sim 10^{-8}$ M), and equilibrium and kinetic studies indicate that the dimer is the form that binds DNA with high affinity. Repressor is present at about 10^{-7} M in ordinary lysogens (about 200 monomers per cell), and the binding constant of the dimer for DNA is about 10^{-13} M (Pirrotta et al. 1970; Chadwick et al. 1971; Sauer and Anderegg 1978; R. T. Sauer, unpubl.).

The complete amino acid sequence of repressor and roughly 80% of the nucleotide sequence of *CI* have been determined; these sequences are colinear (Fig. 2) (Sauer and Anderegg 1978; R. T. Sauer, unpubl.). There is a strong clustering of basic residues at the amino terminus of repressor. Although arginine and lysine constitute about 10% of the total residues, they account for 33% of the 27 amino-terminal residues. There is strong evidence that the amino-terminal third of the molecule is responsible for making specific DNA contacts. A fragment containing the first 92 residues has been generated from highly purified repressor by proteolytic cleavage (R. T. Sauer and C. Pabo, unpubl.). This fragment protects the same bases in the operators from methylation by DMS (see Gilbert et al. 1976; Humayun et al. 1977b) as does whole repressor. The fragment does not dimerize even at high concentrations, and much higher concentrations of fragments, as compared with repressor, are required for protection of the operators (R. T. Sauer, unpubl.). Apparently, the carboxyl two-thirds of the repressor is required for dimer formation and possibly inducer recognition (see below). These conclusions are consistent with the finding that a plasmid which contains only the amino-terminal two-thirds of the repressor gene, and which transcribes that gene fragment at high levels (see below), renders a cell immune to λ (K. Backman, unpubl.). These results also are consistent

<pre>
                                    10   20
NH₂-Ser-Thr-Lys-Lys-Lys-Pro-Leu-Thr-Gln-Glu-Gln-Leu-Glu-Asp-Ala-Arg-Arg-Leu-Lys-Ala-
ATG AGC ACA AAA AAG AAA CCA TTA ACA CAA GAG CAG CT
                                    30   40
    Ile-Tyr-Glu-Lys-Lys-Lys-Asn-Glu-Leu-Gly-Leu-Ser-Gln-Glu-Ser-Val-Ala-Asp-Lys-Met-
                                             GAA TCT GTC GCA GAC AAG ATG
                                    50   60
    Gly-Met-Gly-Gln-Ser-Gly-Val-Gly-Ala-Leu-Phe-Asn-Gly-Ile-Asn-Ala-Leu-Asn-Ala-Tyr-
    GGG ATG GGG CAG TCA GGC GTT GGT GCT TTA TTT AAT GGC ATC AAT GCA TTA AAT GCT TAT
                                    70   80
    Asn-Ala-Ala-Leu-Leu-Ala-Lys-Ile-Leu-Lys-Val-Ser-Val-Glu-Glu-Phe-Ser-Pro-Ser-Ile-
    AAC GCC GCA TTG CTT GCA AAA ATT CTC AAA GTT AGC GTT GAA GAA TTT AGC CCT TCA ATC
                                    90   100
    Ala-Arg-Glu-Ile-Tyr-Glu-Met-Tyr-Glu-Ala-Val-Ser-Met-Gln-Pro-Ser-Leu-Arg-Ser-Glu-
    GC
                                    110   120
    Tyr-Glu-Tyr-Pro-Val-Phe-Ser-His-Val-Gln-Ala-Gly-Met-Phe-Ser-Pro-Glu-Leu-Arg-Thr-
              CCT GTT TTT TCT CAT GTT CAG GCA GGG ATG TTC TCA CCT GAG CTT AGA ACC
                                    130   140
    Phe-Thr-Lys-Gly-Asp-Ala-Glu-Arg-Trp-Val-Ser-Thr-Thr-Lys-Lys-Ala-Ser-Asp-Ser-Ala-
    TTT ACC AAA GGT GAT GCG GAG AGA TGG GTA AGC ACA ACC AAA AAA GCC AGT GAT TCT GCA
                                    150   160
    Phe-Trp-Leu-Glu-Val-Glu-Gly-Asn-Ser-Met-Thr-Ala-Pro-Thr-Gly-Ser-Lys-Pro-Ser-Phe-
    TTC TGG CTT GAG GTT GAA GGT AAT TCC ATG ACC GCA CCA ACG GGC TCC AAG CCA AGC TTT
                                    170   180
    Pro-Asp-Gly-Met-Leu-Ile-Leu-Val-Asp-Pro-Glu-Gln-Ala-Val-Glu-Pro-Gly-Asp-Phe-Cys-
    CCT GAC GGA ATG TTA ATT CTC GTT GAC CCC GAG CAG GCT GTT GAG CCA GGT GAT TTC TGC
                                    190   200
    Ile-Ala-Arg-Leu-Gly-Gly-Asp-Glu-Phe-Thr-Phe-Lys-Lys-Leu-Ile-Arg-Asp-Ser-Gly-Gln-
    ATA GCC AGA CTT GGG GGT GAT GAG TTT ACC TTC AAG AAA CTG ATC AGG GAT AGC GGT CAG
                                    210   220
    Val-Phe-Leu-Gln-Pro-Leu-Asn-Pro-Gln-Tyr-Pro-Met-Ile-Pro-Cys-Asn-Glu-Ser-Cys-Ser-
    GTG TTT TTA CAA CCA CTA AAC CCA CAG TAC CCA ATG ATC CCA TGC AAT GAG AGT TGT TCC
                                    230
    Val-Val-Gly-Lys-Val-Ile-Ala-Ser-Gln-Trp-Pro-Glu-Glu-Thr-Phe-Gly-COOH
    GTT GTG GGG AAA GTT ATC GCT AGT CAG TGG CCT GAA GAG ACG TTT GGC TGA TCG
</pre>

Figure 2 The amino acid sequence of λ repressor and the base sequence of most of *CI* (Humayun 1977; Sauer and Anderegg 1978; R. T. Sauer, unpubl.).

with the finding that *trans*-dominant *CI⁻* mutations are located in the amino-terminal portion of *CI* (Oppenheim and Salomon 1970, 1972; Oppenheim and Noff 1975). These mutations presumably abolish operator affinity of the repressor but not the ability to form dimer, and thus they are analogous to the I^{-d} mutations of the *lacI* gene.

Studies of repressor function and structure have been greatly facilitated by the construction of plasmid DNA molecules, using recombination in vitro, that direct the synthesis of varying amounts of repressor (Backman et al. 1976; Backman and Ptashne 1978). Thus, for example, *CI*-bearing plasmids are available that direct the synthesis of repressor levels in excess of those found in single lysogens by factors of about 5 (pKB158), 50 (pKB252), 100 (pKB280), and 250 (pKB277), respectively. In the latter three cases, *CI* transcription is driven by *lac* promoters. Plasmids pKB280 and pKB277 bear a sequence that encodes a ribosome-binding site for *CI* translation that is a hybrid of λ and *lac* sequences. Strains bearing pKB277, which differs from pKB280 only in regions not carrying the

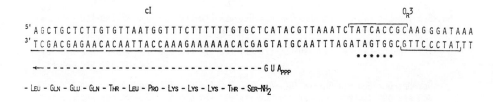

Figure 3 DNA, RNA, and protein sequences in and around the two control regions of phage λ. The repressor binding sites O_L1, O_L2, and O_L3 in O_L (left operator) and O_R1, O_R2, and O_R3 in O_R (right operator) are set off in brackets. The starting points of transcription of genes *N*, *cro*, and *CI* are indicated (Blattner and Dahlberg 1972; Meyer et al. 1975). Also shown are amino-terminal residues of the repressor. Six bases on O_R3, presumed to code for a strong ribosome-binding site for *CI*, are marked with asterisks. The O_L has been reversed from its orientation in Fig. 1. Four mutations that decrease the affinity of DNA for repressor are indicated. The DNA and *CI* mRNA sequences are reported in Maniatis et al. (1974b, 1975a,b), Pirrotta (1975), and Humayun et al. (1976). See Fig. 2 for the amino acid sequence of repressor.

CI-lac fusion, produce some 2–3% of their protein as repressor, and repressor may readily be purified to homogeneity (R. T. Sauer and C. Pabo, unpubl.).

THE OPERATORS

The most striking aspect of the λ operators is that each contains three repressor-binding sites ($O_L1,2,3$; $O_R1,2,3$). The sequences specifically recognized are 17 base pairs long and are separated by spacers, rich in A (adenine) and T (thymine), 3–7 base pairs long. The terminal binding sites O_L1 and O_R1, which are adjacent to the repressor-controlled genes *N* and *cro*, bind repressor with a higher affinity than do the remaining sites. The complete nucleotide sequences of the λ operators are shown in Figure 3. Figure 4 shows a diagram of these sequences that emphasizes several important features. The evidence for the preceding statements may be summarized as follows:

1. At each operator, repressor protects from pancreatic deoxyribonu-
   clease digestion fragments roughly 25, 50, and 80 base pairs in length
   (Ptashne et al. 1976). The size of the protected fragment increases in
   steps as the ratio of repressor to operator in the digestion mix is

Figure 3 (continued)

increased. The smallest fragment from each operator corresponds to O_L1 or O_R1, plus a few adjacent nucleotides, as shown by analysis of pyrimidine tracts (Maniatis and Ptashne 1973a; Humayun et al. 1977a).

2. Various restriction endonucleases cleave within each operator. For example, the enzyme HindII cuts once in each operator. Four of the fragments produced by HindII cleavage of λ DNA bear different portions of O_L and O_R, and each of these binds repressor (Maniatis and Ptashne 1973b). These experiments show directly that each operator contains more than one site that can independently bind repressor.

3. Virulent mutants of phage λ grow in λ lysogens. These mutants have lost their sensitivity to repressor in vivo. Mutations that decrease the repressibility of phage have been located within the sequences O_L1, O_L2, O_R1, and O_R2. Each of these mutations decreases the affinity of a binding site for repressor in vitro (Ptashne and Hopkins 1968; Ordal 1971; Hopkins and Ptashne 1971; Steinberg and Ptashne 1971; Ordal and Kaiser 1973; Maniatis et al. 1974a; Maniatis et al. 1975a; Flashman 1976). Mutations in the spacers have no effect on repressor affinity, but they do affect the action of RNA polymerase at the corresponding promoter (Maurer et al. 1974; Meyer et al. 1975; Kleid et al. 1976). Various operator mutations are identified in Figure 5 and its legend, and four of these mutations are shown in Figure 3.

4. There is a striking similarity between the sequences of the binding sites. In Figure 5 the six sites are aligned and the frequency with which a given base appears at each position is tabulated. The bases changed by various operator mutations are boxed. Each site contains elements of twofold rotational symmetry (Maniatis and Ptashne 1976; Maniatis et al. 1975b), but it is highly unlikely that this symmetry results in the formation of hairpin loops that are recognized by repressor (Maniatis

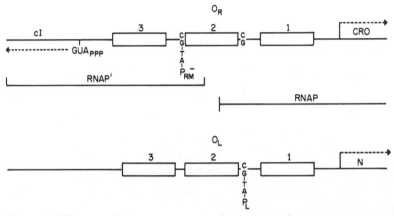

Figure 4 Diagram of the λ operators and a portion of genes *N, cro, CI,* and *rex.* The boxes show the positions of the 17-base-pair repressor-binding sites. The starting points of *cro-, N-,* and P_{RM}-directed *CI* transcription are indicated. The approximate positions of the RNA-polymerase-binding sites at P_L, P_R, and P_{RM}, defined as the DNA protected by polymerase from digestion with λ exonuclease and S_1 (Ptashne et al. 1976), are shown. The line labeled RNAP shows approximately the sequence covered by polymerase bound to P_R or to P_L. The line labeled RNAP' shows the region covered by polymerase when bound to P_{RM}. Mutations that decrease the activity of P_{RM} and P_L, respectively, are indicated (Blattner and Dahlberg 1972; Yen and Gussin 1973; Maurer et al. 1974; Walz and Pirrotta 1975; Meyer et al. 1975).

and Ptashne 1973). Each repressor-binding site consists (on one side) of the sequence 5'-TATCACCGC-3' (C is cytosine; G is guanine), or a sequence differing by two bases, plus (on the other side) a related but more variable sequence. The operator symmetries may correspond to symmetric features of the repressor oligomer, but it is not yet clear whether the detailed interaction of repressor with operator is symmetric. Operator mutations change bases that are largely conserved among the various sites.

5. Kawashima et al. (1978) have synthesized the DNA duplex

$$\begin{bmatrix} TATCACCGCCGGTGATA \\ ATAGTGGCGGCCACTAT \end{bmatrix}$$

and, although no precise estimate of the binding constant has been made, they find that the fragment binds with high affinity to λ repressor. This sequence contains two "perfect half-sites" and does not correspond exactly to any single proposed operator sequence.

6. The extent of methylation of G and A residues in DNA by dimethylsulfate may be used to identify those bases protected by a bound protein (Gilbert et al 1976). The ring nitrogen (N-7) methylated

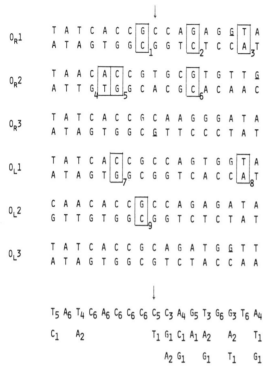

T_5 A_6 T_4 C_6 A_6 C_6 C_6 C_6 C_5 C_3 A_4 G_5 T_3 G_6 G_3 T_6 A_4

C_1 $\quad$ A_2 $\qquad\qquad$ T_1 G_1 C_1 A_1 A_2 $\quad$ A_2 $\quad$ T_1

$\qquad\qquad\qquad\qquad$ A_2 G_1 $\quad$ G_1 $\quad$ T_1 $\quad$ G_1

Figure 5 The six repressor-binding sites in the λ operators. The frequency with which a given base appears in each position is tabulated. Thus, for example, in position 1, T appears five times, C once. The sites have been oriented to reveal their similarities. The arrows indicate the axis of partial twofold symmetry in each site. Base pairs changed by mutations that decrease repressor affinity are boxed. The subscripts correspond to the following mutational changes (see Flashman 1976): (1) V_3: $\frac{G}{C}\to\frac{T}{A}$; (2) V_s326: $\frac{G}{C}\to\frac{T}{A}$; (3) V_R18: $\frac{T}{A}\to\frac{C}{G}$; (4) V_3C: $\frac{A}{T}\to\frac{C}{G}$; (5) V_1, V_H: $\frac{C}{G}\to\frac{A}{T}$; (6) V_N, V_c34: $\frac{C}{G}\to\frac{T}{A}$; (7) V_2: $\frac{G}{C}\to\frac{T}{A}$, V_{003}: $\frac{C}{G}\to\frac{T}{A}$; (8) V_{101}: $\frac{T}{A}\to\frac{C}{G}$; (9) V_{305}: $\frac{C}{G}\to\frac{T}{A}$.

on G lies in the major groove of the helix, whereas the N-3 methylated position on A lies in the minor groove. Lambda repressor protects G's but not A's from methylation and, as expected, only those G's located within the designated repressor-binding sites (Humayun et al. 1977b) (see Fig. 5). This result also suggests that λ repressor specifically contacts DNA in the major groove.

PROMOTER STRUCTURE

A promoter is defined as a DNA sequence necessary for recognition and binding of RNA polymerase and for initiation of transcription. The promoters P_L, P_R, and P_{RM} denote, respectively, promoters for genes *N*, *cro*, and *CI*. At each promoter RNA polymerase protects a fragment of DNA from digestion by DNase. In each case the protected fragment is 45 base pairs long when pancreatic DNase is used, and where examined (P_R), transcription begins roughly in the middle of this protected sequence (Walz and Pirrotta 1975; B. J. Meyer and R. Maurer, unpubl.). When the DNase used is a combination of λ exonuclease and S_1 instead of pancreatic DNase, the protected fragment is roughly 65 base pairs long. The 65-base-pair fragments, unlike the shorter fragments, bind polymerase and direct transcription (Ptashne et al. 1976; B. J. Meyer, unpubl.). Figure 4 shows the approximate location of each promoter as defined by the DNase (S_1 and exonuclease) digestion experiments.

Two promoter mutations have been sequenced (Meyer et al. 1975; Kleid et al. 1976). One, located in the spacer between O_L1 and O_L2, damages P_L. The other, located in the spacer between O_R2 and O_R3, damages P_{RM}. The former is 31 and the latter 33 base pairs from the respective start points of transcription, and each changes the sole G·C in a spacer to A·T. We also know that a promoter mutation occurs in P_R within a few base pairs of the position analogous to that of the P_L mutation, but the exact base change has not been determined (Maurer et al. 1974). The 65-base-pair promoter, unlike the shorter one, includes the region of DNA in which these promoter mutations lie.

I now turn to the five phenomena outlined in the introduction.

Heterogenous Regulation by Repressor

As implied in Figure 4, repressor blocks transcription of *N* and *cro* by preventing binding of RNA polymerase to the corresponding promoters P_L and P_R. The figure shows that the region of DNA covered by bound polymerase overlaps O_R1 and part of O_R2 at P_R and O_L1 and part of O_L2 at P_L. The same region of DNA may be covered either by polymerase or by repressor, and experiments performed in vitro confirm the expectation that bound polymerase is not affected by subsequent addition of repressor (for review, see Ptashne et al. 1976).

Analysis of virulent mutants confirms that the two terminal repressor-binding sites in O_R (O_R1 and O_R2) and in O_L (O_L1 and O_L2) mediate repression of *cro* and *N*, respectively. Mutations that render *cro* transcription constitutive, that is, mutations that reduce repression at the operator, have been found in O_R1 and O_R2; mutations with a similar effect on *N* transcription have been found in O_L1 and O_L2. At each operator, mutation of two sites has a more dramatic effect on repression than does mutation on either site alone. The most virulent mutant analyzed thus far bears mutations in O_L1, O_L2, O_R1, and O_R2. Apparently, repressor bound to two sites excludes polymerase more efficiently than does repressor bound to a single site (Flashman 1976; Ptashne et al. 1976).

Autogenous Regulation

The properties of a hybrid operon, constructed by recombination in vitro, directly illustrate both positive and negative regulation of transcription by repressor. In this hybrid operon, which is carried on a transducing phage (λ112), CI, trpA, and lacZ are all transcribed from the promoter that directs transcription of CI in a lysogen, namely, P_{RM}. The lac and trp promoters are missing from this phage, but their respective ribosome-binding sites are present, and at least in the case of lacZ, we expect that mRNA read from P_{RM} would be translated as efficiently as ordinary lac mRNA. We can conveniently assay the function of P_{RM} in lysogens of this phage by assaying β-galactosidase, and we can compare this function directly with that of the wild-type lac promoter.

To measure the function of P_{RM} in the absence of repressor, we have crossed into this phage a λCI mutation. As indicated in Figure 6, the transducing phage carries repressor genes from two different phages (λ and 21), and because the λ repressor does not control lytic function in this phage, λCI mutants lysogenize normally. Finally, we are able to study the effect of high concentrations of repressor on P_{RM} function by adding the repressor-overproducing plasmid, pKB252, to lysogens of the transducing phage.

The β-galactosidase levels in various lysogens of our transducing phage reflect autogenous regulation at P_{RM} (see Table 1, line 1). The results are qualitatively as follows: In the absence of repressor, only a low level of β-galactosidase is made; the presence of one gene dosage of repressor greatly increases enzyme production, and excess repressor turns down enzyme synthesis. Evidence that λ repressor enhances its own synthesis was presented previously by others (see Reichardt and Kaiser 1971; Reichardt 1975). Pastrana and Brammar (1976) presented evidence indicating that the repressor synthesized by the λ-related phage, λimm^{434}, activated transcription originating at the corresponding P_{RM}.

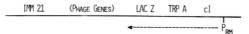

Figure 6 Prophage map of transducing phage (λ112) bearing a lac gene whose transcription is directed by P_{RM}. The phage carried intact lacZ, trpA, and λCI genes. In a lysogen, all three are transcribed only from P_{RM}. This phage was constructed by joining three DNA fragments in vitro, with the use of polynucleotide ligase. One fragment was the left half of a phage bearing the trp-lac fusion W205 (Barnes et al. 1974; Mitchell et al. 1975). This fragment was generated by cleavage with HindIII, which cuts in the trpB gene. The second fragment was the right half of a derivative of λimm^{21}, whose only EcoRI site is to the left of the phage attachment site (kindly provided by R. Pastrana and W. Brammar 1976). The third and shortest fragment, which contains λ's CI and P_{RM}, extends from the HindIII site in rex to a HaeIII site in cro. This HaeIII site was converted to an EcoRI site (Backman et al. 1976).

Table 1 Effects of wild-type and mutant rightward operators (O_R) on P_{RM}-directed synthesis of β-galactosidase

	Repressor source		
	none[a]	CI^+ prophage[b]	pKB252[c]
$\lambda 112O_R{}^+$	100	2,500	250
$V_S 326$	100	100	100
$V_1 V_3$	100	100	100
V_N	100	100	100
V_{3c}	100	1,000	250
$\Delta O_R 1$	100	100	100
p*lac* 5	13,000	13,000	13,000

Lysogens of the fusion phage shown in Fig. 6 as well as lysogens of variants differing at O_R were grown in the presence of three different cellular levels of repressor and assayed for β-galactosidase activity. Each phage derivative was constructed as described in Fig. 6 using DNA bearing the appropriate configuration at O_R. The value for p*lac* 5 is included as a measure of the strength of the *lac* promoter. Results are given in the units of Miller (1972).

[a]No repressor: the phage bore either a *CI* amber mutation or itself produced an insignificant amount of repressor.

[b]A single lysogen level of repressor, supplied by a λ prophage installed at a different site in the chromosome.

[c]A repressor level 50-fold greater than the level in a single lysogen, supplied by the plasmid pKB252.

Our current understanding of the mechanism of negative autogenous regulation of *CI* may be deduced from Figure 4. Transcription of *CI* begins 11 bases to the left of $O_R 3$, and RNA polymerase bound to P_{RM} covers all of $O_R 3$ and part of $O_R 2$ (Meyer et al. 1975; Walz et al. 1976). This relationship implies that repressor competes with polymerase for binding at P_{RM}, as is also true at P_L and P_R. Experiments performed in vitro show that repressor blocks transcription of *CI* only if added to the template before addition of polymerase (Meyer et al. 1975). We do not yet have mutants in $O_R 3$ to confirm the surmise that $O_R 3$ plays a key role in mediating negative autogenous regulation of *CI*, but mutants in $O_R 1$ and in $O_R 2$ apparently have no effect on this negative control as measured in vitro (Meyer et al. 1975).

The mechanism of positive autogenous regulation of *CI* is less clear. Experiments performed in vitro indicate that repressor must bind to $O_R 1$ to enhance *CI* transcription. Thus, appropriate concentrations of repressor increase *CI* transcription about five- to tenfold if and only if the template bears a wild-type $O_R 1$ (Meyer et al. 1975; Walz et al. 1976). This conclusion is reinforced and extended by the properties, in vivo, of *CI-lac* hybrids such as that in Figure 6, but bearing operator mutations in various sites in O_R (see Table 1). Deletion of $O_R 1$ eliminates repressor activation, as does a mutation in $O_R 1$ ($V_S 326$) that decreases the affinity of that site for repressor. The effect of two O_R2 mutations on P_{RM} functions has been measured (see Table 1). The mutation V_{3c}, located in the left half of O_R2 some 40 base pairs upstream from the starting point of transcription, is activated by repressor about half as efficiently as is wild type. We believe it likely that V_{3c} affects the efficiency of P_{RM} per se and not the activating effect of repressor. (The basal value of 100 units seen in the absence of repressor may not reflect transcription initiating at P_{RM}, and it is possible that a mutation of that promoter would not decrease this basal level.) In surprising contrast to the result with V_{3c}, the mutation V_N abolishes repressor activation of P_{RM}. This mutation is located 46 base pairs upstream from the P_{RM} transcriptional starting point in the right half of O_R2. It is possible that V_N damages P_{RM} directly. Alternatively, it is possible that maximal function of P_{RM} requires that repressor be bound to O_R1 (probably as a dimer) and to part of O_R2 (perhaps as a monomer) (B. J. Meyer, unpubl.).

Our analysis indicates that the pattern of positive and negative autogenous regulation of repressor synthesis depends on the order of affinity of the three repressor-binding sites in O_R. Thus, at low repressor concentrations, repressor would bind predominantly to O_R1, thereby turning down *cro* transcription and activating *CI* transcription. At higher repressor concentrations, O_R3 would be filled and repressor transcription shut down. We remain uncertain as to the precise role of O_R2.

Granted that repressor bound to O_R1 (and perhaps to part of O_R2) enhances *CI* transcription, we might imagine various mechanisms for this enhancement. One possibility is the competing-polymerase model, in which it is imagined that polymerase bound to P_R would hinder polymerase binding to P_{RM}. Repressor, a much smaller molecule than polymerase, would then activate *CI* transcription simply by preventing polymerase binding to P_R. An experiment that argues against this possibility is the following: A *CI-lac* hybrid similar to that of Figure 5 was constructed, except that P_R was deleted by elimination of operator (promoter) sequences beginning 1 base pair to the right of O_R2 in Figure 3. In this hybrid, the wild-type sequence is maintained for 51 base pairs to the right of the start point of transcription of *CI*, and presumably P_{RM} is intact. Nevertheless, P_{RM} is inactive in this deletion hybrid, suggesting that the absence of polymerase bound to P_R does not suffice to activate P_{RM}; rather, there is apparently a requirement that repressor be bound to O_R1 (B. J. Meyer, unpubl.). A simple view would be that appropriately positioned repressor contacts polymerase and stabilizes its binding to P_{RM}.

CI: One Gene, Two Messages

We have noted that when repressor is transcribed in lysogens from its promoter P_{RM}, rather low levels of repressor are produced. In contrast, when λ infects a nonlysogen, a burst of repressor is synthesized utilizing a transcript that is not autogenously regulated and that begins at promoter P_{RE}. The precise location of P_{RE} is unknown, but it is believed to lie some hundreds of base pairs to the right of P_{RM} (Reichardt and Kaiser 1971; Echols and Green 1971; Spiegelman et al. 1972). We now believe that an important factor regulating differential repressor synthesis from these promoters is differential translation of the two messengers.

On the CI mRNA read from P_{RM}, the codon corresponding to the amino terminus of repressor is found immediately adjacent to the 5' terminal AUG (Ptashne et al. 1976; Walz et al. 1976). This is remarkable in that all messages analyzed heretofore contain leaders of variable length preceding the AUG or GUG translational start signals. These leaders invariably contain Shine-Dalgarno sequences that promote binding to ribosomes, and hence efficient translation, presumably by pairing with bases at the 3' end of 16S ribosomal RNA (Shine and Dalgarno 1974; Steitz and Jakes 1975). These considerations suggest that the CI mRNA read from P_{RM} would be translated quite inefficiently. The experiment of Table 1 indicates that this is indeed the case. When the $lacZ$ gene and its associated ribosome-binding sequence are transcribed from P_{RM}, roughly 2000 monomers of β-galactosidase are found per cell. (Comparison of lines 2 and 4 show that P_{RM} directs the synthesis of about 25% as much β-galactosidase as does a wild-type lac promoter, which maintains a β-galactosidase concentration of about 10,000 monomers per cell when fully induced.) This value is about tenfold higher than that expected from the level of repressor ordinarily maintained by P_{RM} in lysogens. Apparently, P_{RM} functions at a high level when stimulated by repressor, but the message ordinarily read from P_{RM} is translated inefficiently because it lacks an appropriate leader. It remains a formal possibility that a leader is ligated to the P_{RM} message in vivo, albeit infrequently.

In contrast to CI mRNA read from P_{RM}, that read from P_{RE} should be translated at high efficiency. We expect this because the DNA preceding (to the right of CI in Fig. 3) contains a sequence predicted to be an excellent Shine-Dalgarno sequence (see starred bases in O_R3 in Fig. 3). In conclusion, perhaps the chief reason repressor is synthesized at a higher rate from P_{RE} than from P_{RM} is that in the former case the message is attached to a leader and is translated efficiently, whereas in the latter the message lacks a leader and is translated inefficiently.

The cro Gene and Its Product

The protein encoded by the cro gene has been isolated (Folkmanis et al. 1976). Its amino acid sequence and the colinear sequence of the gene are shown in Figure 7. There are no obvious homologies between the sequences of cro protein and repressor (T. M. Roberts et al. 1977; Hsiang et al. 1978). Mutations that decrease the affinity of DNA for repressor, at least

~~~~~~~~~~~~~~~~~~~→ MetGluGlnArgIleThrLeuLysAspTyrAlaMetArgPhe
ATGTACTAAGGAGGTTGTATGGAACAACGCATAACCCTGAAAGATTATGCAATGCGCTTT
TACATGATTCCTCCAACATACCTTGTTGCGTATTGGGACTTTCTAATACGTTACGCGAAA

GlyGlnThrLysThrAlaLysAspLeuGlyValTyrGlnSerAlaIleAsnLysAlaIle
GGGCAAACCAAGACAGCTAAAGATCTCGGCGTATATCAAAGCGCGATCAACAAGGCCATT
CCCGTTTGGTTCTGTCGATTTCTAGAGCCGCATATAGTTTCGCGCTAGTTGTTCCGGTAA

HisAlaGlyArgLysIlePheLeuThrIleAsnAlaAspGlySerValTyrAlaGluGlu
CATGCAGGCCGAAAGATTTTTTTAACTATAAACGCTGATGGAAGCGTTTATGCGGAAGAG
GTACGTCCGGCTTTCTAAAAAAAATTGATATTTGCGACTACCTTCGCAAATACGCCTTCTC

ValLysProPheProSerAsnLysLysThrThrAla-COOH
GTAAAGCCCTTCCCGAGTAACAAAAAAACAACAGCATAAAT
CATTTCGGGAAGGGCTCATTGTTTTTTTGTTGTCGTATTTA

Figure 7 The amino acid sequence (Hsiang et al. 1978) of *cro*-product and the base sequence of the *cro* gene (T. M. Roberts et al. 1977). Also shown is the start point of transcription of *cro*.

in most cases, decrease the effect of *cro* protein in vivo (Ordal and Kaiser 1973; Echols et al. 1973; Berg 1974). Some of these operator mutations also affect the affinity of DNA for *cro* protein in vitro. *Cro* protein binds to λ DNA with an affinity at least an order of magnitude lower than that of repressor (Takeda et al. 1977). We (Johnson et al. 1978) have recently studied the mechanism of action of *cro* protein by measuring protection of DNA against methylation by dimethylsulfate and by transcription experiments performed in vitro. We found that, at O_R, *cro* protein protects from methylation only G residues within the sites O_R1, O_R2, and O_R3. Moreover, *cro* protein protects a subset of those G residues protected by repressor: one (at O_R3) or two (at O_R1 and O_R2) fewer G's are protected by *cro* protein than by repressor (see Fig. 8). Apparently both *cro* protein and λ repressor contact DNA primarily in the major groove. In vitro, *cro* protein, like the λ repressor, blocks transcription of *CI* and *cro* from P_{RM} and P_R respectively. However, transcription of *CI* is turned off at lower *cro* protein concentrations than is transcription of *cro*, whereas the opposite order of repression is obtained with λ repressor. Moreover, the concentration of *cro* protein required to repress *CI* transcription is the same whether or not that transcription is stimulated by λ repressor. The results of the DMS protection experiments suggest, and the transcription experiments confirm, that the relative affinities of λ repressor and *cro* protein for the three operator sites in O_R are different: whereas repressor binds with an affinity $O_R1 > O_R2 > O_R3$, the order for *cro* protein is $O_R3 > (O_R1, O_R2)$.

The results of Johnson et al. (1978) outlined above, taken with other work discussed in this review, indicate how two repressor proteins can bind to the same three adjacent sites in DNA with markedly different physiological consequences. As discussed λ repressor first binds to O_R1, stimu-

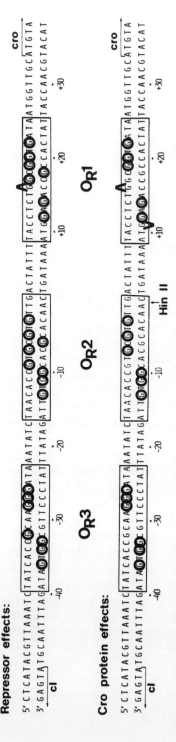

Figure 8 The effects of λ repressor and *cro* protein on the methylation of purines in O_R. Guanines which are protected from methylation are circled, and those whose reaction rate is increased are indicated by a carat. The top sequence shows the effects of repressor on the methylation of O_R (Humayun et al. 1977a). The bottom sequence indicates the effects of the *cro* protein (Johnson et al. 1978). The bases are numbered starting from the *Hin*II cleavage site in O_R.

lating *CI* transcription at P_{RM} and repressing *cro* transcription at P_R. At higher concentrations it binds to O_R3 and turns off transcription of *CI*. In contrast, *cro* protein binds with highest affinity to O_R3. At low concentrations, therefore, *cro* protein turns off *CI* transcription, and at higher concentrations in the absence of repressor, it fills O_R1 and turns off transcription of its own gene, *cro*. *Cro* protein, like the λ repressor, exerts its negative regulatory functions by excluding binding of RNA polymerase. The negative effect of *cro* protein on *CI* transcription is epistatic to the stimulatory effect of λ repressor on that transcription.

Prophage Induction

The λ repressor is inactivated, and the prophage induced, when lysogens are treated with any of a variety of agents, including UV light and mitomycin (see Moreau et al. 1976, ref. 9–11). In general, any activated carcinogen will induce λ, and λ induction has been shown to be a sensitive assay for carcinogens (Moreau et al. 1976). Repressor is cleaved upon induction (Roberts and Roberts 1975), but it is not known whether this is the cause or consequence of repressor inactivation. Repressor inactivation (cleavage) requires a functional product of the *recA* gene. Mutants with certain lesions in *recA* (called *tif*) cause repressor inactivation when grown at high temperature (Goldthwait and Jacob 1964). Extracts of cells bearing the *tif* and other important mutations (Mount et al. 1976) contain an activity that will cleave λ repressor in vitro, a process that requires adenosine triphosphate (ATP) (J. W. Roberts et al. 1977). The product of the *recA* gene is the protein previously called the X protein (McEntee 1978; Little and Kleid 1977); its level increases dramatically upon induction (Gudas and Pardee 1975). It is possible that the *recA* protein is (an ATP-dependent) protease that cleaves the λ repressor, as well as other repressors that control a variety of cellular functions (Radman 1975); Witkin 1976).

RATIONALIZATION

Why is repressor autogenously regulated, both positively and negatively? We imagine that it is to the lysogen's advantage to maintain fairly constant repressor levels and to be able to adjust to shifts up or down in growth rates. This would ensure that, on the one hand, prophage would not induce capriciously and, on the other, that repressor concentrations would never reach levels that would prevent complete inactivation by the inducing machinery. This argument suffices to justify negative autogenous control, but it does not explain positive autogenous control. The former mechanism will maintain constant repressor levels, but the latter can only destabilize the system. One possibility is that positive autogenous regulation ensures efficient induction upon treatment with an inducer. In the absence of positive autogenous regulation, the rate of repressor synthesis would increase as the repressor was inactivated; the imposition of positive autogenous regulation ensures that once a certain amount of repressor has been inactivated, repressor synthesis will rapidly fall to zero. To evaluate these ideas, we will have to learn more about the magnitude of the positive and negative effects of repressor under various physiological conditions.

We have previously argued that a requirement for maintaining repressor levels constant over even very short time periods might explain why transcription from P_{RM} yields a mRNA that lacks a leader and is translated inefficiently. We noted that there is a general problem in maintaining low concentrations of a gene product in a bacterial cell. In the *lacI* gene, for example, apparently only one or two transcripts are produced per generation; and these are translated quickly several times and then degraded. The consequence is that *lac* repressor levels must fluctuate during the cell cycle. The λ repressor levels might not be subject to such fluctuations, however, because *CI* mRNA is produced at a constant and high rate. Presumably, a small but constant fraction of these *CI* mRNA molecules is translated throughout the cell cycle.

ACKNOWLEDGMENTS

I wish to thank Alexander Johnson, Russell Maurer, Barbara Meyer, Carl Pabo, and Robert Sauer, graduate students, and Ricardo Pastrana, Thomas M. Roberts, and Michael Ross, postdoctoral fellows in the Department of Biochemistry and Molecular Biology, for unpublished information and for comments on the manuscript.

REFERENCES

Backman, K. and M. Ptashne. 1978. Maximizing gene expression on a plasmid using recombination *in vitro*. *Cell* **13**:65.

Backman, K., M. Ptashne, and W. Gilbert. 1976. Construction of plasmids carrying the *cI* gene of bacteriophage λ. *Proc. Natl. Acad. Sci.* **73**:4174.

Barnes, W. M., R. B. Siegel, and W. S. Reznikoff. 1974. The construction of λ transducing phages containing deletions defining regulatory elements of the *lac* and *trp* operons in *E. coli. Mol. Gen. Genet.* **129**:201.

Berg, D. E. 1974. Genes of phage λ essential for λdv plasmids. *Virology* **62**:224.

Blattner, F. R. and J. E. Dahlberg. 1972. RNA synthesis start-points in bacteriophage λ: Are the promoter and operator transcribed? *Nat. New Biol.* **237**:227.

Chadwick, P., V. Pirrotta, R. Steinberg, N. Hopkins, and M. Ptashne. 1971. The λ and 434 phage repressor. *Cold Spring Harbor Symp. Quant. Biol.* **35**:283.

Echols, H. and L. Green. 1971. Establishment and maintenance of repression by bacteriophage lambda: The role of the cI, cII, and cIII proteins. *Proc. Natl. Acad. Sci.* **68**:2190.

Echols, H., L. Green, A. B. Oppenheim, A. Oppenheim, and A. Honigman. 1973. Role of the cro gene in bacteriophage λ development. *J. Mol. Biol.* **80**:203.

Eisen, H. and M. Ptashne. 1971. Regulation of repressor synthesis. In *The bacteriophage lambda* (ed. A. D. Hershey), p. 239. Cold Spring Harbor Laboratory, Cold Spring Harbor, New York.

Flashman, S. M. 1976. "The relation between structure and function in the operators of bacteriophage lambda: An analysis using O^c mutations." Ph.D. thesis, Harvard University, Cambridge, Massachusetts.

Folkmanis, A., Y. Takeda, J. Simuth, G. Gussin, and H. Echols. 1976. Purification and properties of a DNA-binding protein with characteristics expected for the Cro protein of bacteriophage λ, a repressor essential for lytic growth. *Proc. Natl. Acad. Sci.* **73**:2249.

Gilbert, W., A. Maxam, and A. Mirzabekov. 1976. Contact between the lac repressor and DNA revealed by methylation. In *In control of ribosome synthesis* (ed. N. O. Kjelgaard and O. Maaløe), p. 139. Munksgaard, Copenhagen.

Goldthwait, D. and F. Jacob. 1964. Sur le méchanisms de l'induction du dévelopment du prophage chez les bactéries lysogènes. *C. R. Acad. Sci.* **D259**:661.

Gudas, L. J. and A. B. Pardee. 1975. Model for regulation of *Escherichia coli* DNA repair function. *Proc. Natl. Acad. Sci.* **72**:2330.

Herskowitz, I. 1973. Control of gene expression in bacteriophage lambda. *Annu. Rev. Genet.* **7**:289.

Hopkins, N. and M. Ptashne. 1971. Genetics of virulence. In *The bacteriophage lambda* (ed. A. D. Hershey), p. 571. Cold Spring Harbor Laboratory, Cold Spring Harbor, New York.

Hsiang, M. W., Y. Takeda, R. D. Cole, and H. Echols. 1978. Amino acid sequence of the Cro regulatory protein of bacteriophage λ. *Nature* **270**:275.

Humayun, Z. 1977. DNA sequence at the ends of the cI gene in bacteriophage λ. *Nucleic Acids Res.* **4**:2137.

Humayun, Z., A. Jeffrey, and M. Ptashne. 1977a. Completed DNA sequences and organization of repressor-binding sites in the operators of phage lambda. *J. Mol. Biol.* **112**:265.

Humayun, Z., D. Kleid, and M. Ptashne. 1977b. Sites of contact between λ operators and λ repressor. *Nucleic Acids Res.* **4**:1595.

Humayun, Z., B. Meyer, R. Sauer, K. Backman, and M. Ptashne. 1976. Transcriptional and translational (?) control of the λ repressor gene (cI). In *Molecular mechanisms in the control of gene expression* (ed. D. P. Nierlich et al.), p. 67. Academic Press, New York.

Johnson, A., B. J. Meyer, and M. Ptashne. 1978. Mechanism of action of the cro protein of bacteriophage λ. *Proc. Natl. Acad. Sci.* **75**:1783.

Kawashima, E., T. Gadek, and M. H. Caruthers. 1978. IV. Chemical and enzymatic synthesis of bacteriophage lambda pseudo operator DNA. In *Studies on gene control regions* (in press).

Kleid, D., Z. Humayun, A. Jeffrey, and M. Ptashne. 1976. Novel properties of a restriction endonuclease isolated from *Haemophilus parahaemolyticus*. *Proc. Natl. Acad. Sci.* **73**:293.

Little, J. W. and D. G. Kleid. 1977. *Escherichia coli* protein X is the *recA* gene product. *J. Biol. Chem.* **252**: 6251.

Maniatis, T. and M. Ptashne. 1973a. Structure of the λ operators. *Nature* **246**: 133.

———. 1973b. Multiple repressor binding at the operators in bacteriophage λ. *Proc. Natl. Acad. Sci.* **70**: 1531.

———. 1976. A DNA operator-repressor system. *Sci. Am.* **234**: 64.

Maniatis, T., A. Jeffrey, and D. G. Kleid. 1975a. Nucleotide sequence of the rightward operator of phage λ. *Proc. Natl. Acad. Sci.* **72**: 1184.

Maniatis, T., M. Ptashne, and R. Maurer. 1974a. Control elements in the DNA of bacteriophage λ. *Cold Spring Harbor Symp. Quant. Biol.* **38**: 857.

Maniatis, T., M. Ptashne, B. G. Barrell, and J. Donelson. 1974b. Sequence of a repressor-binding site in the DNA of bacteriophage λ. *Nature* **250**: 394.

Maniatis, T., M. Ptashne, K. Backman, D. Kleid, S. Flashman, A. Jeffrey, and R. Maurer. 1975b. Recognition sequences of repressor and polymerase in the operators of bacteriophage lambda. *Cell* **5**: 109.

Maurer, R., T. Maniatis, and M. Ptashne. 1974. Promoters are in the operators in phage lambda. *Nature* **249**: 221.

McEntee, K. 1978. Protein X is *recA*. *Proc. Natl. Acad. Sci.* (in press).

Meyer, B. J., D. G. Kleid, and M. Ptashne. 1975. λ Repressor turns off transcription of its own gene. *Proc. Natl. Acad. Sci* **72**: 4785.

Miller, J. H., ed. 1972. *Experiments in molecular genetics.* Cold Spring Harbor Laboratory, Cold Spring Harbor, New York.

Mitchell, D. H., W. S. Reznikoff, and J. R. Beckwith. 1975. Genetic fusions defining *trp* and *lac* operon regulatory elements. *J. Mol. Biol.* **93**: 331.

Moreau, P., A. Bailone, and R. Devoret. 1976. Prophage λ induction in *Escherichia coli* K12 *envA uvrB*: A highly sensitive test for potential carcinogens. *Proc. Natl. Acad. Sci.* **73**: 3700.

Mount, D. W., C. K. Kosel, and A. Walker. 1976. Inducible error-free DNA repair in *ts1 recA* mutants of *E. coli. Mol. Gen. Genet.* **146**: 37.

Oppenheim, A. B. and D. Noff. 1975. Deletion mapping of *trans* dominant mutations in the λ repressor gene. *Virology* **63**: 553.

Oppenheim, A. B. and D. Salomon. 1970. Studies on partially virulent mutants of lambda bacteriophage. I. Isolation and general characterization. *Virology* **41**: 151.

———. 1972. Studies on partially virulent mutants of lambda bacteriophage. II. The mechanism of overcoming repression. *Mol. Gen. Genet.* **115**: 101.

Ordal, G. W. 1971. Supervirulent mutants and the structure of operator and promoter. In *The bacteriophage lambda* (ed. A. D. Hershey), p. 565. Cold Spring Harbor Laboratory, Cold Spring Harbor, New York.

Ordal, G. W. and A. D. Kaiser. 1973. Mutations in the right operator of bacteriophage lambda: Evidence for operator-promoter interpretation. *J. Mol. Biol.* **79**: 709.

Pastrana, R. and W. J. Brammar. 1976. Control of *cI* gene expression in bacteriophage λ*imm*[434], studies in an immunity/*trp* fusion made *in vitro*. *Mol. Gen. Genet.* **146**: 191.

Pirrotta, V. 1975. Sequence of the O_R operator of phage λ. *Nature* **254**: 114.

Pirrotta, V., P. Chadwick, and M. Ptashne. 1970. Active form of two coliphage repressors. *Nature* **227**: 41.

Ptashne, M. 1971. Repressor and its action. In *The bacteriophage lambda* (ed. A.

D. Hershey), p. 221. Cold Spring Harbor Laboratory, Cold Spring Harbor, New York.

Ptashne, M. and N. Hopkins. 1968. The operators controlled by the λ phage repressor. *Proc. Natl. Acad. Sci.* **60**: 1282.

Ptashne, M., K. Backman, M. Z. Humayun, A. Jeffrey, R. Maurer, B. Meyer, and R. T. Sauer. 1976. Autoregulation and function of a repressor in bacteriophage lambda. *Science* **194**: 156.

Radman, M. 1975. SOS repair hypothesis: Phenomenology of an inducible DNA repair which is accompanied by mutagenesis. In *Molecular mechanisms for repair of DNA* (ed. P. Hanawalt and R. B. Setlow), part A, p. 355. Plenum Press, New York.

Reichardt, L. F. 1975. Control of bacteriophage lambda repressor synthesis after phage infection: The role of the *N*, *c*II, *c*III, and *cro* products. *J. Mol. Biol.* **93**: 267.

Reichardt, L. and A. D. Kaiser. 1971. Control of λ repressor synthesis. *Proc. Natl. Acad. Sci.* **68**: 2185.

Roberts, J. W. and C. W. Roberts. 1975. Proteolytic cleavage of bacteriophage lambda repressor in induction. *Proc. Natl. Acad. Sci.* **72**: 147.

Roberts, J. W., C. W. Roberts, and D. W. Mount. 1977. Inactivation and proteolytic cleavage of phage λ repressor *in vitro* in an ATP-dependent reaction. *Proc. Natl. Acad. Sci.* **74**: 2283.

Roberts, T. M., H. Shimatake, C. Brady, and M. Rosenberg. 1977. The nucleotide sequence of the *cro* gene of bacteriophage lambda. *Nature* **270**: 274.

Sauer, R. T. and R. Anderegg. 1978. Primary structure of the λ repressor. *Biochemistry* **17**: 1092.

Shine, J. and L. Dalgarno. 1974. The 3'-terminal sequence of *Escherichia coli* 16S ribosomal RNA: Complementarity to nonsense triplets and ribosome binding sites. *Proc. Natl. Acad. Sci.* **71**: 1342.

Spiegelman, W. G., L. F. Reichardt, M. Yaniv, S. F. Heinemann, A. D. Kaiser, and H. Eisen. 1972. Bidirectional transcription and the regulation of phage λ repressor synthesis. *Proc. Natl. Acad. Sci. U.S.A.* **69**: 3156.

Steinberg, R. A. and M. Ptashne. 1971. *In vitro* repression of RNA synthesis by purified λ phage repressor. *Nat. New Biol.* **230**: 76.

Steitz, J. A. and K. Jakes. 1975. How ribosomes select initiator regions in mRNA: Base pair formation between the 3' terminus of 16S rRNA and the mRNA during initation of protein synthesis in *Escherichia coli*. *Proc. Natl. Acad. Sci.* **72**: 4734.

Takeda, Y., A. Folkmanis, and H. Echols. 1977. Cro regulatory protein specified by bacteriophage λ. *J. Biol. Chem.* **252**: 6177.

Waltz, A. and V. Pirrotta. 1975. Sequence of the P_R promoter of phage λ. *Nature* **254**: 118.

Walz, A., V. Pirrotta, and K. Ineichen. 1976. λ Repressor regulated the switch between P_R and P_{rm} promoters. *Nature* **262**: 665.

Weisberg, R. A., M. E. Gottesman, and S. Gottesman. 1977. In *Comprehensive virology* (ed. J. Fraenkel-Conrat and R. Wagner), vol. 8, p. 197. Plenum Press, New York.

Witkin, E. M. 1976. Ultraviolet mutagenesis and inducible DNA repair in *Escherichia coli*. *Bacteriol. Rev.* **40**: 869.

Yen, K.-M. and G. N. Gussin. 1973. Genetic characterization of a prm⁻ mutant of bacteriophage λ. *Virology* **56**: 300.

Structure and Function of an Intercistronic Regulatory Region in Bacteriophage Lambda

Martin Rosenberg, Donald Court, Hiroyuki Shimatake, and Catherine Brady
Laboratory of Molecular Biology
National Cancer Institute
National Institutes of Health
Bethesda, Maryland 20014

Daniel Wulff
Department of Biology
University of California
Irvine, California 92664

INTRODUCTION

When bacteriophage λ infects *Escherichia coli*, two possible pathways of development may ensue. The virus may undergo a lytic mode of growth resulting in the formation and release of progeny virus concomitant with lysis of the host cell. Alternatively, the phage may enter a lysogenic state in which the viral DNA integrates into the bacterial genome and concurrently represses expression of viral functions. Crucial to the establishment of lysogeny is the synthesis of two phage functions: the integration protein, which catalyzes the genetic recombination between the viral DNA and the host genome, and the repressor protein, which directly inhibits transcription of phage functions. In simple terms, the viral infection can be considered a competition between the accumulation of those gene products which commit the virus to lytic development and the expression of gene products which turn on synthesis of the phage repressor protein, thereby committing the infection to lysogeny. Under normal growth conditions, a delicate balance is achieved whereby both lytic and lysogenic patterns of development are expressed in a single viral infection (for review, see Weisberg et al. 1977).

Immediately after λ infection, transcription is initiated by the host RNA polymerase from two major promoters, P_R and P_L, located within the phage immunity region (see Fig. 1). At early times the majority of this transcription, both rightward and leftward, is limited to the immunity region by sites of transcription termination, t_{R1} and t_L, respectively (Fig. 1). Efficient transcription distal to these two termination sites depends upon expression of λ N function, the gene product encoded by the early leftward transcript (Taylor et al. 1967; Luzzati 1970; Kourilsky et al. 1971;

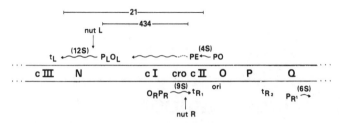

Figure 1 Genetic map of bacteriophage λ showing the location of the *cro-CII* intercistronic boundary (i.e., *Y* region) on the λ chromosome. Locations and relative sizes of the major RNA transcripts and the boundaries of the λ*imm*[434] and λ*imm*[21] immunity substitution regions are indicated.

Heinemann and Spiegelman 1971). Although the mechanism of action of N is not understood, N acts as a positive regulator and allows transcription by RNA polymerase to read through (i.e., antiterminate) termination sites (Roberts 1969; Lozeron et al. 1976; D. Court et al., in prep.). Thus, N protein allows rightward transcription to proceed past the t_{RI} termination site through the *CII*, *O*, and *P* genes and into other genes required for lytic growth. Genes *O* and *P* are also lytic functions in that they promote λ DNA replication. The *CII* gene, however, is a lysogenic function required for the activation of repressor (*CI*) synthesis as well as integration function (Katzir et al. 1976; Reichardt and Kaiser 1971). *CII* (in conjunction with the *CIII* gene product which requires N action on the P_L-initiated leftward transcript; see Fig. 1) activates transcription of repressor at a site called *pre* (*p*romoter for *r*epressor *e*stablishment) somewhere to the right of the *cro* gene (Fig. 1) (Echols and Green 1971). The exact location of the *pre* promoter is still unclear; however, transcription from *pre* proceeds leftward in the opposite (i.e., antisense) direction through the *cro* gene before entering the *CI* gene (Spiegelman et al. 1972). Clearly, this region of the λ genome is somewhat unusual in that transcription can occur in either direction (i.e., both DNA strands serve as templates for transcription). Rightward transcription through this region (from P_R) is predominantly involved in the expression of functions required for lytic development, whereas leftward transcription (from *pre*) is necessary for the synthesis of repressor protein and the establishment of the lysogenic state. It should be noted that *CII* function appears to play an important pivotal role in control of this bidirectional transcription. Expression of *CII* is dependent upon rightward transcription, whereas *CII* function itself is required for activation of leftward transcription.

A variety of mutations have been obtained which genetically map in the intercistronic region between the *cro* and *CII* genes (i.e., the *Y* region) and which affect the ability of λ to establish either lytic or lysogenic patterns of development. These mutations have helped to define a number of related transcriptional and translational regulatory elements positioned in the Y region. Apparently, the potential interactions and structural overlaps of these control elements couple the regulation of bidirectional transcription through this region and, in turn, provide the molecular basis for the decision between lytic and lysogenic growth patterns made by phage λ. Some of the structural and functional features of the Y region are described below.

RHO-MEDIATED TRANSCRIPTION TERMINATION AT t_{R1}

In vitro, transcription of λ DNA by purified *E. coli* RNA polymerase initiates at the same P_L and P_R promoters as in vivo and results in the production of relatively high-molecular-weight (>16S) RNA transcripts which extend well beyond the immunity region and thus beyond the proposed transcription-termination sites t_L and t_{R1} (Roberts 1969). Roberts (1969, 1971) isolated a host-encoded protein factor, rho, which when added to the in vitro transcription system results in termination of the P_L- and P_R-initiated transcripts and production of lower-molecular-weight products of defined size (as determined by sucrose gradient analysis). A 12S RNA product presumably encoding the N function is obtained from the left (*l*-strand template) and a smaller RNA which encodes the *cro* gene product is obtained from the right (*r*-strand template). These products are also observed as discrete 12S and 8S–9S RNAs by electrophoretic separation on polyacrylamide gels (Rosenberg et al. 1975). From these results it has been inferred that the termination events observed in vitro to be rho-factor-dependent might be identical to those responsible for the synthesis of the early mRNAs found in infected cells. This suggests that termination in vivo at t_{R1} requires the bacterial rho factor and that the λ N protein counteracts this rho-dependent termination (i.e., transcriptional attenuation).

In vitro, transcription termination of the P_R-initiated mRNA (8S–9S RNA) occurs within the intercistronic region between the genes for *cro* and *CII* (Y region) and is absolutely dependent on the protein termination factor rho (Fig. 2A). The site on the DNA at which the rho-dependent termination event occurs was exactly positioned by selectively isolating the 3'-terminal oligonucleotide products produced from T₁ RNase fragmentation of the 8S–9S RNA by chromatography on dihydroxyboryl (DBAE)-cellulose (Rosenberg et al. 1978). The 3'-end fragments obtained by this procedure were initially characterized by two-dimensional homochromatography (Fig. 3C). Subsequent analyses of each separately resolved oligonucleotide indicated that they were all sequence-related and differed only by the nucleoside residues occurring at their 3' termini. These same terminal oligonucleotides were detected in the T₁ fingerprint of a 100-nucleotide RNA fragment isolated by direct

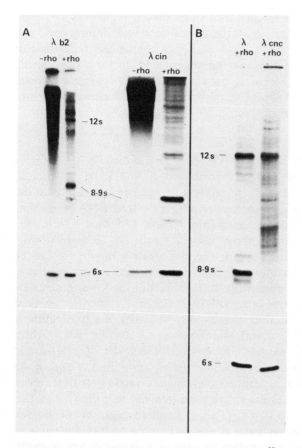

Figure 2   Polyacrylamide gel electrophoresis of ^{32}P-labeled RNA synthesized in vitro from several λ DNA templates in either the presence or absence of rho factor. (*A*) $\lambda b2S7$ ($\lambda b2$) and $\lambda CI857cin1S7$ (λcin); (*B*) $\lambda CI857S7$ (λ) and $\lambda CI857cin1cnc1S7$ (λcnc). DNAs were transcribed and analyzed on 3.5% acrylamide slab gels which contained 8.0 M urea. The $b2$ region of λ accounts for ~50% of the transcription observed in vitro (Roberts 1969). Thus the templates used which contain the $b2$ region (e.g., λ, λcin, and λcnc) have additional transcription products not present in the analysis of the $\lambda b2$ RNA. Adapted from Rosenberg et al. (1978).

hybridization from the 3'-terminal region of the 8S–9S RNA (Fig. 3B, 9a, b, c, d, e). However, when transcription was carried out in the absence of rho and the P_R-initiated mRNA was isolated and fingerprinted (as in Fig. 3D), these 3'-terminal oligonucleotides were not detected. All other T_1 products characteristic of the 3'-terminal region of the rho-terminated transcript were observed in this fingerprint, as well as additional new oligonucleotides which are not present in the 8S–9S mRNA transcript.

These new oligonucleotides represented transcription products that were derived from the region beyond the t_{RI} site of termination (see Fig. 4). One of these (oligonucleotide 9, Fig. 3D) had the sequence CAUACAUUCAAUCAAUUG and was the only oligonucleotide consistent with transcriptional read-through of the termination site. Thus, in vitro, rho-mediated transcription termination in the t_{RI} site occurs heterogeneously over four or five adjacent nucleotide pairs and results in production of a 308–312-nucleotide mRNA which includes 198 nucleotides that encode the 66 amino acids of the *cro* protein (Roberts et al. 1977; Hsiang et al. 1977), the 18-nucleotide leader sequence for the *cro* message (Steege 1977), and 92–96 nucleotide residues (apparently untranslated) beyond the ochre translation-termination triplet for *cro* (Rosenberg et al. 1978) (Figs. 4 and 5A). In the absence of rho, the RNA polymerase reads through the termination site and into the *CII* gene to produce a single, contiguous polycistronic RNA transcript of high molecular weight.

Similar hybridization and fingerprinting methods have been used to monitor *r*-strand transcription throughout the *Y* region under a variety of in vivo and in vitro conditions (Rosenberg et al. 1978; D. Court et al., in prep.). For example, to quantitate the efficiency of transcription termination at t_{RI}, in vitro reactions were carried out in the presence of rifampicin in order to allow only a single round of transcription to initiate from the P_R promoter. This RNA was then selectively isolated by hybridization, and T_1 fingerprints were prepared. Certain T_1 oligonucleotide products are uniquely characteristic for specific regions of the transcript, and their relative intensities are a measure of the amount of transcription in these regions. By determining the molar ratios of the appropriate T_1 products, transcription preceding and distal to t_{RI} was directly compared (see Table 1). The results of these experiments indicate that, in the presence of rho, termination at t_{RI} is approximately 80% effective; 20% of the polymerases transcribe through t_{RI}. In the absence of rho, no termination is detected.

These same procedures were also applied to the isolation and analysis of the P_R-initiated early mRNA species obtained from λ-infected cells pulse-labeled with $[^{32}P]H_3PO_4$ under a variety of different conditions and at varying times after infection (D. Court et al., in prep.). The results indicate that, in vivo, transcription termination of the early *cro* mRNA occurs at the same site and over the same four or five residues as in vitro. In addition, termination at t_{RI} in vivo is completely rho-factor-dependent, and efficient read-through at the site requires expression of the λ N function (Table 1B). In the presence of both N and rho, N (i.e., antitermination) predominates, and in a wild-type infection of normal host cells, termination at t_{RI} is detected only early after infection, prior to N expression. However, in the absence of N function (i.e., infection in the presence of chloramphenicol or with an N mutant), termination is

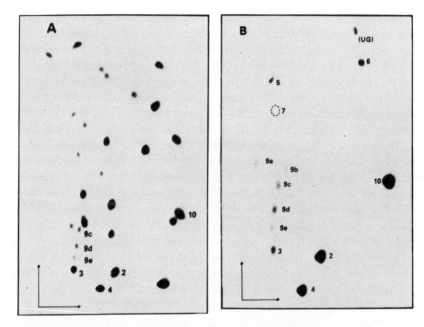

Figure 3 Autoradiographs of two-dimensional fingerprints of RNase T_1 oligo-nucleotide products derived from the P_R-initiated, rightward mRNA transcript. *(Horizontal dimension)* Electrophoresis on cellogel in 8.0 M urea at pH 3.5. *(Vertical dimension)* Ascending thin-layer homochromatography on plates of DEAE-cellulose using homosolvent B (Sanger et al. 1965; Brownlee and Sanger 1969; Barrell 1971). *(A)* T_1 fingerprint of the entire 9S mRNA transcript labeled with $[\alpha\text{-}^{32}P]$UTP and purified by polyacrylamide gel electrophoresis, as shown in Fig. 2. *(B)* T_1 fingerprint of a 100-nucleotide RNA fragment isolated from the 3'-terminal region of the $\lambda b2$ 9S RNA transcript by hybridization. The RNA fragment depicted represents that portion of the P_R-initiated, rho-terminated mRNA transcript which extends beyond the right-hand boundary of the λimm^{434} region of nonhomology (see Figs. 4 and 5A).

50–70% effective at t_{R1}, somewhat less than was found in vitro with rho present. When a host defective in rho is used (e.g., rho_{ts15}), no termination at t_{R1} is detected (Table 1). Thus the results obtained in vitro and in vivo appear to be completely consistent.

A striking analogy exists between the control of transcription termination at t_{R1} and the various polarity effects (both natural and mutational) which have been observed in bacterial operons (for review, see Adhya and Gottesman 1978). For example, the existence of rho-dependent in vitro transcription stop signals has been noted within both the *gal* and *lac* operons (de Crombrugghe et al. 1973). Transcription does not terminate

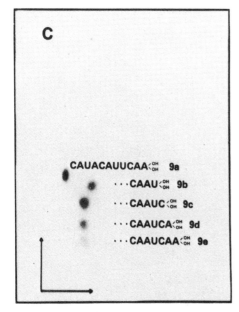

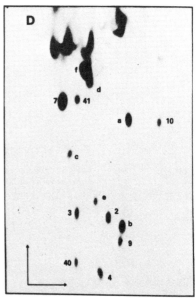

Figure 3 (continued)   (C) Two-dimensional fractionation of the 3′-terminal oligo-nucleotides isolated on DBAE-cellulose (Rosenberg 1974) from the 9S mRNA transcript shown in *A*. (*D*) T_1 fingerprint of an RNA transcript which extends beyond the t_{RI} rho-dependent site of transcription termination (see Fig. 4). The RNA fragments obtained represent that portion of the P_R-initiated transcript which extends beyond the λimm^{434} boundary and spans the *Y* region and part of the *CII* gene. Numbered oligonucleotides indicate characteristic T_1 products which occur in the transcript preceding the t_{RI} rho-dependent termination site (see Fig. 3A). Lettered oligonucleotides represent characteristic RNase T_1 products which occur distal to the t_{RI} site. Adapted from Rosenberg et al. (1978).

at these sites in vivo under normal conditions. However, it has been suggested that these sites become active when translation is inhibited (e.g., by nonsense mutation or chloramphenicol treatment) in the promoter-proximal region of the operon. A direct correlation seems to exist between the degree of the polarity effect and the nucleotide distance between the respective translation and transcription stop sites. Presumably the untranslated RNA is more susceptible to transcription termina-tion. Rho factor is known to play a role in polarity and a variety of Rho mutants have been obtained which suppress polar effects (Richardson et al. 1975; Korn and Yanofsky 1976; Reyes et al. 1976; Das et al. 1976).

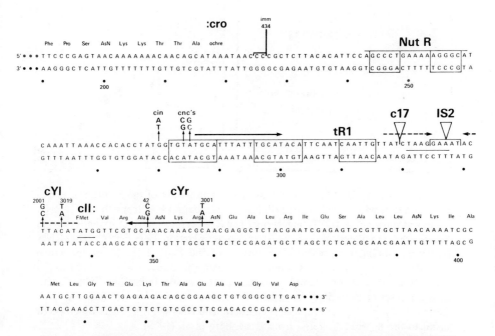

Figure 4 DNA sequence of the intercistronic region between the λ *cro* and *CII* genes, including the sequence generated by a variety of known mutations (↑) within the region (see text). Residue numbers indicate relative position from the start point of transcription of the P_R-initiated mRNA. Only those regions of dyad symmetry (i.e., inverted repeat sequences) pertinent to the discussion in the text are shown. These occur at positions 244–248 and 258–254, 282–289 and 303–296, 286–299 and 359–346, and 317–324 and 338–329; they are denoted either with boxes or with horizontal arrows. Underscored residues at positions 321–327 and 338–340 indicate the presumptive ribosome-binding site and AUG start point of the *CII* protein. The mRNA transcript of this region exhibits the necessary complementarity to the 3′ end of the *E. coli* 16S rRNA (Shine and Dalgarno 1974; Steitz and Jakes 1975). In addition, in vitro translation and ribosome-binding experiments, as well as sequence determination of several point mutations affecting *CII* function, support the positioning of the *CII* coding region (M. Beher et al., in prep.; B. Paterson and M. Rosenberg, in prep.). The right-hand boundary of the 434 immunity-region substitution (Fig. 1) is located to the right of the *cro* gene between residues 224 and 227. Adapted from Rosenberg et al. (1978).

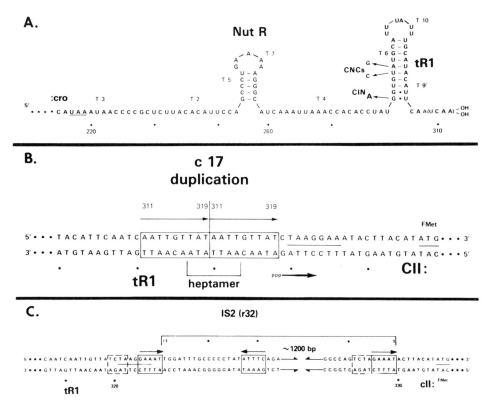

Figure 5 (*A*) The primary and possible secondary structure at the 3' end of the t_{RI}-terminated mRNA. Mutations affecting termination are shown. Residue positions are numbered as in Fig. 4. T_1 ribonuclease products (T#) are those indicated in Fig. 3B. T9' represents the heterogeneous 3'-terminal oligonucleotides 9a, b, c, d, e from Fig. 3*B* and *C*. The secondary structure suggested is based on both thermodynamic considerations (Gralla and Crothers 1973; Tinoco et al. 1973) and relative susceptibility of the structure to partial enzymatic cleavage (D. Court et al., in prep.). The underscored UAA sequence denotes the ochre termination signal of the *cro* gene (Roberts et al. 1977). (*B*) DNA sequence of the *c*17 mutation of phage λ. Note that residue numbers indicated below the sequence differ from those in Fig. 4 beyond the site of the mutation in order to compensate for the additional 9-base-pair duplication. The start point and direction of transcription of the *c*17-initiated mRNA are indicated (see text for details). All other designations are identical to those shown in Fig. 4. (*C*) DNA sequence surrounding the site of IS*2* insertion in phage λ*r*32. The inserted DNA segment (i.e., all nucleotide residues not occurring in the wild-type sequence shown in *A*) is designated by brackets (⌐). Residue numbers which occur below the sequence are identical to those in Fig. 4; residue numbers above the sequence refer only to the inserted DNA segment (+1 to −1). Arrows and boxes indicate both direct and inverted sequence repeats. All other designations are identical to those shown in Fig. 4. Adapted from Rosenberg et al. (1978).

Table 1 Efficiency of transcription termination at the t_{RI} terminator

A. *In vitro*

DNA template	Percent read-through at			
	25 sec	40 sec	55 sec	5 min
λ^+ (+*rho*)	—	—	—	20
$\lambda cin1$ (+*rho*)	—	—	—	5–10
$\lambda cin1cnc1$ (+*rho*)	—	—	—	90
λ^+ (−*rho*)	0	5	15	100
$\lambda cin1cnc1$ (−*rho*)	75	90	—	95

B. *In vivo*

Infecting phage	Percent read-through[a] at 2.5–5.0 min after infection	
	wild-type host (*rho*[+])	*rho*$_{ts15}$ host (*rho*[−])
λN^+	95	—
λN^-	50	100
λ (+*cam*)[b]	35	100
λN^-cin1	15	90
$\lambda N^-cin1cnc1$	90	100
λN^+cin1	45	85
$\lambda N^+cin1cnc1$	100	100

[a]Percent read-through was calculated by comparing the mole ratios of certain T_1 oligonucleotides characteristic for the regions of the template preceding and distal to t_{RI}. (Data adapted from Rosenberg et al. 1978; D. Court et al., in prep.)
[b]λ Infection after initial treatment of cells with chloramphenicol.

Current models suggest that rho factor must first interact with "naked" RNA transcript, prior to its action on RNA polymerase in bringing about the termination event.

Similarly for λ, the transcription termination site t_{RI} results in the polar expression of λ's early rightward functions (i.e., prior to N expression or under N^- conditions, the *cro* gene is transcribed in greater amounts than genes distal to t_{RI}). In vivo, 40–50% of the RNA polymerase molecules which initiate transcription from the P_R promoter transcribe beyond the t_{RI} site, whereas in vitro, read-through efficiency at t_{RI} is only 20%. In either case, inactivation (or removal) of rho function releases the block at t_{RI}, thereby suppressing the polar effect. It is interesting that translation termination of the *cro* gene occurs only 93 nucleotides prior to the site of transcription termination (Figs. 4 and 5A). This distance may be too small for rho function to effectively interact with the untranslated portion of the RNA transcript. Since *cro* translation is actively occurring in vivo, this may account for the reduced efficiency of transcription termination measured at t_{R1} in vivo, as well as account for the discrepancy between the termination efficiencies observed in vivo and in vitro. Support for this contention is suggested by measurements of termination efficiency at t_{R1} carried out in vivo in the presence of chloramphenicol in order to inhibit *cro* translation. Consistently, increased levels of termination (to ~70%) were observed (see Table 1B).

STRUCTURE AT t_{R1}

Certain common structural features have been noted at the 3' termini of RNA transcripts obtained from a variety of different systems and thought to result in vivo and/or in vitro from transcription termination (Lebowitz et al. 1971; Pieczenik et al. 1972; Dahlberg and Blattner 1973; Bertrand et al. 1975; Sogin et al. 1976). These include (1) a run of consecutive uridylate residues at the 3' end of the RNA transcript, (2) a GC-rich region of variable length (4–12 consecutive residues) immediately preceding the uridylates, and (3) a potential RNA stem-and-loop structure near the end of the transcript (reflecting a region of hyphenated dyad symmetry within the DNA template). For those RNAs which can be prepared in vitro, the RNA polymerase apparently recognizes the proper signal and terminates transcription at the appropriate site on the DNA in the absence of any additional factors (i.e., independent transcription termination). The termination factor rho appears to help effect termination at certain of these sites both in vitro (Rosenberg et al. 1975; Howard et al. 1977) and in vivo (Korn and Yanofsky 1976; Bertrand et al. 1978).

Transcription termination at the t_{R1} site clearly differs both structurally and functionally from that at the sites described above. Termination both in vivo and in vitro is completely dependent on rho. The transcript that results does not end in a run of uridylates, although a U-rich region does occur 13–17 residues prior to the actual point of termination (Figs. 4 and 5). There is also no apparent GC-rich region preceding the site. Although these two structural features may be essential in the independent termination reaction, they are not required for the rho-dependent event at t_{R1}. The most striking similarity between the t_{R1} site and other sites of transcription termination is the occurrence of the hyphenated dyad symmetry in the DNA (Fig. 4) preceding the site of termination. The importance of this feature will be dealt with later.

Another rho-dependent site of transcription termination has been defined in vitro beyond the end of the *E. coli* tyrosine tRNA gene (Kupper et al. 1978). As observed for t_{R1}, termination is heterogeneous within the site and no uridylate-rich sequence is found at the 3' end of the transcript. However, the most striking similarity between this site and t_{R1}

is the occurrence of a common sequence, CAATCAA, near the point of termination. The importance, if any, of this sequence to the rho-mediated termination event is unclear. The termination region of the tRNA gene differs in several ways from other known sites of transcription termination. For example, no potential stem-and-loop structure immediately precedes the termination site and an extensive GC-rich region just follows the site. Although little is known about the ability of this site to function in vivo, its occurrence in vitro suggests that various combinations of alternative structural features may be used to effect a termination event. Presumably the structural differences noted among various sites of transcription termination may reflect functional differences such as terminator "strength" and factor dependence (analogous to the differences observed among various sites of transcription initiation).

MUTATIONS AFFECTING TERMINATION

A variety of mutations which affect the ability of λ to grow either lytically or lysogenically map in the Y region (cin, cnc, cY, c17, and IS elements) (Kaiser 1957; Pereira da Silva and Jacob 1968; Dove et al. 1969; Brachet et al. 1970; Wulff 1976; McDermit et al. 1976; M. Beher et al., in prep.). One of these, cin, is a cis-acting mutation which increases λ's ability to lysogenize its host, even in the presence of certain other mutations which alone permit little or no lysogeny (e.g., CII, CIII, cY) (Wulff 1976; McDermit et al. 1976). A secondary set of mutations, cnc, map just to the right of cin and effectively negate the cin phenotype, thereby shifting phage development back toward conditions favoring lysis (McDermit et al. 1976). The proximity of these mutations and their opposing effects on development suggest that the region defined by these and other Y-region mutations encodes information which is critical to the regulation of λ's lytic and lysogenic modes of growth.

The nucleic-acid-sequence changes of the cin and several cnc mutations (Figs. 4 and 5A) have been determined and their effects on rightward transcription in the region surrounding the t_{R1} site have been examined (Rosenberg et al. 1978). Hybridization and fingerprint analyses were again used to monitor transcription in both the in vitro and in vivo systems. The cin mutation occurs 30 residues 5' to the point of termination and increases rho-dependent transcription termination at t_{R1}. The relative efficiencies of transcription termination at t_{R1} using $\lambda+$ and λ cin DNA templates were compared (Table 1). In contrast to the 80% termination efficiency observed for the wild-type template in vitro, the cin DNA exhibited >90% termination efficiency in the presence of rho; less than 10% of the transcripts were extended beyond t_{R1}. In vivo, the effect of cin was even more pronounced (Table 1) (D. Court et al., in prep.).

Termination at t_{RI} is normally detectable only at early times after λ infection (i.e., prior to N expression). In contrast, in strains carrying the *cin* mutation, transcription terminates at t_{RI} with relatively high efficiency (approximately 60%) even after N expression. If N is mutated (e.g., λ*NN⁻cin*), only 10% of the polymerases that reach t_{RI} are able to transcribe through; 90% of rightward transcription is terminated. These results are similar to those obtained in vitro. By using a rho-defective host, it was shown that all termination at the site remains dependent on rho factor (D. Court et al., in prep.).

The *cin* mutation has at least two structural effects at the t_{RI} site: (1) The single base change extends the region of hyphenated, dyad symmetry within the DNA and, hence, the potential length and stability of the RNA (or DNA) stem-and-loop structure which can form near the t_{RI} site (Fig. 5A). The increase in stability of the stem region contributed by the additional A-U base pair is relatively small. If, however, this region of the RNA or DNA were involved in multiple interactions (see below), then relatively small changes in stability might result in structural equilibrium shifts large enough to have major functional effects. In this case at least one such effect would be an increase in rightward termination efficiency at the t_{RI} site. (2) A "heptamer" sequence, TATGGTG (positions 277–283, Fig. 4), similar to those involved in the formation of stable RNA polymerase preinitiation complexes at sites of transcriptional initiation (Pribnow 1975), occurs 27–33 residues upstream of the termination site. The *cin* mutation also alters the central purine position of this sequence, G → A (Fig. 4). If this heptamer sequence is important to the termination event, then the mutation may affect (e.g., by stabilizing) the interaction of RNA polymerase with this site in such a way as to increase rho-dependent transcription termination at t_{RI}.

Three independently isolated *cnc* mutations have been examined (Rosenberg et al. 1978). The sequence changes of two of these are shown in Figures 4 and 5A; the third has a different but still undetermined base change and occurs between positions 284 and 287 in the sequence. All of the *cnc* mutations interfere with rho-dependent transcription termination at t_{RI}. In vitro, in the presence or absence of rho, little, if any, termination is detected at the *cnc*-altered t_{RI} site (Fig. 2B; Table 1). In vivo, similar results are obtained both in the presence and in the absence of N function (D. Court et al., in prep.) (Table 1). The *cnc* mutations are located 4–6 base pairs to the right of *cin* (Figs. 4 and 5A) adjacent to, not within, the heptamer sequence. Most strikingly, these base changes all reduce the dyad symmetry of the DNA in this region and thus correspondingly reduce the stability of the potential stem-and-loop structure which can form within the termination site. The absence of rho-dependent termination in strains carrying the *cnc* mutation may result from their interference with this structure.

Thus the phenotypically opposing *cin* and *cnc* mutations are alterations in the t_{RI} termination region which have opposite effects on termination function and correspondingly opposite effects on the stability of the potential secondary structure within this region. Comparisons of the various stem-and-loop structures occurring at all the known transcription termination sites indicate no obvious primary sequence homologies. However, the independent termination sites (sites at which RNA polymerase stops independently of added factors) have base-paired stem structures of greater stability (i.e., more potential base pairing and/or more G-C pairs) than the rho-dependent t_{RI} site. Perhaps differences in the overall efficiency and factor dependence of the termination sites are reflected, in part, by the stability of this structural feature.

RNA POLYMERASE PAUSE SITE

Termination of transcription is thought to consist of a number of discrete steps. Prior to release of the RNA transcript and dissociation of the RNA polymerase from the DNA, the polymerase presumably stops or pauses at some specific signal encoded in the DNA template. Gilbert (1976) has suggested that a GC-rich region found 10 base pairs (i.e., one turn of the helix) upstream from a termination site may impede the progress of the RNA polymerase. The ability of RNA polymerase (initiated at the P_R promoter) to move through the region surrounding t_{RI} in the absence of rho factor was examined in kinetically controlled in vitro transcription reactions. Aliquots were withdrawn from an in vitro transcription reaction (carried out in the presence of rifampicin at 37°C with a relatively high triphosphate concentration, $\geq 100 \, \mu M$) at 15-second intervals after initiation of transcription. The RNA was isolated and fingerprinted, and the relative intensities (i.e., mole ratios) of the appropriate oligonucleotides proximal and distal to t_{RI} were monitored as described earlier. The results (Table 1) (Rosenberg et al. 1978) indicate that, even in the absence of rho factor, RNA polymerase undergoes a substantial kinetic "pause" within the t_{RI} site before it transcribes the distal *CII* region. The signal specifying the pause at t_{RI} is presumably encoded in the template and does not appear to require a region of extensive G-C base pairs.

Similar experiments were carried out with the *cnc* mutations, which eliminate rho-dependent termination at t_{RI} (see above). Little, if any, pause in transcription was detected with these mutations (Table 1) (Rosenberg et al. 1978). The results suggest that the pause may be a necessary step in the termination event. Since in the absence of rho the pause at t_{RI} is only transient, in contrast to other sites of transcription termination which have been studied, one major functional difference between various termination signals may be the overall efficiency with which the RNA polymerase can be slowed or stopped at those sites.

N RECOGNITION SITES (*nut*)

The N product of λ allows extension of transcription from both the P_L and P_R promoters beyond their respective termination signals (Kourilsky et al. 1971; Heinemann and Spiegelman 1971). The N product of phage λ will not function in the transcription of phage 21, nor will the N analog of phage 21 work with λ (Friedman et al. 1973). In contrast, the heteroimmune phage λimm^{434} and λ have the same functional N gene. This suggests that N may recognize a region in the genome between the boundaries of λimm^{434} and λimm^{21} (Fig. 1). Indeed, for leftward transcription from P_L, a site of N recognition (*nutL*) has been genetically defined to the left of λimm^{434}, between the startpoint of leftward transcription, S_L, and the gene N (Salstrom and Szybalski 1976, 1978). Mutations at this site are defective in recognition of the N-gene product and thereby prevent antitermination of leftward transcription (initiated from P_L) at various terminator regions within the left arm of the λ genome. These mutations, however, produce a normal N-gene product which acts to antiterminate transcription initiated at P_R.

For rightward transcription from P_R, N prevents termination at t_{R1} (D. Court et al., in prep.). This suggests a possible recognition signal for N upstream (5') from the t_{R1} site of action but to the right of the λimm^{434} boundary (Figs. 1 and 4). Comparison of the nucleic acid sequence of this region with the sequence determined by Dahlberg and Blattner (1975) for the 5'-terminal region of the P_L-initiated transcript indicates the occurrence in each region of almost identical sequences (16 of 17 consecutive nucleotides) appropriately positioned in the same orientation relative to the direction of transcription (Fig. 6). Both sequences display a hyphenated, twofold rotational symmetry that gives rise to a potential stem-and-loop structure in the RNA transcripts of these regions. In addition, these sequences contain a rather striking asymmetrical arrangement of purine and pyrimidine residues (i.e., nine contiguous purines in the RNA transcript, five of which would comprise the entire loop structure).

More recently, the sequence changes that occur in several independently isolated λ*nutL* mutations have been determined (M. Rosenberg et al., in prep.). These mutations were found to occur at two different sites within the 17-nucleotide sequence (Fig. 6). Note that the *nutL63* and *nutL44* mutations occur at the same position within the site and that neither base change disrupts the symmetry element (i.e., potential stem-and-loop feature) of the sequence. In fact, the *nutL63* mutation is a transversion (G-C→T-A) which increases the dyad symmetry feature of the site. The *nutL44* mutation, however, is a transition (G-C→A-T) which does not affect either the symmetry of the site or the arrangement of purine and pyrimidine residues within the site. Both mutations appear equally defective in N recognition. The data clearly suggest that these two

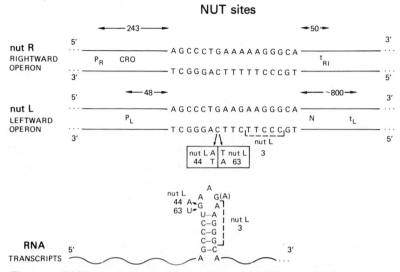

Figure 6 DNA sequence identities and potential RNA secondary structure of the regions in the P_L and P_R operons which encode the sites of N recognition (*nut*). *NutL* mutations are indicated. Although the sequence change(s) associated with the *nutL3* mutation is still unknown, RNA sequence analysis indicates that it occurs within the designated (⌐---¬) region of the pancreatic RNase digestion product GAAGAAGGGC. All other designations are identical to those used in Fig. 4. Adapted from M. Rosenberg et al. (in prep.).

sequences (one on the left and one on the right of the λ immunity region) are in some way involved in N recognition prior to N action at downstream terminators. It is not yet known whether recognition involves structure in the DNA or RNA.

TERMINATOR AND PROMOTER—λc17

The *c17* mutation of bacteriophage λ lies in the intercistronic region between the *cro* and *CII* genes (Pereira da Silva and Jacob 1968). This mutation is thought to be a small DNA insertion (Allet and Solem 1974) which creates a new promoter site for rightward transcription by RNA polymerase from within the *Y* region of λ. Although *CII* function (necessary for repressor establishment) is expressed in the mutant (Reichardt 1975), the phage cannot lysogenize its host, presumably due to constitutive expression of the DNA replication functions *O* and *P* (Packman and Sly 1968).

The nucleic acid sequence of the *c17* mutation has been determined and in vitro RNA transcription in the region surrounding the mutation has been examined (Figs. 4 and 5B) (Rosenberg et al. 1978). Structural analysis indicates that the mutation results from an exact DNA duplication of 9 consecutive base pairs occurring within and adjacent to the t_{RI} site (positions 311–319 of the wild-type sequence). This small duplication, which may well result from a DNA replication error rather than a DNA insertion mutation, extends an AT-rich segment of the DNA (eight of the nine residues are A-T) and creates a heptamer sequence (TATAATT) (Pribnow 1975) at the junction of the repeat (Fig. 5B). Transcription studies indicate that, in vitro, RNA polymerase will bind efficiently at this site and initiate transcription 6 base pairs to the right of the heptamer at residue position 329 (Shimatake and Rosenberg 1978). Thus, the $c17$-initiated transcript atypically contains a template-specified 5′-cytidine triphosphate (CTP). Although potential purine start points occur at residue positions 327 and 331 (4 and 8 base pairs, respectively, from the heptamer), little if any initiation occurs from these positions. This suggests that at the $c17$ promoter the steric constraints on promoter function outweigh the necessity for RNA polymerase to initiate transcription with a purine triphosphate. Under typical in vitro transcription conditions, the $c17$ promoter was found to be somewhat weaker (three- to fourfold) than the P_R promoter (M. Rosenberg, unpubl.). This was also suggested from in vivo studies (Mark 1973; Friedman and Ponce-Campos 1975). Perhaps the relative inefficiency of the $c17$ promoter is a direct result of the pyrimidine triphosphate initiation requirement. The $c17$ duplication and its promoter activity do not appear to disrupt the function of the rho-dependent t_{RI} terminator site. Transcription initiated normally from the P_R promoter of $λc17$ is still sensitive to rho termination at the appropriate t_{RI} site in vitro (M. Rosenberg, unpubl.). However, it is not known whether polymerase entry and initiation at the $c17$ promoter affect proper transcriptional regulation at the t_{RI} site in vivo.

Although the heptamer sequence created by the duplication probably accounts for formation of the tight-binding site for RNA polymerase, the 9-base-pair duplication does not encode all the information sufficient for specifying promoter function. DNA structure 35–40 base pairs upstream from RNA polymerase initiation sites has been implicated in proper polymerase recognition (Schaller et al. 1975; Dickson et al. 1975; Gilbert 1976). This suggests that part of the information required for polymerase recognition and entry at the $c17$ promoter must be derived from the DNA region surrounding the $c17$ mutation. RNA polymerase protection studies carried out on DNA restriction fragments containing the $c17$ promoter indicate that the t_{RI} terminator region, appropriately positioned 20–50 residues 5′ to the $c17$ initiation site, also serves as a recognition signal for those RNA polymerase molecules which initiate transcription at the $c17$ promoter (Shimatake and Rosenberg 1978). This implies that certain common features (both structural and functional) may occur between sites of transcription termination and RNA polymerase entry and initiation sites. The possible existence of overlapping promoter and terminator signals in bacteriophage φX174 has also been noted (Sanger et al. 1977).

INSERTION ELEMENT—IS2

The phage λr32 contains an IS2-type insertion element in the Y region (Brachet et al. 1970; Fiandt et al. 1972). This ~1200-base-pair DNA segment occurs as a normal component in the bacterial chromosome, as well as in extrachromosomal plasmids, and appears to be involved in the transposition of genetic information within the bacterial cell (Shapiro et al. 1977). When inserted into a gene, the IS2 acts as a mutation and may exert polar effects on the expression of distally located genes (Shapiro 1969). In λr32 the IS insertion interferes directly with the expression of CII function and also exerts a polar effect (in the absence of N function) on the expression of the adjacent genes, O and P.

The exact site of insertion of the IS2 element in λr32 has been identified and the DNA structure at each end of the insertion element determined (Figs. 4 and 5C) (Rosenberg et al. 1978). The sequence information obtained is consistent with the contention that the IS2 DNA segment inserts between two adjacent base pairs (i.e., within a single internucleotide linkage) without deleting any of the original DNA structure. However, a direct sequence repeat of 5 base pairs (GAAAT) is found at each end of the insertion (Fig. 5C). Since this sequence occurs only once in the phage DNA, the repeat must either come from the IS2 element itself or else result from a duplication of structure at the time of the insertion event. A second site of IS2 insertion has been defined near the start point of transcription of the gal operon (i.e., λgal490; R. Musso, unpubl.). The nucleotide sequence into which this IS2 element has inserted is different from that found in λr32, although some similarities can be noted (Musso and Rosenberg 1978). The nature and extent of any sequence repetition occurring at the ends the IS2 inserted into gal is still not known. Similar to IS2 insertion, sequence repeats 9 base pairs in length have been found at sites of IS1 insertion (Calos et al. 1978; Grindley 1978). Among the various sites of IS1 insertion that have been examined, the duplicated nucleotide sequence is always different. The data suggest similar mechanisms for IS1- and IS2-type insertions.

The IS2 insertion in phage λr32 does not occur within the structural coding region of the CII gene (Rosenberg et al. 1978); however, the phage is defective in CII function (Brachet et al. 1970). The insertion does occur within the presumptive ribosome-binding region of CII and thus presumably interferes with ribosome recognition and translation initiation of the CII gene (see legend to Fig. 4 for evidence establishing the position of the CII coding region). Due to the sequence repetition occurring at each end of the IS2 element, the insertion does not appreciably alter the nucleotide sequence for 19 base pairs immediately preceding the ATG start point of the *CII* protein (compare Figs. 4 and 5C). In fact, the insertion results only in an apparent deletion of two residues in that part of the sequence exhibiting complementarity to the 3' end of the 16S ribosomal RNA (implicated in ribosome recognition by Shine and Dalgarno [1974]). In addition, it is known that the transcript initiated at residue position 320 (Fig. 4) from the *c*17 promoter of phage λ*c*17 contains only 18 residues preceding the AUG start point of the *CII* gene (see above) and is translated into *CII* protein (Reichardt 1975). Thus it appears likely that the 2-base-pair alteration in the Shine and Dalgarno sequence is responsible for the *CII* defect in phage λ*r*32. It is of interest that the IS*2* insertion which occurs near the start point of the *gal* operon (described above) also interferes with expression of the *gal* epimerase (*E*) gene without affecting the structural coding region of *E*. Apparently the IS again has inserted into and affected proper recognition of a ribosome-binding site.

CONTROL OF REPRESSOR ESTABLISHMENT—c*Y* REGION

λ*cY* mutations, which lie within the *Y* region, interfere with repressor synthesis during the establishment of lysogeny (Kaiser 1957; M. Beher et al., in prep.). These closely linked, *cis*-acting mutations apparently define a site of regulation whose function is required for repressor expression. One suggestion is that the *cY* region is a promoter site (*pre*; Fig. 1) for leftward transcription into the *CI* gene (Reichardt and Kaiser 1971; Echols and Green 1971; Court et al. 1975). Alternatively, it has been suggested that the *pre* promoter for *CI* transcription is, in fact, the promoter for "*oop*" RNA transcription, P_o, which lies to the right of the *CII* gene (Honigman et al. 1976) (see Fig. 1). If this is the case, then the *cY* region would in some way regulate the elongation of this mRNA transcript initiated several hundred base pairs upstream (perhaps via an attenuator-type mechanism). The primary structure of this region alone does not allow us to discriminate between these two possibilities.

Genetically, a fine-structure map of the *Y* region produces two distinct but tightly linked clusters of *cY* mutations (M. Beher et al., in prep.). The sequence changes associated with seven independently obtained *cY* mutants have been determined (Fig. 7), two from the left cluster (cY_L) and five from the right (cY_R) (Rosenberg et al. 1978; M. Beher et al., in prep.). Each mutation results from a single base-pair alteration and confirms the relative genetic locations of these mutations. The nature of the *cY* base changes and their relative positions do not appear analogous to classical promoter-type mutations (for review, see Gilbert 1976). If the *cY* region does promote leftward transcription of repressor, then this promoter and its regulation must be different from those previously examined. Separation of the *cY* mutations into two groups is further

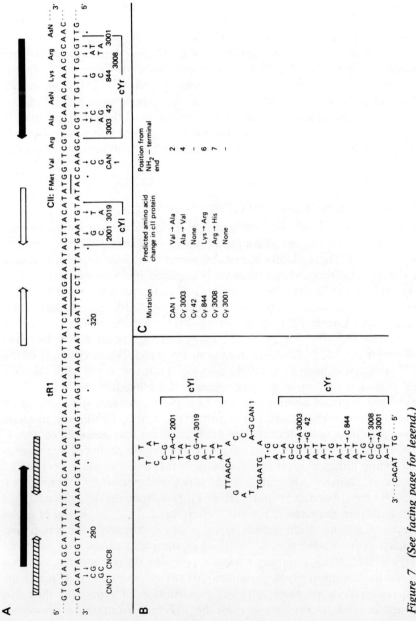

Figure 7 (See facing page for legend.)

suggested by the occurrence and location of the λ*can*1 mutation (Jones and Herskowitz 1978). Sequence analysis identifies this mutation as a single base change occurring between the cY_L and cY_R mutations (Fig. 7A,B) (M. Beher et al., in prep.). Although this mutation occurs within the cY region, the mutant appears to have a functional cY regulatory system which remains normally dependent upon *CII* function (see legend to Fig. 7 for discussion of the Can1 phenotype).

Structurally, the cY mutants also appear to define two adjacent but separate sites (Fig. 7). The cY_L mutations are located to the left of the indicated *CII* structural gene, within a short, imperfect, inverted repeat sequence (positions 331–338 are rotationally symmetrical with positions 317–324; Fig. 7) which occurs just to the right of t_{R1}. These mutations occur within the presumptive ribosome-binding region of the *CII* protein, three and six residues, respectively, preceding the *CII* AUG initiation codon. However, these mutations appear normal in *CII* function.

The cY_R mutations are located within the coding region of the indicated *CII* protein. Two of these mutations (*cY42* and *cY3001*) result in third (wobble)-position codon changes which would not alter the amino acid sequence of the *CII* protein. Three of the mutations, however, would give rise to changes in the amino acid sequence of *CII* (Fig. 7A,C). Nevertheless, all of the cY_R mutations are phenotypically equivalent, and all appear normal in *CII* function. Apparently the three missense mutations do not appreciably affect *CII* protein function. Note that in

Figure 7 (*A*) DNA sequence of the λ cY region and several cY mutations. Regions of dyad symmetry pertinent to the discussion in the text are indicated by horizontal arrows. The *can*1 mutation is also shown. This λ mutant has the ability to efficiently establish lysogeny in the absence of the *CIII*-gene product (Jones and Herskowitz 1978). It was suggested that the *can*1 mutation might increase either the level or the activity of *CII* protein. Sequence analysis (M. Beher et al., in prep.) indicates that the mutation would result in a change in the second position of the second codon of the *CII* cistron (i.e., Val→Ala change in the second amino acid of the *CII* protein). The possibility exists that this alteration directly affects the activity of the protein. However, Weissman et al. (1978) have recently found that a mutation in the first base of the second codon of the coat protein cistron of RNA phage Qβ significantly affects ribosome binding and, in turn, translation efficiency of this protein. Analogously, the *can*1 mutation may be affecting translation efficiency of *CII* protein, rather than the activity of the protein. All other designations are identical to those shown in Fig. 4. (*B*) Potential secondary structure of the *l*-strand DNA of λ which spans the t_{R1}-cY region and serves as template for rightward RNA transcription. Similar structures can be drawn for the complementary *r*-strand DNA, as well as for the RNA transcript(s) which traverse this region. The cY and *can*1 mutations are indicated. (*C*) Amino acid changes expected in the *CII* protein resulting from the cY and *can*1 mutations. (Adapted from M. Beher et al., in prep.).

each case the amino acid resulting from the mutation has similar properties (e.g., charge, hydrophobicity) to the corresponding amino acid it replaces from the wild-type sequence (Fig. 7C).

The most striking feature of the region defined by the cY_R mutations is again one of structural symmetry. The region encompasses a 14-base-pair nucleotide sequence (residues 346–359; Fig. 7) which is repeated in 12 of 14 consecutive positions in the opposite orientation within the t_{R1} site (residues 286–299). The length and relative positions of these inverted repeat sequences (one comprising a site, cY, controlling transcriptional expression leftward into the immunity region and the other contained in a site, t_{R1}, regulating early rightward transcription) suggest the possibility of some common control mechanism which functionally links the two opposing regulatory sites. For example, the potential exists for a direct interaction of the sites resulting from the formation of base-paired secondary structure which might occur in either strand of the DNA template or in the RNA transcripts which span this region in both directions (an example of one such potential structure is shown in Fig. 7B). Note that the cY mutations would result in the destabilization of such a structure. Alternatively, the similarity in sequence of the two sites may denote two separate but related recognition sites of a common control protein. In fact, genetic experiments suggest that the region defined by the cY_R mutations is the site of action of the CII protein (M. Beher et al., in prep.). Thus, CII may act at a site which concomitantly encodes its own structural information and, in doing so, may mediate (i.e., either promote or interfere with) structural interactions between the t_{R1} and cY regions.

Earlier, another inverted repeat sequence was described which occurs within the t_{R1} termination site and which was thought to be important in the control of terminator function. The sequences involved in the formation of this "termination structure" overlap with that implicated in the cY interaction. Thus the additional possibility exists that the t_{R1}-cY region may exhibit alternative structural conformations, each exclusive of the other. Furthermore, it may be the equilibrium between the multiple conformations and the factors (both viral and host) affecting this equilibrium which couples the regulation of bidirectional transcription through this region. A somewhat analogous form of transcriptional control based on alternative potential secondary structures has been postulated for attenuator control of the tryptophan operon (Lee and Yanofsky 1977).

CONCLUSION

A set of regulatory elements which control transcriptional and translational expression within the Y region of phage λ have been defined. These elements apparently function in the regulation of both the lytic and lysogenic modes of viral development. The structure and relative positioning of these sites suggest that regulation of this region may be a function of the molecular overlaps and potential structural interactions which occur between the various control sequences. We have already discussed the possibility of direct and/or indirect interactions occurring between the t_{RI} and cY control regions, as well as the occurrence of overlapping promoter and terminator sites in the phage λc17. In addition, the proximity of the recognition site for N function ($nutR$) and the t_{RI} termination site allows for the possibility of some direct interaction between N protein and RNA polymerase while each is situated at its respective site. Yet another example involves the overlap between the cY region and the presumptive site for ribosome recognition and initiation of translation of CII protein. It has been suggested that CII protein, while acting within the cY region, concomitantly regulates its own expression (Court et al. 1975; M. Beher et al., in prep.). Although overlapping functions may simply reflect an evolutionary mechanism for conservation of genetic coding potential, clearly these overlaps may also have important regulatory significance. What certainly becomes evident is the number and complexity of potential molecular interactions that may occur within the λ Y region. These interactions and their temporal control ultimately lead to the delicate balance achieved by λ in expressing both lytic and lysogenic patterns of development in a single vital infection.

ACKNOWLEDGMENTS

We thank Alana Muto for typing and editing the manuscript and Ray Steinberg for help with the illustrations.

REFERENCES

Adhya, S. and M. Gottesman. 1978. Control of transcription termination. *Annu. Rev. Biochem.* **47:** (in press).

Allet, B. and B. Solem. 1974. Separation and analysis of promoter sites in bacteriophage *lambda* DNA by specific endonucleases. *J. Mol. Biol.* **85:** 475.

Barrell, B. G. 1971. Fractionation and sequence analysis of radioactive nucleotides. In *Procedures in Nucleic Acids Research* (ed. G. Cantoni and D. Davies), vol. 2, p. 751. Harper and Row, New York.

Bertrand, K., L. Korn, F. Lee, and C. Yanofsky. 1978. The attenuator of the tryptophan operon of *Escherichia coli*. *J. Mol. Biol.* (in press).

Bertrand, K., L. Korn, F. Lee, T. Platt, C. L. Squires, C. Squires, and C. Yanofsky. 1975. New features of the regulation of the tryptophan operon. *Science* **189:** 22.

Brachet, P., H. Eisen, and A. Rambach. 1970. Mutations of coliphage λ affecting the expression of replicative functions *O* and *P*. *Mol. Gen. Genet.* **108:** 266.

Brownlee, G. G. and F. Sanger. 1969. Chromatography of ^{32}P-labelled oligonucleotides on thin layers of DEAE-cellulose. *Eur. J. Biochem.* **11:** 395.

Calos, M., L. Johnsrud, and J. Miller. 1978. DNA sequence at the integration sites of the insertion element IS*1*. *Cell* **13**:411.

Court, D., L. Green, and H. Echols. 1975. Positive and negative regulation by the *C*II and *C*III gene products of bacteriophage λ. *Virology* **63**:484.

Dahlberg, J. E. and F. R. Blattner. 1973. Sequence of a self-terminating RNA made near the origin of DNA replication of phage *lambda*. *Fed. Proc.* **32**:664.

————. 1975. Sequence of the promoter-operator proximal region of the major leftward RNA of bacteriophage *lambda*. *Nucleic Acids Res.* **2**:1441.

Das, A., D. Court, and S. Adhya. 1976. Isolation and characterization of conditional lethal mutants of *Escherichia coli* defective in transcription termination factor *rho*. *Proc. Natl. Acad. Sci.* **73**:1959.

de Crombrugghe, B., S. Adhya, M. Gottesman, and I. Pastan. 1973. Effect of *rho* on transcription of bacterial operons. *Nat. New Biol.* **241**:260.

Dickson, R., J. Abelson, W. Barnes, and W. Reznikoff. 1975. Genetic regulation: The *lac* control region. *Science* **187**:27.

Dove, W. F., E. Hargrove, M. Ohashi, F. Haugli, and A. Guha. 1969. Replicator activation in *lambda*. *Jpn. J. Genet.* (Suppl. 1) **44**:11.

Echols, H. and L. Green. 1971. Establishment and maintenance of repression by bacteriophage *lambda*: The role of the *C*I, *C*II, and *C*III proteins. *Proc. Natl. Acad. Sci.* **68**:2190.

Fiandt, M., W. Szybalski, and M. H. Malamy. 1972. Polar mutations in *lac*, *gal* and phage λ consist of a few IS-DNA sequences inserted with either orientation. *Mol. Gen. Genet.* **119**:223.

Friedman, D. I. and R. Ponce-Campos. 1975. Differential effect of phage regulator functions on transcription from various promoters: Evidence that the P22 gene 24 and the λ gene *N* products distinguish three classes of promoters. *J. Mol. Biol.* **98**:537.

Friedman, D. I., G. S. Wilgus, and R. J. Mural. 1973. Gene *N* regulator function of phage λ*imm*21: Evidence that a site of *N* action differs from a site of *N* recognition. *J. Mol. Biol.* **81**:505.

Gilbert, W. 1976. Starting and stopping sequences for the RNA polymerase. In *RNA Polymerase* (ed. R. Losick and M. Chamberlin), p. 193. Cold Spring Harbor Laboratory, Cold Spring Harbor, New York.

Gralla, J. and D. M. Crothers. 1973. Free energy of imperfect nucleic acid helices. II. Small hairpin loops. *J. Mol. Biol.* **73**:497.

Grindley, N. 1978. IS*1* insertion generates duplication of a nine base pair sequence at its target site. *Cell* **13**:419.

Heinemann, S. F. and W. G. Spiegelman. 1971. Role of the gene *N* product in phage *lambda*. *Cold Spring Harbor Symp. Quant. Biol.* **35**:315.

Honigman, A., S. L. Hu, R. Chase, and W. Szybalski. 1976. 4S *oop* RNA is a leader sequence for the immunity-establishment transcription in coliphage λ. *Nature* **262**:112.

Howard, B., B. de Crombrugghe, and M. Rosenberg. 1977. Transcription *in vitro* of bacteriophage *lambda* 4S RNA: Studies on termination and *rho* protein. *Nucleic Acids Res.* **4**:827.

Hsiang, M., Y. Takeda, R. Cole, and H. Echols. 1977. Amino acid sequence of Cro regulatory protein of bacteriophage *lambda*. *Nature* **270**:275.

Jones, M. O. and I. Herskowitz. 1978. Mutants of bacteriophage lambda which do not require the *c*III gene for efficient lysogenization. *Virology* (in press).

Kaiser, A. D. 1957. Mutations in a temperate bacteriophage affecting its ability to lysogenize *Escherichia coli*. *Virology* **3**:42.

Katzir, N., A. Oppenheim, M. Belfort, and A. Oppenheim. 1976. Activation of *lambda* int gene by the *c*II and *c*III gene products. *Virology* **74**:324.

Korn, L. and C. Yanofsky. 1976. Polarity suppressors defective in transcription termination at the attenuator of the tryptophan operon of *Escherichia coli* have altered *rho* factor. *J. Mol. Biol.* **106**:231.

Kourilsky, P., M. F. Bourguignon, and F. Gros. 1971. Kinetics of viral transcription after induction of prophage. In *The bacteriophage lambda* (ed. A. D. Hershey), p. 647. Cold Spring Harbor Laboratory, Cold Spring Harbor, New York.

Küpper, H., T. Sekiya, M. Rosenberg, J. Egan, and A. Landy. 1978. A ρ-dependent termination site in the gene coding for tyrosine tRNA su3 of *E. coli*. *Nature* **272**:423.

Lebowitz, P., S. Weissman, and C. M. Radding. 1971. Nucleotide sequence of a ribonucleic acid transcribed in vitro from λ phage deoxyribonucleic acid. *J. Biol. Chem.* **246**:5120.

Lee, F. and C. Yanofsky. 1977. Transcription termination at the *trp* operon attenuators of *Escherichia coli* and *Salmonella typhimurium*: RNA secondary structure and regulation of termination. *Proc. Natl. Acad. Sci.* **74**:4365.

Lozeron, H. A., J. E. Dahlberg, and W. Szybalski. 1976. Processing of the major leftward mRNA of coliphage *lambda*. *Virology* **71**:262.

Luzzati, D. 1970. Regulation of λ exonuclease synthesis: Role of the *N* gene product and λ repressor. *J. Mol. Biol.* **49**:515.

Mark, K. 1973. Effect of the *N*-bypass mutations *nin* and *byp* on the rightward transcription in coliphage *lambda*. *Mol. Gen. Genet.* **124**:291.

McDermit, M., M. Pierce, D. Staley, M. Shimaji, R. Shaw, and D. L. Wulff. 1976. Mutations masking the *lambda* Cin-1 mutation. *Genetics* **82**:417.

Musso, R. and M. Rosenberg. 1977. Nucleotide sequences at two sites for IS*2* DNA insertion. In *DNA insertion elements, plasmids, and episomes* (ed. A. I. Bukhari et al.), p. 597. Cold Spring Harbor Laboratory, Cold Spring Harbor, New York.

Packman, S. and W. S. Sly. 1968. Constitutive λ DNA replication by λC17, a regulatory mutant related to virulence. *Virology* **34**:778.

Pereira da Silva, L. and F. Jacob. 1968. Étude génétique d'une mutation modifiant la sensibilité a l'immunité chez le bactériophage *lambda*. *Ann. Inst. Pasteur* **115**:145.

Pieczenik, G., B. G. Barrell, and M. Gefter. 1972. Bacteriophage φ80-induced low molecular weight RNA. *Arch. Biochem. Biophys.* **152**:152.

Pribnow, D. 1975. Nucleotide sequence of an RNA polymerase binding site at an early T7 promoter. *Proc. Natl. Acad. Sci.* **72**:784.

Reichardt, L. F. 1975. Control of bacteriophage *lambda* repressor synthesis after phage infection: The role of the *N*, *c*II, *c*III and *cro* products. *J. Mol. Biol.* **93**:267.

Reichardt, L. F. and A. D. Kaiser. 1971. Control of λ repressor synthesis. *Proc. Natl. Acad. Sci.* **68**:2185.

Reyes, O., M. Gottesman, and S. Adhya. 1976. Suppression of polarity of insertion mutations in the *gal* operon and *N* mutations in bacteriophage *lambda*. *J. Bacteriol.* **126**:1108.

Richardson, J. P., C. Grimley, and C. Lowery. 1975. Transcription termination factor *rho* activity is altered in *Escherichia coli* with *suA* gene mutations. *Proc. Natl. Acad. Sci.* **72**:1725.

Roberts, J. W. 1969. Termination factor for RNA synthesis. *Nature* **224**:1168.

———. 1971. The ρ factor: Termination and anti-termination in *lambda*. *Cold Spring Harbor Symp. Quant. Biol.* **35**:121.

Roberts, T., H. Shimatake, C. Brady, and M. Rosenberg. 1977. Sequence of *cro* gene of bacteriophage *lambda*. *Nature* **270**:274.

Rosenberg, M. 1974. Isolation and sequence determination of the 3'-terminal regions of istopically labelled RNA molecules. *Nucleic Acids Res.* **1**:653.

Rosenberg, M., B. de Crombrugghe, and S. Weissman. 1975. Termination of transcription in bacteriophage λ. *J. Biol. Chem.* **250**:4755.

Rosenberg, M., D. Court, H. Shimatake, C. Brady, and D. L. Wulff. 1978. The relation between function and DNA sequence in an intercistronic regulatory region in phage λ. *Nature* **272**:414.

Salstrom, J. S. and W. Szybalski. 1976. Phage *lambda nutL* mutants unable to utilize *N* product for leftward transcription. *Fed. Proc.* **35**:1538.

———. 1978. Coliphage λ*nutL⁻*: A unique class of mutants defective in the site of *N* utilization for antitermination of leftward transcription. *J. Mol. Biol.* (in press).

Sanger, F., G. G. Brownlee, and B. G. Barrell. 1965. A two-dimensional fractionation procedure for radioactive nucleotides. *J. Mol. Biol.* **13**:373.

Sanger, F., G. M. Air, B. G. Barrell, N. L. Brown, A. R. Coulson, J. C. Fiddes, C. A. Hutchison III, P. M. Slocombe, and M. Smith. 1977. Nucleotide sequence of bacteriophage φX174 DNA. *Nature* **265**:687.

Schaller, H., C. Gray, and K. Herrmann. 1975. Nucleotide sequence of an RNA polymerase binding site from the DNA of bacteriophage fd. *Proc. Natl. Acad. Sci.* **72**:737.

Shapiro, J. A. 1969. Mutations caused by the insertion of genetic material into the galactose operon of *Escherichia coli*. *J. Mol. Biol.* **40**:93.

Shapiro, J. A., S. Adhya, and A. Bukhari. 1977. Introduction: New pathways in the evolution of chromosome structure, pp. 3–11. In *DNA insertion elements, plasmids, and episomes* (ed. A. I. Bukhari et al.), p. 3. Cold Spring Harbor Laboratory, Cold Spring Harbor, New York.

Shimatake, H. and M. Rosenberg. 1978. The *c17* mutation of bacteriophage *lambda*—An unusual promoter. *Fed. Proc.* **37**:1499.

Shine, J. and L. Dalgarno. 1974. The 3'-terminal sequence of *Escherichia coli* 16S ribosomal RNA: Complementarity to nonsense triplets and ribosome binding sites. *Proc. Natl. Acad. Sci.* **71**:1342.

Sogin, M., N. Pace, M. Rosenberg, and S. Weissman. 1976. Nucleotide sequence of a 5S ribosomal RNA precursor from *Bacillus subtilis*. *J. Biol. Chem.* **251**:3480.

Spiegelman, W. G., L. F. Reichardt, M. Yaniv, S. F. Heinemann, A. D. Kaiser, and H. Eisen. 1972. Bidirectional transcription and the regulation of phage λ repressor synthesis. *Proc. Natl. Acad. Sci.* **69**:3156.

Steege, D. A. 1977. A ribosome binding site from the P_R RNA of bacteriophage *lambda*. *J. Mol. Biol.* **114**:559.

Steitz, J. A. and K. Jakes. 1975. How ribosomes select initiator regions in mRNA:

Base pair formation between the 3' terminus of 16S rRNA and the mRNA during initiation of protein synthesis in *Escherichia coli. Proc. Natl. Acad. Sci.* **72:** 4734.

Taylor, K., Z. Hradecna, and W. Szybalski. 1967. A symmetric distribution of the transcribing regions on the complementary strands of coliphage λ DNA. *Proc. Natl. Acad. Sci.* **57:** 1618.

Tinoco, I., Jr., P. N. Borer, B. Dengler, M. D. Levine, O. C. Uhlenbeck, D. M. Crothers, and J. Gralla. 1973. Improved estimation of secondary structure in ribonucleic acids. *Nat. New Biol.* **246:** 40.

Weisberg, R. A., S. Gottesman, and M. E. Gottesman. 1977. Bacteriophage λ: The lysogenic pathway. *Comprehensive Virology* **8:** 197.

Weissman, C., T. Taniguchi, E. Domingo, D. Sabo, R. A. Flavell. 1978. Site-directed mutagenesis as a tool in genetics. In *Proceedings of Ninth Miami Winter Symposium.* Academic Press (in press).

Wulff, D. L. 1976. Lambda *cin*-1, a new mutation which enhances lysogenization by bacteriophage lambda, and the genetic structure of the lambda *cY* region. *Genetics* **82:** 401.

Regulation in the *hut* System

Boris Magasanik
Department of Biology
Massachusetts Institute of Technology
Cambridge, Massachusetts 02139

INTRODUCTION

Although the ability to degrade L-histidine is widely distributed among bacteria, nature has not seen fit to bestow this ability on *Escherichia coli*. However, enteric organisms related to *E. coli*, such as *Klebsiella aerogenes* (Magasanik and Bowser 1955) and some strains of *Salmonella typhimurium* (Meiss et al. 1969), are capable of degrading histidine to an equimolar mixture of ammonia, L-glutamate, and formamide. A comparison of the *hut* (histidine utilization) system with *lac* is therefore reasonable, particularly since it has been possible to introduce the *hut* genes of *K. aerogenes* (Tyler and Goldberg 1976) and of *S. typhimurium* (Smith 1971) into *E. coli*, where they function essentially as they do in the strains from which they were derived (Parada and Magasanik 1975; Goldberg et al. 1976).

The comparison between *hut* and *lac* reveals striking similarities. Both systems are negatively controlled by a specific repressor. In both systems the physiological inducer, L-histidine or β-D-lactose, is converted by an enzyme of the respective system, histidase or β-galactosidase, to the actual inducer, urocanate or allolactose. Both systems contain an inducer-destroying enzyme, urocanase or β-galactosidase. Both systems consist of two linked units of transcription: in each case one of the units contains the structural gene for the repressor. At least one unit of transcription of either system is subject to regulation by catabolite repression.

The differences between *hut* and *lac* are equally striking. In *hut*, the unit of transcription containing the structural gene for the repressor contains, in addition, the structural genes for two enzymes of the system and is subject to regulation by the repressor; thus, the synthesis of the repressor responds to autogenous regulation, the first unambiguous example of this process. In *lac*, this unit of transcription contains only the structural gene for the repressor and is not subject to regulation. Starvation for ammonia overcomes, in *K. aerogenes* and in *E. coli*, the effects of catabolite repression on *hut*, but not on *lac*, because the expression of the *hut* operons is subject to positive control by a protein which also plays an important role in cellular metabolism, the enzyme glutamine synthetase.

373

The similarities and differences in the regulation of *hut* and *lac* reflect the physiological roles of the substrates and enzymes of the two systems. Lactose is not produced by enteric organisms and serves only as a source of carbon and energy. Histidine, on the other hand, is produced by these cells and plays an essential role in protein synthesis; it also serves, thanks to the *hut* system, as a source of carbon and energy as well as a source of nitrogen. The regulatory apparatus of each system is designed to deal with these properties of lactose and of histidine.

ENZYMES

K. aerogenes has the ability to form the enzymes histidase (E. C. 4.3.1.3), urocanase (E. C. 4.2.1.49), imidazolonepropionase (IPase) (E. C. 3.5.3.8), and formiminoglutamase (FGase) (E. C. 3.5.3.8). The cellular levels of these enzymes are increased 50–100-fold by the addition of histidine to the growth medium containing ammonia and a poor carbon source, such as succinate or citrate, but the addition of glucose to such a histidine-containing medium results in an approximately tenfold reduction of the levels of these enzymes (Revel and Magasanik 1958; Magasanik et al. 1965). Omission of ammonia from the glucose- and histidine-containing medium results in cells with high levels of these enzymes (Neidhardt and Magasanik 1957). Thus, these enzymes are inducible and require for their expression either energy starvation (no glucose) or nitrogen starvation (no ammonia).

The four enzymes acting in series catalyze the conversion of histidine to ammonia, L-glutamate, and formamide (Fig. 1). Mutants lacking any one of the four enzymes lose the ability to use histidine as a source of carbon

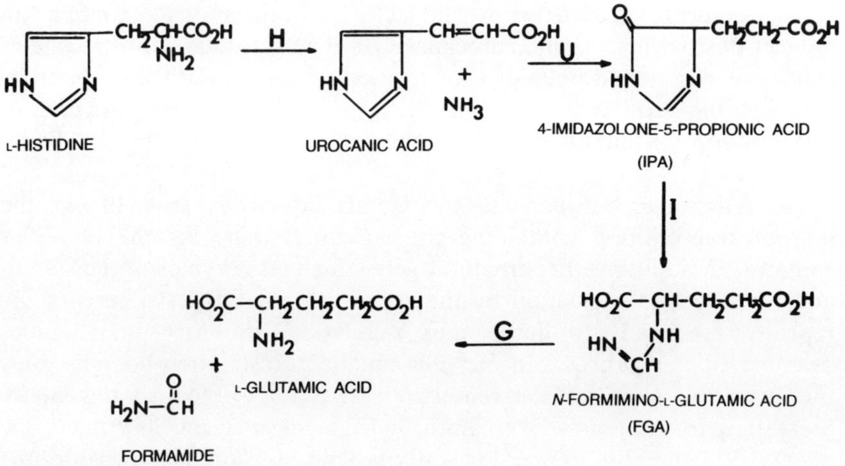

Figure 1   The pathway of histidine degradation.

(Schlesinger et al. 1965). Since no adenosine triphosphate (ATP) is generated in the reactions catalyzed by these enzymes, it is apparent that the building blocks and the ATP required for growth are generated by the further aerobic degradation of glutamate. The degradation does not require glutamate dehydrogenase (E. C. 1.4.1.4), but rather the successive action of aspartate aminotransferase (E. C. 2.5.1.1) and of aspartase (E. C. 4.3.1.1); however, the formation of these enzymes is not specifically induced by histidine (Magasanik et al. 1965).

The ammonia formed in the first step of histidine degradation and the glutamate formed in the last step are utilized by the cell for the formation of nitrogen-containing constituents. This is apparent from the observation that cells growing with glucose as the major source of carbon and histidine as the sole source of nitrogen excrete neither ammonia nor glutamate into the growth medium (Neidhardt and Magasanik 1957). On the other hand, the formamide is not used, but accumulates in an amount equivalent to degraded histidine in the medium (Magasanik and Bowser 1955). It can be shown that 1 mole of histidine as a source of nitrogen yields the same cell mass as 2 moles of NH_3 (Friedrich and Magasanik 1978).

The same four enzymes are also responsible for the utilization of histidine by *S. typhimurium*. However, as discussed in later sections, neither of the two strains of *S. typhimurium* studied is fully competent to utilize histidine: in strain LT-2 the levels of the *hut* enzymes are so low that histidine fails to serve as either a source of energy or a source of carbon; in strain 15-59 the levels of the *hut* enzymes are high enough to permit histidine to be a source of nitrogen, but not of carbon. For either strain it is possible to obtain in two separate steps mutants that resemble *K. aerogenes* in the levels of the *hut* enzymes and in the ability to use histidine as a source of carbon and nitrogen (Meiss et al. 1969; Brill and Magasanik 1969; Smith et al. 1971).

The properties of the *hut* enzymes of *K. aerogenes* and of *S. typhimurium* have not been studied in great detail. This histidase of *S. typhimurium* has been purified to homogeneity; it appears to be a tetramer composed of four identical subunits of molecular weight 65,000 (Hagen et al. 1974). It resembles in its properties the more thoroughly studied histidase of *Bacillus subtilis* and *Pseudomonas* (Magasanik et al. 1971; Rechler and Tabor 1971).

The urocanase of *K. aerogenes* has been partially purified (Revel and Magasanik 1958); in this case too, the corresponding enzymes of *B. subtilis* and *Pseudomonas* have been more thoroughly characterized (Magasanik et al. 1971; Phillips and George 1971).

The properties of the crude IPase of *S. typhimurium* have been described (Smith et al. 1971). This enzyme of *Pseudomonas fluorescens* has been partly purified (Rao and Greenberg 1961).

The FGase of *K. aerogenes* has been partly purified (Lund and Magasanik 1965). It resembles in its properties the more highly purified enzyme from *B. subtilis* (Magasanik et al. 1971).

In addition to the enzymes required for the degradation of histidine, *K. aerogenes* can be induced by histidine to produce a permease for urocanate which is also capable of transporting imidazolepropionate (Schlesinger and Magasanik 1965). It is this permease that enables *K. aerogenes* to use urocanate as a source of carbon or nitrogen. *S. typhimurium* lacks this inducible permease and is consequently unable to utilize urocanate (Meiss et al. 1969). It is possible to isolate mutants of *S. typhimurium* capable of using urocanate as source of nitrogen; however, these mutants do not appear to possess an inducible specific urocanate permease (Brill and Magasanik 1969). No histidine-specific permease is induced by histidine.

OPERONS

Most of the information concerning the genetic organization of the *hut* system comes from an intensive study of *S. typhimurium* 15-59. However, there is sufficient information to conclude that the *hut* systems of *S. typhimurium* LT-2 and of *K. aerogenes* have essentially the same structure.

The mutations affecting the utilization of histidine occur in a cluster of genes shown by transduction with phage P376 (a close relative of P22) to be located on the chromosome between *gal* and *bio* (Brill and Magasanik 1969). The *hut* genes could be integrated into the chromosome of *E. coli* K12 by mating (Smith 1971) and into an F′ *gal* episome derived from *E. coli* by transduction (Smith and Magasanik 1971a). The fact that the attachment site for phage λ is located between *gal* and *bio* made it possible to isolate λ phages carrying the *hut* genes (Smith 1971). The availability of F′*hut* and λp*hut* was essential for the genetic analysis of the *hut* system.

The order of the individual *hut* genes, shown in Figure 2, was determined by multiple factor crosses and confirmed by deletion analysis.

The structural genes for the four enzymes responsible for histidine degradation are *hutH* (histidase), *hutU* (urocanase), *hutI* (IPase), and *hutG* (FGase). Mutations in any one of these genes lead to the loss of the ability to use histidine as a source of nitrogen and to a deficiency in the corresponding enzyme. The growth of mutants lacking IPase is inhibited by histidine due to the toxicity of imidazolonepropionate (Hagen et al. 1975).

Mutations in *hutC* have a pleiotropic effect: the expression of all four

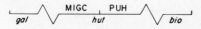

Figure 2 Map of the *hut* region of *S. typhimurium* and of *K. aerogenes*.

enzymes no longer requires induction (Brill and Magasanik 1969). The constitutive phenotype of some *hutC* mutations can be suppressed by the amber suppressor and is recessive to the inducible phenotype determined by the normal *hutC* gene (Smith and Magasanik 1971a,b). Furthermore, HutC mutants lack a protein, present in the normal strain, which is able to interact with *hut*-specific DNA and with the inducer of the *hut* enzymes (Hagen and Magasanik 1973). These observations clearly identify the *hutC* product as the *hut* repressor.

Other mutations with pleiotropic effects occur in the *hutP* site. These mutations can give rise to three different phenotypes and affect only *hutU* and *hutH*, located *cis* to the mutated gene (Brill and Magasanik 1969; Smith and Magasanik 1971a). One phenotype, HutP, is unable to utilize histidine because of an almost complete loss of histidase and urocanase. Another phenotype, HutR, acquires the ability to produce histidase and urocanase in the presence of glucose and in all media at levels higher than that of the parent strain. The strong catabolite repression of histidase in the normal organism prevents it from utilizing histidine as a source of carbon and energy. HutR mutants are selected for their ability to grow on glucose-histidine. Histidase and urocanase are inducible in HutR mutants; but the same selection also results in the isolation of strains with mutations in *hutP* whose histidase and urocanase are partially constitutive, as well as insensitive to catabolite repression (HutQ). It is of particular interest that, among revertants of HutP mutants selected for their ability to grow on succinate-histidine, one finds a considerable number of organisms with the HutR phenotype and some organisms with the HutQ phenotype. Together these observations indicate that *hutP* is the site of the promoter for the right-hand operon consisting of *hutU* and *hutH*, and also the target of catabolite repression. It thus corresponds to the promoter site of the *lac* operon (Silverstone et al. 1969, 1970). However, the mutation resulting in the HutQ phenotype, which combines insensitivity to catabolite repression and constitutivity, has no parallel in *lac*. So far, mutants which are operator-constitutive but catabolite-sensitive, corresponding to *lac* operator mutants, have not been isolated. The inability of *S. typhimurium* LT-2 to utilize histidine as a source of nitrogen is due to a defect in *hutP*; rare mutants of this organism, which have acquired the ability to grow on succinate-histidine, carry a mutation at a site corresponding to the *hutP* site in *S. typhimurium* 15-59 and have the HutR phenotype (Meiss et al. 1969).

Neither the wild-type strain of *S. typhimurium* nor HutR mutants can use histidine as the sole source of carbon and energy. It has not been possible to isolate from the wild-type strain mutants capable of growing on histidine; however, such mutants can be isolated from HutR mutants. The mutation responsible for the ability to use histidine as carbon source is at *hutM* and results in increased expression of *hutI*, *hutG*, and *hutC*, located *cis* to the mutated gene (Smith et al. 1971; Smith and Magasanik 1971a). Apparently, in the wild-type strain, the levels of IPase and FGase are too low to allow the conversion of histidine to glutamate at a rate sufficient to supply carbon and energy for growth. The increased production of the repressor, the product of the *hutC* gene, could be demonstrated by direct measurement (Hagen and Magasanik 1973), as well as by the observations that strains with *hutM* mutations produced less histidase and urocanase than strains with normal *hutM* and that this deficiency could be corrected by further mutations in either *hutC* or *hutP* resulting in constitutive expression of the right-hand operon (Smith and Magasanik 1971b). These observations identify *hutM* as the site of the promoter for the left-hand operon and *hutC* as a member of the operon. As expected, a deletion removing *hutM* as well as a portion of *hutI*, but leaving at least a portion of *hutG* and all of *hutC*, results in constitutive expression of the right-hand operon (Smith and Magasanik 1971b). In the next section, we shall consider the physiological consequences of the autogenous regulation of the synthesis of the *hut* repressor.

The different pleiotropic mutations affect primarily the transcription of the respective operons, as demonstrated by the measurement of *hut*-specific RNA produced by the wild-type strain and mutants grown in a variety of media (Cooper and Tyler 1977). In addition, the DNA strand used as template for the synthesis of *hut*-specific RNA could be identified; the direction of transcription of the *hut* genes established by these observations is an agreement with the functions of *hutM* and *hutP* as promoters of the two operons (Cooper and Tyler 1977).

The order of the structural *hut* genes in *K. aerogenes* is identical with that observed in *S. typhimurium* (Goldberg and Magasanik 1975). However, this organism produces all enzymes at levels as high as or higher than *S. typhimurium* carrying "promoter-up" mutations in *hutM* and *hutP* and therefore grows readily on histidine as the sole source of carbon and energy (Magasanik et al. 1965). Furthermore, as discussed later, *K. aerogenes* grows readily on glucose-histidine (Neidhardt and Magasanik 1957). It has therefore not been possible to isolate mutations in the putative promoter sites. Nevertheless, the fact that histidase and urocanase show a different response to regulation than do IPase and FGase is strong evidence for the view that in this organism, too, the genes for these groups of enzymes are in separate operons.

It is perhaps of interest to note that in an organism unrelated to these enteric bacteria, *B. subtilis*, the *hut* genes appear to be organized as a single operon (Kimhi and Magasanik 1970; Kaminskas and Magasanik 1970).

NEGATIVE CONTROL

The *hut* system, like *lac*, is subject to negative control exerted by the repressor, the product of the *hutC* gene. The repressor exerts its effect by binding to the operator regions of two operons and can be released from them by the inducer, urocanate (Hagen and Magasanik 1973, 1976). A nonsense mutation in *hutC* results in the constitutive synthesis of the enzymes of both operons (HutC⁻) (Smith and Magasanik 1971b). A missense mutation giving rise to a repressor unable to be released from the operators by the inducer renders the enzymes of both operons uninducible (HutCˢ) (Hagen et al. 1975). In the appropriate merodiploids, HutC⁺ is dominant to HutC⁻ and HutCˢ is dominant to both HutC⁻ and HutCˢ (Smith and Magasanik 1971a; Hagen et al. 1975).

We can see that in these respects the *hutC* gene and the *lacI* gene show close correspondence. However, in contrast to the *lac* repressor, the *hut* repressor regulates two operons and its structural gene is a member of one of them.

In *S. typhimurium*, the *hut* repressor has greater affinity for the right-hand operator than for the left-hand operator (Hagen and Magasanik 1976). As a result, relative to the fully induced levels, the basal levels of the components of the left-hand operon are considerably higher than those of the components of the right-hand operon. In this connection it is interesting that of two HutCˢ repressors, neither of which had affinity for the inducer, one had *increased* affinity for both operators (*hutC183*) and the other *decreased* affinity for both operators (*hutC161*) (Hagen et al. 1975). In the former case, the left-hand operon was more severely repressed; this resulted because of autogenous regulation in a lowered repressor level, which was nevertheless sufficient for almost complete repression of the right-hand operon. In the latter case, the left-hand operon was not repressed at all; this resulted because of autogenous regulation in an increased repressor level, which in spite of the decreased affinity of the repressor for the operator was adequate to ensure almost complete repression of the right-hand operon. As expected in the appropriate merodiploid the HutC⁻ phenotype of the *hutC161* mutation is recessive to HutC⁺, but the HutCˢ phenotype of the right-hand operon is dominant to HutC⁺.

The lower affinity of the repressor for the left-hand operator has the consequence that a lower level of inducer is required for the induction of the left-hand operon than for the right-hand operon (Parada and Magasanik 1975). In strains carrying a mutation in *hutM*—the left-hand promoter, resulting in increased transcription of the left-hand operon—the induced level of the repressor is so high that the intracellular concentration of inducer is not sufficient for full induction of the right-hand operon (Smith and Magasanik 1971b).

The regulation of the two operons by the repressor is similar for *S. typhimurium* and *K. aerogenes*, though in the latter organism the left-hand operon is more tightly controlled than in the former. The systems in the two organisms are sufficiently similar to allow the repressor of each organism to regulate in merodiploid strains the *hut* operons of the other species. The repression exerted by the homologous repressor on the left-hand operon is, in both organisms, stronger than that exerted by the heterologous repressor (Gerson and Magasanik 1975).

Urocanate (the product of histidase) and not histidine (its substrate) is the inducer of the *hut* operons: urocanate, but not histidine, prevents binding of the repressor to *hut*-specific DNA (Hagen and Magasanik 1973). It is therefore not surprising that strains with *hutH* mutations can be induced by urocanate or by its analog imidazolepropionate, but not by histidine, to form the remaining enzymes of the *hut* system; furthermore, strains with *hutU* mutations produce the remaining enzymes of the *hut* system in the absence of any exogenously added inducer (Schlesinger et al. 1965; Brill and Magasanik 1969). This apparently constitutive synthesis is due to induction by endogenous urocanate. A portion of the endogenously synthesized histidine is converted by the small amount of histidase present in the uninduced cells to urocanate, which, in the absence of urocanase, accumulates and inactivates the repressor. The induction of histidase results in more rapid accumulation of urocanate and finally in full induction of histidase, IPase, and FGase.

It is interesting that this diversion of histidine to the formation of urocanate does not lower the histidine level of the cells sufficiently to bring about derepression of the *his* operon. It appears that in cells growing on minimal medium without added histidine the levels of the enzymes of the *his* operon are sufficiently high to allow the production of twice as much histidine as is actually produced. The actual rate of histidine production is lowered by feedback inhibition exerted by histidine on the first enzyme of histidine biosynthesis (Schlesinger et al. 1965).

The fact that urocanate is the inducer of the *hut* enzymes casts histidase in the role of an inducer-producing enzyme and urocanase in the role of an inducer-destroying enzyme. It is therefore essential for the cell to regulate the activities of these two enzymes with regard to each other, and this is ensured by the fact that *hutU* and *hutH* are members of the same operon. The necessity for this regulation is illustrated by a mutation in *hutH* which is *trans*-dominant in preventing the utilization of histidine as a source of nitrogen (Hagen et al. 1974). The histidase produced by the diploid strain containing the mutation as well as a normal *hutH* gene has one-half the activity of normal histidase; however, the preponderance of urocanase over histidase in the diploid cell makes it impossible for histidine to serve as inducer.

It is interesting to speculate why urocanate rather than histidine has been selected as inducer. One possible explanation is that the organism has guarded itself against induction resulting from a transient increase in the level of histidine, an essential metabolite; with urocanate as inducer, only a rise in the histidine level sufficiently sustained to allow the accumulation of urocanate will result in induction. However, as we have already discussed, even induction of the *hut* system in the absence of histidine does not result in a dangerous depletion of the endogenously produced histidine and is therefore not disastrous to the cell. Moreover, in another organism, *B. subtilis*, histidine and not urocanate is the actual inducer of the *hut* enzymes (Chasin and Magasanik 1968).

POSITIVE CONTROLS

The formation of the histidine-degrading enzymes is subject to control by catabolite repression exerted by glucose. The fact that addition of cyclic AMP (cAMP) to the glucose-containing medium stimulates the synthesis of histidase suggested the catabolite-activating protein (CAP) charged with cAMP to be an activator of the transcription of *hut*. This role of CAP-cAMP was confirmed by the observation that *crp* mutants of *K. aerogenes* fail to grow in a medium containing histidine as the source of carbon and fail to produce histidase when grown in a glucose-limited chemostat. Mutants defective in adenylate cyclase (*cya*) behave similarly, except that their ability to produce histidase can be restored by the addition of cAMP (Prival and Magasanik 1971; Parada and Magasanik 1975). Finally, it has been shown that the transcription of *S. typhimurium hut* DNA by purified RNA polymerase is stimulated by the addition of CAP together with cAMP (Tyler et al. 1974).

The *hut* operons of *S. typhimurium* and of *K. aerogenes* respond in a somewhat different manner to catabolite repression when they find themselves in a heterologous cytoplasm. Each histidase is repressed by glucose to approximately the same degree in its own cytoplasm; however, the *Salmonella* histidase is more severely repressed in the *Klebsiella* cytoplasm, and the *Klebsiella* histidase is not repressed at all in the *Salmonella* cytoplasm (Parada and Magasanik 1975; Goldberg et al. 1976). It would appear that in *Klebsiella* glucose metabolism results in a stronger repression signal than in *Salmonella* and that the homologous *hut* system is adjusted to make the proper response.

The relatively weak repression exerted by glucose on the left-hand *hut* operon is not antagonized by the addition of cAMP (Parada and Magasanik 1975). There is no definitive evidence that activation of transcription of the left-hand operon requires CAP and cAMP.

The *hut* system differs from *lac* in that its transcription can be activated not only by CAP charged with cAMP, but also by glutamine synthetase (GS) (E. C. 1.4.1.4). This activation is responsible for the ability of *K. aerogenes* to grow in a medium containing glucose as a source of energy and histidine as the sole source of nitrogen.

In most experiments establishing the role of glutamine synthetase in the regulation of histidine degradation, a constitutive (HutC) mutant of *K. aerogenes* was used. It could be shown that this mutant contained a low level of histidase when cultured in a medium containing glucose and ammonia in excess, but high levels of histidase when cultured in chemostats limited either on glucose or on ammonia. In similar experiments, the level of β-galactosidase induced by IPTG was found to be increased by glucose limitation but decreased by ammonia limitation. Mutants with defects in *crp* failed to produce β-galactosidase under all conditions and histidase when limited on glucose; however, they produced histidase readily during ammonia limitation. Thus the activation of histidase synthesis by ammonia starvation did not appear to require CAP charged with cAMP (Prival and Magasanik 1971).

The responsibility of glutamine synthetase (GS) for the activation of histidase production was suggested by the observations that in normal strains of enteric organisms the level of GS increases upon ammonia starvation, that mutants of *K. aerogenes* lacking GS fail to produce histidase upon ammonia starvation, and that mutants with a high level of GS in ammonia excess also produce histidase in that condition (Prival et al. 1973). Finally, it could be shown that the transcription of *hut*-specific DNA by purified RNA polymerase can be activated not only by CAP-cAMP, but also by highly purified GS (Tyler et al. 1974).

A few words need be said at this point about an unexpected difference in the response of *hut* in *K. aerogenes* and in *S. typhimurium*. As mentioned earlier, in contrast to *K. aerogenes*, *S. typhimurium* 15-59 is unable to grow on glucose-histidine. Apparently, in this organism, starvation for ammonia fails to bring about the activation of the transcription of the *hut* genes. Nevertheless, when present in the cytoplasm of *K. aerogenes* or *E. coli*, the *hut* genes of *S. typhimurium* respond to ammonia starvation (Prival and Magasanik 1971; Goldberg et al. 1976). In fact, in the experiment demonstrating the activation of *hut* transcription by GS, *hut*-specific DNA from *S. typhimurium* was used. It is known that in *S. typhimurium* ammonia starvation causes an increase in the level of GS. Moreover, it has recently been shown that in an *E. coli* strain which harbors the *hut*-specific DNA of *S. typhimurium* and whose structural gene for GS has been replaced by that of *S. typhimurium*, histidase formation is stimulated by starvation for ammonia. It would appear, therefore, that *S. typhimurium* lacks a factor which is required for the stimulation of *hut* transcription by GS (Bloom et al. 1977).

The *hut* enzymes are not the only ones whose synthesis can be stimulated by GS. The formation of most enzymes or enzyme systems capable of supplying *K. aerogenes* with ammonia or glutamate is stimulated by the increase in the level of GS which results from ammonia starvation. Some of the enzyme systems act on compounds able, like histidine, to serve the cell as sources of nitrogen as well as of energy. Among these systems are those responsible for the degradation of proline, arginine, and agmatine. The synthesis of these enzymes requires specific induction and is subject to catabolite repression. Other enzymes whose synthesis is activated by GS, such as urease, the low-K_m asparaginase of *K. aerogenes*, and the nitrogenase of *K. pneumoniae*, do not require induction and are not subject to catabolite repression. These enzymes contribute to the nitrogen metabolism, but not to the energy metabolism of the cell (Magasanik 1977).

The choice of GS as activator of the synthesis of enzymes capable of supplying the cell with ammonia or glutamate is explained by the role these enzymes play in the assimilation of ammonia. It was shown by Tempest and coworkers (1970) that when the concentration of ammonia in the medium is less than 1 mM, the equilibrium of the reaction catalyzed by glutamate dehydrogenase is not adequate for the synthesis of glutamate:

$$NH_3 + \alpha\text{-ketoglutarate} + NADPH + H^+ \rightleftharpoons glutamate + NADP^+ + H_2O.$$

In that case, the utilization of ammonia for the formation of glutamate depends on the action of two enzymes, GS and glutamate synthase:

$$glutamate + NH_3 + ATP \longrightarrow glutamine + ADP + P_i$$
$$glutamine + \alpha\text{-ketoglutarate} + NADPH + H^+ \longrightarrow 2 \ glutamate + NADP^+$$

$$\overline{\phantom{NH_3 + ATP + \alpha\text{-ketoglutarate} + NADPH + H^+ \longrightarrow glutamate + NADP^+ + H_2O + ADP + P_i}}$$

$$NH_3 + ATP + \alpha\text{-ketoglutarate} + NADPH + H^+ \longrightarrow$$
$$glutamate + NADP^+ + H_2O + ADP + P_i$$

As expected, mutants of *K. aerogenes* lacking glutamate synthase fail to grow when the concentration of NH_3 in the medium is lower than 1 mM (Brenchley et al. 1973).

This essential role of GS in the assimilation of ammonia present in low concentrations is presumably responsible for the elaborate regulation of the activity and level of GS in response to the ammonia concentration of the growth medium. It has been shown that GS of *E. coli* is converted by the attachment of an adenylyl group to each of its 12 identical subunits from the form capable of catalyzing the synthesis of glutamine to an inactive form (Kingdon et al. 1967). Three proteins, ATase, P_{II}, and UTase-UR, are responsible for the activation and inactivation of GS, as shown in Figure 3. UTase is activated by α-ketoglutarate and inhibited by glutamine. Consequently, when the α-ketoglutarate-glutamine ratio is high, P_{II} is converted by the action of UTase to its uridylylated form, P_{II}-UMP, which in combination with ATase stimulates deadenylylation of GS. Conversely, when the α-ketoglutarate-glutamine ratio is low, UTase is inactive and P_{II}-UMP is converted to P_{II}, which in combination with ATase stimulates adenylylation of GS. In addition, the ATase-P_{II} complex is activated by glutamine and inhibited by α-ketoglutarate, further enhancing adenylylation of GS when the α-ketoglutarate-glutamine ratio is low.

In the growing cell, the α-ketoglutarate-glutamine ratio reflects the

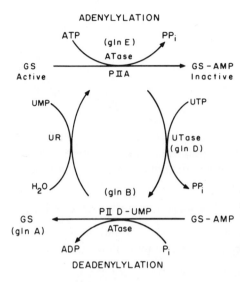

ADENYLYLATION

Figure 3 Adenylylation and deadenylylation of glutamine synthetase adapted from Ginsburg and Stadtman (1973). GS is glutamine synthetase; ATase is adenylylation enzyme; UTase is uridylyltransferase enzyme; UR is uridyl-removing enzyme (probably identical with UTase); *gln* indicates genes controlling production of GS.

availability of ammonia. When ammonia is present in excess, this ratio is low, since the activity of GS ensures a high level of glutamine and the α-ketoglutarate is converted to glutamate by glutamate dehydrogenase and glutamate synthase. Conversely, when ammonia is present in low concentration, the level of α-ketoglutarate is high and the level of glutamine is low. Thus, an excess of ammonia favors inactivation of GS, and ammonia deficiency favors activation of GS.

In addition to regulating the activity of GS, the availability of ammonia also regulates the level of GS. The total level of GS, active and inactive, varies more than 100-fold with the composition of the growth medium. It would appear that GS synthesis is subject to autogenous regulation, with GS-AMP playing the role of repressor and GS the role of activator of GS synthesis (Magasanik 1977).

The key role of GS in ammonia assimilation requires this elaborate regulation of its activity and synthesis. As a consequence of this careful regulation, the level of nonadenylylated GS is a precise gauge of the availability of ammonia and glutamate. It therefore makes good sense for the cell to use GS to regulate the synthesis of enzymes capable of supplying the cell with ammonia and glutamate. A low level and high adenylylation state of GS is an indication that additional ammonia or glutamate is not required. A high level of nonadenylylated GS indicates that more ammonia and glutamate would be of use. In fact, the activation of the synthesis of the *hut* enzymes is stimulated only by nonadenylylated GS, and not by GS-AMP, and requires an intracellular level of GS three to four times higher than that found in cells growing with an excess of ammonia (Prival et al. 1973; Tyler et al. 1974).

OPERATION

We have shown that the expression of the *hut* operons of *K. aerogenes* requires removal of the specific *hut* repressor and activation either by CAP charged with cAMP or by nonadenylylated GS. This combination of one negative and two positive control mechanisms ensures operation of the *hut* system according to the needs of the cell.

Cells of *K. aerogenes* growing in a medium containing glucose, ammonia, and histidine require neither the energy and carbon building blocks nor the ammonia and glutamate the degradation of histidine would provide. In these cells, neither CAP charged with cAMP nor nonadenylylated GS is present in an amount sufficient for the activation of the transcription of the *hut* operons. Should these cells use up their glucose, the level of CAP charged with cAMP would increase sufficiently to bring about transcription of the *hut* operons. Similarly, should the cells use up their ammonia while glucose is still available, the level of nonadenylylated GS would increase sufficiently to bring about transcription of the *hut* operons. Finally, should the cells use up the histidine supplied in the medium, they would no longer be able to inactivate the *hut* repressor and the useless transcription of the *hut* operon would not take place, regardless of the need of the cells for energy or ammonia.

ACKNOWLEDGMENTS

This investigation was supported by U.S. Public Health Service research grants GM-07446 from the National Institute of General Medical Sciences and AM-13894 from the National Institute of Arthritis, Metabolism, and Digestive Diseases, and by grant PCM 75-03398 from the National Science Foundation.

REFERENCES

Bloom, F. R., S. L. Streicher, and B. Tyler. 1977. Regulation of enzyme synthesis by glutamine synthetase of *Salmonella typhimurium*: A factor in addition to glutamine synthetase is required for activation of enzyme formation. *J. Bacteriol.* **130**:983.

Brenchley, J. E., M. J. Prival, and B. Magasanik. 1973. Regulation of the synthesis of enzymes responsible for glutamate formation in *Klebsiella aerogenes*. *J. Biol. Chem.* **248**:6122.

Brill, W. J. and B. Magasanik. 1969. Genetic and metabolic control of histidase and urocanase in *Salmonella typhimurium*, strain 15-59. *J. Biol. Chem.* **244**:5392.

Chasin, L. A. and B. Magasanik. 1968. Induction and repression of the histidine-degrading enzymes of *Bacillus subtilis*. *J. Biol. Chem.* **243**:5165.

Cooper, T. G. and B. Tyler. 1977. Transcription of the *hut* operons of *Salmonella typhimurium*. *J. Bacteriol.* **130**:192.

Friedrich, B. and B. Magasanik. 1978. Utilization of arginine by *Klebsiella aerogenes*. *J. Bacteriol.* **133**:680.

Gerson, S. L. and B. Magasanik. 1975. Regulation of the *hut* operons of *Salmonella typhimurium* and *K. aerogenes* by heterologous *hut* repressors. *J. Bacteriol.* **124**:1269.

Ginsburg, A. and E. R. Stadtman. 1973. Regulation of glutamine synthetase in *Escherichia coli*. In *The enzymes of glutamine metabolism* (ed. S. Prusiner and E. R. Stadtman), p. 9, Academic Press, New York.

Goldberg, R. B. and B. Magasanik. 1975. Gene order of the histidine utilization (*hut*) operons in *K. aerogenes*. *J. Bacteriol.* **122**:1025.

Goldberg, R. B., F. R. Bloom, and B. Magasanik. 1976. Regulation of histidase synthesis in intergeneric hybrids of enteric bacteria. *J. Bacteriol.* **127**:114.

Hagen, D. C. and B. Magasanik. 1973. Isolation of the self-regulated repressor protein of the *hut* operons of *Salmonella typhimurium*. *Proc. Natl. Acad. Sci.* **70**:808.

———. 1976. Deoxyribonucleic acid-binding studies on the *hut* repressor and mutant forms of the *hut* repressor of *Salmonella typhimurium*. *J. Bacteriol.* **127**:827.

Hagen, D. C., S. L. Gerson, and B. Magasanik. 1975. Isolation of super-repressor mutants in the histidine utilization system of *S. typhimurium*. *J. Bacteriol.* **121**:583.

Hagen, D. C., P. J. Lipton, and B. Magasanik. 1974. Isolation of *trans*-dominant histidase-negative mutant of *Salmonella typhimurium*. *J. Bacteriol.* **120**:906.

Kaminskas, E. and B. Magasanik. 1970. Sequential synthesis of histidine degrading enzymes in *Bacillus subtilis*. *J. Biol. Chem.* **245**:3549.

Kimhi, Y. and B. Magasanik. 1970. Genetic basis of histidine degradation in *Bacillus subtilis*. *J. Biol. Chem.* **245**:3545.

Kingdon, H. S., B. M. Shapiro, and E. R. Stadtman. 1967. Regulation of glutamine synthetase. VIII. ATP:glutamine synthetase adenylyltransferase, an enzyme that catalyzes alterations in the regulatory properties of glutamine synthetase. *Proc. Natl. Acad. Sci.* **58**:1703.

Lund, P. and B. Magasanik. 1965. N-formimino-L-glutamate formiminohydrolase of *Aerobacter aerogenes*. *J. Biol. Chem.* **240**:4316.

Magasanik, B. 1977. Regulation of bacterial nitrogen assimilation by glutamine synthetase. *Trends Biochem. Sci.* **2**:9.

Magasanik, B. and H. R. Bowser. 1955. The degradation of histidine by *Aerobacter aerogenes*. *J. Biol. Chem.* **213**:571.

Magasanik, B., E. Kaminskas, and Y. Kimhi. 1971. Histidine degradation (*Bacillus subtilis*). *Methods Enzymol.* **17B**:45.

Magasanik, B., P. Lund, F. C. Neidhardt, and D. T. Schwartz. 1965. Induction and repression of the histidine-degrading enzymes in *Aerobacter aerogenes*. *J. Biol. Chem.* **240**:4320.

Meiss, H. K., W. J. Brill, and B. Magasanik. 1969. Genetic control of histidine degradation in *Salmonella typhimurium*, strain LT-2. *J. Biol. Chem.* **244**:5382.

Neidhardt, F. C. and B. Magasanik. 1957. Reversal of the glucose inhibition of histidase biosynthesis in *Aerobacter aerogenes*. *J. Bacteriol.* **73**:253.

Parada, J. L. and B. Magasanik. 1975. Expression of the *hut* operons of *S. typhimurium* in *K. aerogenes* and in *E. coli*. *J. Bacteriol.* **124**:1263.

Phillips, A. T. and D. Y. George. 1971. Urocanase (*Pseudomonas putida*). *Methods Enzymol.* **17B**:63.

Prival, M. J. and B. Magasanik. 1971. Resistance to catabolite repression of histidase and proline oxidase during nitrogen-limited growth of *Klebsiella aerogenes*. *J. Biol. Chem.* **246**:6288.

Prival, M. J., J. E. Brenchley, and B. Magasanik. 1973. Glutamine synthetase and the regulation of histidase formation in *Klebsiella aerogenes*. *J. Biol. Chem.* **248**:4334.

Rao, D. R. and D. M. Greenberg. 1961. Studies on the enzymic decomposition of urocanic acid. IV. Purification and properties of 4(5)-imidazolone-5(4)-propionic acid hydrolase. *J. Biol. Chem.* **236**:1758.

Rechler, M. M. and H. Tabor. 1971. Histidine ammonia lyase (*Pseudomonas*). *Methods Enzymol.* **17B**:63.

Revel, H. R. B. and B. Magasanik. 1958. The enzymatic degradation of urocanic acid. *J. Biol. Chem.* **233**:930.

Schlesinger, S. and B. Magasanik. 1965. Imidazolepropionate, a non-metabolizable inducer for the histidine-degrading enzymes in *Aerobacter aerogenes*. *J. Biol. Chem.* **240**:4325.

Schlesinger, S., P. Scotto, and B. Magasanik. 1965. Exogenous and endogenous induction of the histidine-degrading enzymes in *Aerobacter aerogenes*. *J. Biol. Chem.* **240**:4331.

Silverstone, A. E., R. R. Arditti, and B. Magasanik. 1970. Catabolite insensitive revertants of *lac* promoter mutants. *Proc. Natl. Acad. Sci.* **66**:773.

Silverstone, A. E., B. Magasanik, W. S. Reznikoff, J. H. Miller, and J. R. Beckwith. 1969. Catabolite sensitive site of the *lac* operon. *Nature* **221**:1012.

Smith, G. R. 1971. Specialized transduction of the *Salmonella hut* operons by coliphage λ: Deletion analysis of the *hut* operons employing λp*hut*. *Virology* **45**:208.

Smith, G. R. and B. Magasanik. 1971a. The two operons of the histidine utilization system in *Salmonella typhimurium*. *J. Biol. Chem.* **246**:3330.

———. 1971b. Nature and self-regulated synthesis of the repressor of the *hut* operons in *Salmonella typhimurium*. *Proc. Natl. Acad. Sci.* **68**:1493.

Smith, G. R., Y. S. Halpern, and B. Magasanik. 1971. Genetic and metabolic control of enzymes responsible for histidine degradation in *Salmonella typhimurium*. *J. Biol. Chem.* **246**:3320.

Tempest, D. W., J. L. Meers, and C. M. Brown. 1970. Glutamine (amide): 2-oxoglutarate aminotransferase oxido-reductase (NADP), an enzyme involved in the synthesis of glutamate by some bacteria. *J. Gen. Microbiol.* **64**:187.

Tyler, B. and R. B. Goldberg. 1976. Transduction of chromosomal genes between enteric bacteria by bacteriophage P1. *J. Bacteriol.* **125**:1105.

Tyler, B., A. B. Deleo, and B. Magasanik. 1974. Activation of transcription of *hut* DNA by glutamine synthetase. *Proc. Natl. Acad. Sci.* **71**:225.

Molecular Aspects of *ara* Regulation

Nancy Lee
Department of Biological Sciences
University of California
Santa Barbara, California 93106

THE *ara* REGULON

In *Escherichia coli*, the metabolism of L-arabinose involves the expression of six genes, *araA* through *araF* (Englesberg 1971; Englesberg and Wilcox 1974). These genes are located at three different regions on the *E. coli* chromosome (Fig. 1). Genes *araA*, *araB*, *araC*, and *araD* are located between the threonine and leucine operons, at approximately 1 minute (min) on the circular linkage map of *E. coli* (Gross and Englesberg 1959; Englesberg 1961; Englesberg et al. 1962; Bachman et al. 1976). The *araE* gene is located at about 61 min between *thyA* and *serA* (Novotny and Englesberg 1966), and the *araF* gene has been tentatively mapped at 44–45 min, close to the structural genes for the histidine operon and the galactose binding protein (R. Hogg, pers. comm.).

Genes *araB*, *araA*, and *araD*, together with their controlling sites *araI* and *araO*, constitute a single unit of transcription, the *araBAD* operon (Englesberg 1971; Englesberg and Wilcox 1974; Schleif and Lis 1975). The structural genes code for L-ribulokinase (*araB*) (Lee and Englesberg 1962; Lee and Bendet 1967; Lee and Patrick 1970), L-arabinose isomerase (*araA*) (Lee and Englesberg 1962; Patrick and Lee 1968, 1969), and L-ribulose 5-phosphate 4-epimerase (*araD*) (Lee et al. 1968), the first three enzymes of L-arabinose catabolism (Fig. 1). Genes *araE* and *araF* are both involved in active transport of L-arabinose (Novotny and Englesberg 1966; Hogg and Englesberg 1969; Schleif 1969). The *araE* gene may code for a membrane protein (R. Hogg, pers. comm.), whereas the *araF* gene codes for a periplasmic protein which binds L-arabinose (Hogg and Englesberg 1969; Schleif 1969; Brown and Hogg 1972; Parsons and Hogg 1974). There is a single regulatory gene, *araC*, whose protein product (Irr and Englesberg 1971; Zubay et al. 1971; Greenblatt and Schleif 1971; Wilcox 1972) is required for the expression of *araBAD*, *araE*, and *araF*.

The *araC* gene can exist in a number of allelic forms: C^+, the wild-type allele, confers upon the cell inducibility of the *ara* regulon by L-arabinose; C^-, which results from the nonsense (Englesberg 1971) and deletion (Sheppard and Englesberg 1967b; Kessler and Englesberg 1969) mutations in *araC*, is characterized by noninducibility. C^c, the allele for

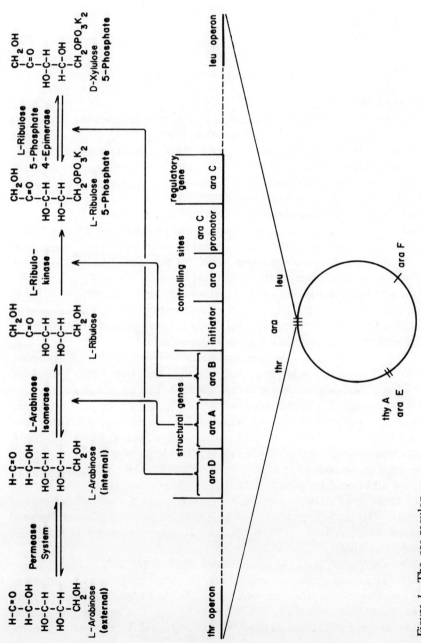

Figure 1 The *ara* regulon.

constitutivity, is the result of missense mutations (Irr and Englesberg 1971; Nathanson and Schleif 1975) and abolishes the requirement for L-arabinose for induction (Englesberg et al. 1965). C^c mutants may be sensitive (Englesberg 1971), resistant (Englesberg et al. 1965), or dependent (Doyle et al. 1972) in their responses to the competitive anti-inducer D-fucose. Mutations in *araC* can also alter the sensitivity of the *ara* regulon to catabolite repression. C^i mutants have a decreased sensitivity (Heffernan et al. 1976; Heffernan and Wilcox 1976), whereas C^h mutants are hypersensitive (Gendron and Sheppard 1974; Sheppard and Eleuterio 1976).

Through a series of studies employing temporary (Helling and Weinberg 1963) and permanent (Sheppard and Englesberg 1967a,b) merodiploids in *araC*, Englesberg and coworkers have demonstrated that the product of the *araC* gene plays a positive role in regulation (Englesberg et al. 1965; Sheppard and Englesberg 1967a). These findings were the first indication that positive as well as negative control was utilized in gene regulation in *E. coli*.

The *araC* protein, functionally a positive regulator, is capable of repressing the *araBAD* operon. Discovery of the repressor activity of *araC* and the operator *araO* was made during an analysis of the effect of a C$^+$ or C$^-$ allele in *trans* position to *araC* deletions (Englesberg et al. 1969). This divides the regulatory region for *araBAD* into two parts: the region *araO*, which is required for the expression of the repressor function of *araC*, the region *araI*, which is required for the initiation of *araBAD* transcription by the activities of RNA polymerase, *araC* activator, and the catabolite gene activator (CGA) proteins. The finding that the protein coded by the *araC* gene can positively and negatively control the *araBAD* operon has led to the proposal by Englesberg that the *araC* protein exists in two conformational states, both biologically active (Englesberg et al. 1969). The repressor form of *araC* protein, P1, interacts with the operator *araO* and reduces the level of *araBAD* expression. The activator form, P2, in conjunction with CGA protein and 3',5'-cyclic AMP (cAMP), potentiates transcription of *araBAD*. It is postulated that two regulatory events take place upon the addition of L-arabinose. First, P1 is removed from the operator by a shift in the equilibrium between P1 and P2 in the direction of P2. Second, P2 activates transcription of *araBAD*. In addition, the expression of *araBAD* is sensitive to catabolite repression (Katz and Englesberg 1971; Lis and Schleif 1973), and mutations affecting the production of either cAMP or CGA protein give rise to Ara$^-$ phenotypes (Zubay et al. 1970). Wild-type cells growing on L-arabinose are "self-catabolite-repressed" (Katz and Englesberg 1971), so that the level of *araBAD* enzymes is about 50% that of strains with missense mutations in *araB* or *araA*. The enzyme levels of various strains are given in Table 1.

Table 1 Expression of *araBAD* in various
strains of *E. coli* B/r

Strain	Monomers per cell[a]
Wild type (induced)	12,000
araA⁻ (missense; induced)	24,000
araB⁻ (missense; induced)	24,000
Wild type	30
araCᶜ	1,500–16,000
araIᶜaraCΔ	600– 1,200
araIᶜaraCΔ/F′araC⁺	100– 140
araIᶜaraC⁺	100– 140
araIᶜaraC⁺	12,000± 750
araCΔ	30
araCΔ/F′araC⁺	30
araCΔaraOΔ	30
araCΔaraOΔ/F′araC⁺	500
araIᶜaraCΔaraOΔ	600– 1,200
araIᶜaraCΔaraOΔ/F′araC⁺	650– 2,500
araXᶜaraCΔ	2,000
araIᶜXᶜaraCΔ	4,000– 6,000

[a]The enzyme monomers per cell are based on the activities of cell extracts prepared from exponential-phase cultures in minimal salt medium supplemented with 1% casamino acids. The inducer L-arabinose is absent in all cases, except where stated. The number of monomers was calculated based on the following: (1) The molecular weights of *araB*, *araA*, and *araD* gene products are 50,000, 60,000, and 35,000, respectively. (2) The activities of the enzymes are 2,500, 12,000, and 2,200 units/mg enzyme, respectively. (3) A single cell contains 1.8×10^{-13} g of solubilizable protein under our conditions of extraction. Where assays were performed on merodiploid strains, the expression of *araBAD* enzymes was determined by the activity of the enzyme produced by the endogenote. For example, for the merodiploid *araIᶜaraCΔ/ F′ araC⁺*, the episome is *araA2* and the extract was assayed for *araA*.

With the development of in vitro systems of DNA-directed protein and RNA synthesis, most aspects of the model elaborated by Englesberg and his coworkers have received direct confirmation. The presence of *araC* protein plus L-arabinose was shown to be required for the in vitro synthesis of L-ribulokinase (*araB*) and L-arabinose isomerase (*araA*). The *araC* protein could be supplied either in the form of an extract of C⁺ cells (Greenblatt and Schleif 1971; Yang and Zubay 1973; Wilcox et al. 1974c) or in the form of DNA from a transducing bacteriophage, φ80iᐱd*ara*, carrying a wild-type *araC* gene (Yang and Zubay 1973; Wilcox et al. 1974c; Zubay et al. 1971). In the latter case, *araC* protein was made in vitro. The synthesis of *araBAD* messenger RNA with purified RNA polymerase demonstrated conclusively that the transcription of *araBAD* showed an absolute requirement for the presence of *araC* protein, L-arabinose, CGA protein, and cAMP (Lee et al. 1974; Hirsch and Schleif 1977), confirming the idea that both positive regulators acted at the level of transcription (Englesberg 1971; Power and Irr 1973; Wilcox et al. 1971a). In these studies it was also shown that D-fucose antagonized the stimulatory effect of L-arabinose in a competitive manner (Greenblatt and Schleif 1971; Wilcox et al. 1974c; Lee et al. 1974). The repressor activity of *araC* was shown by the finding that the in vitro constitutive synthesis of L-arabinose isomerase, directed by DNA from the transducing phage $\phi80i^Adara I^c110I^c44C\Delta766$, was reduced by the addition of an ammonium sulfate fraction of a C^+ extract in the absence of L-arabinose (Wilcox et al. 1974c).

The specific binding of *araC* repressor to DNA containing *araO* was measured by the retention of ^{32}P-labeled $\phi80i^Adara$ DNA on nitrocellulose filters (Wilcox et al. 1971a) after extensive purification of the *araC* protein by affinity chromatography (Wilcox 1972; Wilcox et al. 1971b; Wilcox et al. 1974a; Wilcox and Clementson 1974) in the absence of L-arabinose. The amount of radioactivity retained by the filter after subtraction of the amount nonspecifically bound to ^{32}P-labeled helper DNA was found to be greatly reduced by the addition of unlabeled $\phi80i^Adara$ DNA, but not by the addition of unlabeled helper DNA, and only minimally by the addition of unlabeled $\phi80i^Adara$ DNA containing deletions which excised *araO*. Surprisingly, neither the direct binding nor the equilibrium competition was affected by the presence of L-arabinose. The possibility that this preparation of *araC* protein has lost its ability to undergo the change from the repressor to the activator form has not been ruled out (Wilcox et al. 1974a).

The ability of *araC* protein to undergo a conformational change in the presence of inducer has been suggested by fluorescence spectroscopy (Wilcox 1974). The addition of L-arabinose to a solution of *araC* protein caused a quenching of its intrinsic fluorescence, and this quenching was reduced by the addition of the anti-inducer D-fucose. Since L-arabinose and D-fucose bind to the same site on *araC* protein, as suggested by the competitive nature of D-fucose inhibition both in vivo (Doyle et al. 1972; Beverin et al. 1971) and in vitro (Wilcox 1974c; Lee et al. 1974), it was deduced that the quenching produced by L-arabinose was indicative of a conformational change in the protein rather than the masking of a tryptophan residue at the binding site (Wilcox 1974).

Presently, several laboratories are analyzing the detailed biochemical mechanism or specific role of each of the macromolecular components involved in the expression of the *araBAD* operon. Work directed towards the isolation and characterization of the proteins and nucleic acids of *ara* regulation necessary for this analysis is summarized below.

THE CLONING OF *ara* DNA

The first cloning of *ara* DNA was described by Gottesman and Beckwith (1969). The *araCOIBAD* region from *E. coli* B/r was transposed to a region on the *E. coli* K12 chromosome close to the attachment site of the bacteriophage $\phi80$. This strain, made lysogenic for $\phi80$, gave rise to defective transducing phages which carried *araCOIBAD* in either orientation with respect to phage genes. To facilitate obtaining large quantities of phage, the temperature-sensitive repressor (*CI*857) and lysis-inhibition (S⁻) markers from a lambda phage were crossed into these $\phi80$d*ara* phages (Gottesman 1971). A similar $\phi80$-lambda hybrid phage was constructed independently by Schleif et al. (1971) from a $\phi80$d*ara* (Gottesman 1971). These hybrid $\phi80i^{\lambda}CI857S^{-}$d*ara* transducing phages carried the entire *araCOIBAD* region from *E. coli* B/r and have been used extensively in in vitro studies (Zubay et al. 1971; Greenblatt and Schleif 1971; Yang and Zubay 1973; Wilcox et al. 1974b,c; Lee et al. 1974; Lee and Carbon 1977).

Portions of *araCOIBAD* from *E. coli* B/r (Boulter and Lee 1975) and from *E. coli* K12 (Lis and Schleif 1975) have been cloned with lambda phage. Secondary-site lysogens with prophage inserted in *araB* or *araC* could be directly selected in a Cᶜ strain deleted for the normal attachment site for lambda (Shimada et al. 1972) by resistance to ribitol inhibition (Katz 1970) or in a D⁻ strain by resistance to arabinose inhibition (Englesberg et al. 1962). Boulter and Lee have obtained integration of the prophage with opposite orientations at two different sites in the *araB* gene and at a single site in the *araC* gene in *E. coli* B/r. Various λ*ara* transducing phages have been isolated from these secondary-site lysogens. These carried various portions of *araCOIBAD*, and one defective phage carried the *leu* operon as well (Boulter and Lee 1975). They have been used to determine the polarity of transcription of the *araC* gene (Wilcox et al. 1974a) and to provide assays of *araBAD* and *araC* messenger RNA (Lee and Carbon 1977; Lee et al. 1974; N. Lee, unpubl.).

Lis and Schleif (1975) have obtained λ*ara* transducing phages which carried portions of *araCOIBAD* from *E. coli* K12. In this case, the selection yielded secondary-site lysogens at a single site in *araB* and a single site in *araC*. Lysogens were used to obtain an extensive set of *ara* deletions (Schleif 1972). The λ*ara* transducing phages derived from these lysogens have been used in the physical mapping of *ara* controlling sites by electron microscopy (Lis and Schleif 1975; Hirsh and Schleif 1976, 1977).

The development of bacterial plasmids as cloning agents afforded yet another means of enrichment of *ara* genes (Clarke and Carbon 1975; Kaplan et al. 1978). These agents can be used to amplify select restriction fragments of *ara* DNA. When used in conjunction with well-characterized genetic mutations, these should soon provide information on the structure-function relationships in the *ara* regulatory region.

THE *ara* CONTROLLING SITES

The *araBAD* operon and the *araC* gene are transcribed in opposite directions, and their controlling sites are located between *araC* and *araB* (Wilcox et al. 1974a). Determination of the structure and function of this region is currently being pursued, and extensive sequence information has recently become available for *E. coli* K12 and *E. coli* B/r. In addition, several classes of mutations have been described which map within the controlling region. Elucidation of the altered sequences would provide valuable insights into the functional aspects of the *ara* regulatory region.

Nucleotide Sequence of the *ara* Controlling Region

The nucleotide sequence of the *ara* regulatory region has been determined for *E. coli* K12 by B. Smith and R. Schleif (unpubl.) and for *E. coli* B/r by L. Greenfield and G. Wilcox (unpubl.). Both groups have utilized the DNA sequencing techniques described by Maxam and Gilbert (1977). The 5′-nucleotide sequence of *araBAD* operon messenger RNA, as well as the N-terminal amino acid sequence of the product of the first cistron (*araB*), is known (Lee and Carbon 1977). The results of these studies closely agree and are shown in Figure 2.

As shown in Figure 2, transcription of *araBAD* mRNA is initiated at position +1 with A, and the transcript contains a noncoding or leader region of 27 nucleotides that precedes the starter AUG codon for the *araB* gene. Within this leader region there is a purine-rich sequence (+13 to +20) containing the sequence G-G-A-G (+17 to +20) which is complementary to a four-base sequence at the 3′ end of *E. coli* 16S ribosomal RNA, strongly suggesting a role in ribosomal recognition (Steitz and Jakes 1975).

Another feature within the leader region is a stretch of seven consecutive uridyl residues (+6 to +12). A similar sequence has been shown to be associated with transcription termination (Squires et al. 1976). It is not known at present whether this region in *ara* serves as an attenuator of transcriptional activity, since the 5′ fragment preceding this region is too short to permit detection by the DNA-RNA hybridization methods employed to isolate *ara* messenger RNA.

None of the *cis*-dominant regulatory mutations of the I^c or X^c type (see below) tested appears to lie within the leader region. A comparison of the transcripts from five different I^c and $I^c X^c$ templates with that of the wild type shows that they have identical sequences in the first 69 nucleotides at the 5′ end (Lee and Carbon 1977; N. Lee, unpubl.).

The nucleotide sequence to the right of *araBAD* messenger RNA must contain the sites for RNA polymerase interaction as well as the putative sites for interaction with *araC* (both the activator P2 form and the repressor P1 form) and with the CGA protein. The assignment of regions

```
   -90          -100        -110          -120         -130          -140        -150
   .            .           .   T         .            .             .           .
GTGTGACGCCGTGCAAATAATCAATGTGGACTTTTCTGCCGTGATTATAGACACTTTTGTTACGCGTTTTTGT
CACACTGCGGCACGTTTATTAGTTACACATGAAAAGACGGCACTAATATCTGTGAAAACAATGCGCAAAAACA
                                  C
```

```
                       40          30          20          10         !         -10
                       .           .           .           .                     .
                C A A T T G C A A T C G C C A T C G T T T C A C T C C A T C C A A A A A A A A C G G G T A T G G A G A A A C A G T A G A
                G T T A A C G T T A G C G G T A G C A A A G T G A G G T A G G T T T T T T T G C C C A T A C C T C T T T G T C A T C T
```

(U)GUCUUAGUGACGGUUUUUAGCUCCGGUUAACGUUAGCGGUAGCAAAGUGAGGUAGGUUUUUUUGCCCA 5' araBAD mRNA

Val Ser Asp Ser Gly Phe Asp Leu Gly Ile Ala Ile Ala–NH$_2$ L–Ribulokinase

Figure 2 Nucleotide sequence of the *ara* controlling sites, showing the K12 DNA sequence from −207 to +47 (B. Smith and R. Schleif, unpubl.), the B/r DNA sequence from −149 to +43 (L. Greenfield and G. Wilcox, unpubl.), and the B/r RNA sequence at the 5′ end of *araBAD* operon mRNA (Lee and Carbon 1977). The B/r and K12 sequences are identical except at position −113, where K12 has a G-C and B/r has a T-A. The sequence of U's in *ara* mRNA has been corrected from eight to seven.

to specific functions awaits the results of studies now in progress on the changes in nucleotide sequences in DNA from mutants. Comparison of the *ara* sequence with those of *lac* and *gal* reveals some interesting analogies. The sequence from − 35 to − 29, A-C-G-C-T-T-T, is strikingly similar to the sequence A-C-G-C-T-T-T located from −36 to −30 in *gal* (Musso et al. 1977) and from −33 to −27 in *lac* (Dickson et al. 1975). Gilbert (1976) has proposed that this region is involved in RNA polymerase recognition. There is a heptanucleotide sequence from −16 to −10 which bears close resemblance to similar sequences in other promoters (Pribnow 1975). A 13-base palindrome of yet unknown significance occurs from −82 to −68.

The Function of *ara* Controlling Sites

The *ara* controlling region has been characterized at the functional level by the study of mutants. For the purpose of this discussion, the entire region is divided into three segments as shown in Figure 3. The region adjacent to *araB* is designated the initiator region for *araBAD* and is defined as that segment of DNA which is required for the *araC*-activator–CGA-protein-dependent initiation of *araBAD* transcription (Lee et al. 1974). The region next to *araC* is designated the promoter region for *araC* and is defined as the segment of DNA required for the initiation of *araC* transcription. The *araO* region is the segment of DNA required for the repressor (P1) function of *araC* (Englesberg et al. 1969).

```
      -160        -170        -180        -190        -200
CATGGCTTTGGTCCCGCTTTGTTACAGAATGCTTTTAATAAGCGGGGTTA  3'
GTACCGAAACCAGGGCGAAACAATGTCTTACGAAAATTATTCGCCCCAAT  5'



      -20      -30       -40       -50       -60       -70       -80
GAGTTGCGATAAAAAGCGTCAGGTAGGATCCGCTAATCTTATGGATAAAAATGCTATGGCATAGCAAA
CTCAACGCTATTTTTCGCAGTCCATCCTAGGCGATTAGAATACCTATTTTTACGATACCGTATCGTTT
```

Figure 2   (continued)

The ordering of the three regions is based on the following observations. A pair of mutants contain deletions *ara718* and *ara719*, which extend into the *ara* controlling sites (Fig. 2). The Ara719 phenotype is such that it has lost the sensitivity to P1 (Englesberg et al. 1969). In the presence of L-arabinose and an episomal *trans araC* gene, the *araBAD* operon is expressed at the wild-type level and the strain retains its requirement for the GCA protein–cAMP system (Bass et al. 1977). Therefore, the initiator region for *araBAD* is intact in strains carrying *ara719*. The *ara718* strain, on the other hand, produces *araC* protein and complements all *araC* mutations, including *ara719*. Thus, the promoter region of *araC* is functional in strains with *ara718*. That the ends of these deletions approach each other and may in fact overlap is suggested by the finding that it is not possible to obtain wild-type recombinants between them by transduction with bacteriophage P1 (E. Englesberg, pers. comm.). These two deletions must therefore both terminate in a region between the initiator for *araBAD* and the promoter for *araC*. The absence of *araO* in strains with *ara719* (Englesberg et al. 1969) and the failure of either deletion to compete for specific binding of P1 to *ara* DNA (Wilcox et al. 1974a)

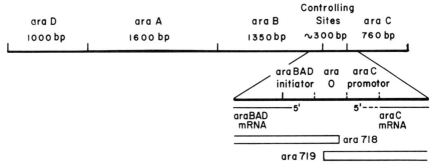

Figure 3 The *ara* controlling sites. *Ara719* and *ara718* are a pair of deletions which extend into this region from *araC* and *araB*, respectively. The broken lines indicate positions that are uncertain.

indicate that both deletions excise at least part of the binding site, placing the promoter for *araC* to the right of *araO*.

This proposed order of *araC* promoter and *araO* is tentative. Conceivably, the promoter for *araC* may be located to the left of *araO* and the expression of *araC* in *ara718* may be the result of linking *araC* to an upstream promoter. If this were true, one might expect (1) the maximal level of *araC* expression to be altered in *ara718* and (2) the *araC* transcript from *ara718* to bear an altered nucleotide sequence at the 5' end. Both of these predictions are undergoing testing in the author's laboratory. It should perhaps be noted that an intact promoter for *araC* may exist without retention of a complete regulatory region for this gene, just as *araO* may be deleted from the *aracOIBAD* operon without affecting its ability to promote transcription.

The initiation region for *araBAD* has been assigned the function of interaction with RNA polymerase and the two positive regulators–*araC* activator and the CGA protein (Englesberg 1971; Englesberg and Wilcox 1974; Lee et al. 1974; Bass et al. 1977). These processes are conceptually discrete events and have been assigned the respective interaction sites *araI* (initiator site for the activator form of the *araC* protein), *ara(CGA)* or *araX* (catabolite-sensitivity site for the CGA protein and cAMP), and *araP* (promoter site for RNA polymerase). The locations of these sites are being analyzed by both genetic and physical approaches.

The *araI* Mutations

Mutations in the initiator region designated I^c were isolated as Ara$^+$ revertants of strains deleted for the *araC* gene after diethylsulfate (Englesberg et al. 1969) or 2-aminopurine (Gielow et al. 1971) mutagenesis. These mutants, deleted for the *araC* gene, synthesize *ara* enzymes constitutively at about 5–10% of the rate in L-arabinose-induced wild-type cells (Table 1). The constitutivity applies to *araBAD* genes *cis* to the *araI* mutation. When the *araC* gene is restored either by crossing out the deletion in *araC* or by introducing an episome which carries a wild-type *araC* allele, these mutants produce *ara* enzymes in the presence of L-arabinose at the wild-type level (Englesberg et al. 1969; Gielow et al. 1971).

The response to P1 is retained in these I^c strains. If the *araO* region *cis* to the *araI* mutation is not removed by deletion, then the introduction of a *trans* C^+ allele, in the absence of inducer, reduces the constitutive expression of *araBAD* enzymes five- to tenfold (Englesberg et al. 1969; Gielow et al. 1971).

The response to the small quantity of P2 present in a C^+ cell in the absence of inducer is also seen in I^c strains. If *araO* *cis* to the *araI* mutation is removed by deletion, then a *trans* C^+ allele, in the absence of inducer, raises the level of *araBAD* enzymes four- to fivefold (Englesberg et al. 1969; Gielow et al. 1971).

The retention of a normal inducible level of *araBAD* expression in I^c mutants, in addition to their sensitivity to P1 and P2 forms of the *araC* protein in the uninduced cell, seems to argue against extensive modification of the regulatory region in AraI mutants, such as deletions joining *araBAD* to an upstream promoter or the introduction of an extraneous segment of DNA which carries a foreign promoter in the correct orientation. The observation that the frequency of *araI* mutations is increased by treatment with base analogs (Gielow et al. 1971) and the fact that none of the transducing phages which carry I^c mutations exhibited altered density in equilibrium centrifugation in CsCl gradients (N. Lee, unpubl.) seem to support such a view.

To date, mutations of the I^c and X^c types (see below) have been reported only in B/r strains. However, extremely slow-growing Ara⁺ revertants can be obtained on minimal arabinose plates for a K12 *araC* strain after aminopurine mutagenesis (P. Frieden and N. Lee, unpubl.).

A group of mutations which may be designated I^o have been described by Eleuterio et al. (1972). These spontaneous mutations, located between the end of the deletion *ara719* and the most proximal point mutation in *araB*, are *cis*-acting mutations which abolish the expression of the whole *araBAD* operon. Interestingly, three of these mutations are cross-suppressible by extragenic suppressor mutations (whose effect on other transcription termination signals has not yet been tested). As pointed out by Eleuterio et al. (1972), it is difficult to exclude the possibility of insertion mutations, and the question of whether an i^o phenotype can arise as a result of a single base change can only be resolved by DNA sequencing.

The *araX* Mutations

A second class of mutations within the initiator region of *araBAD* is designated *araX* (Colomè et al. 1977), *araI* (Wilcox et al. 1974c; Lee et al. 1974), or *ara(CGA)* (Bass et al. 1977). The *araX* mutations have been isolated from parental cells with $I^c\Delta C$ by selecting for faster growth on 0.4% minimal L-arabinose media. The parent strain grew slowly on minimal L-arabinose and formed minute (0.1-mm dia) colonies after 2 days at 37°C (Colomè et al. 1977). Under the same conditions, $I^c X^c$ mutant colonies measured 0.7–0.9 mm in diameter. The *araX* mutations further augment the level of constitutive synthesis of *araBAD* enzymes and, like I^c mutations, are *cis*-dominant. The level of constitutive enzymes rises from 5 to 10% that of the wild type in the parental *araIaraC* to about 30–50% that of the wild type in the *araIaraXaraC* triple mutants (Table 1). In addition, these X^c mutations result in a pronounced reduction in the sensitivity of the *araBAD* operon to catabolite repression, both in vivo (Colomè et al. 1977) and in vitro (N. Lee, unpubl.).

The *araX* mutations do not affect the level of *araBAD* enzymes if the *araC* activator is supplied by a wild-type *C*⁺ allele plus L-arabinose. Under these conditions, the level of *araBAD* expression is identical to that of the wild-type strain (Colomè et al. 1977) (Table 1).

The *araX* mutations also retain sensitivity to P1. In the absence of L-arabinose, the level of *araBAD* in a $C^+I^cX^c$ strain is reduced four- to fivefold below that of the homologous $C^-I^cX^c$ strain. The response to small quantities of P2 found in uninduced C⁺ cells has not been tested with *araX* mutants.

The most striking property of *araX* mutations is their reduced sensitivity to catabolite repression. Four independently isolated *araX* mutations, selected for higher constitutive levels of *araBAD* enzymes than the I^c parents, have all acquired this property as an unselected character. The parental strains, I^cC^-, were all wild type in *cya* and *crp* genes and sensitive to catabolite repression (Bass et al. 1977). If these four *araX* mutations were the result of single mutational events, this would suggest that on *ara* DNA a single modification may abolish the requirement for both positive regulators. The phenotype of insensitivity to catabolite repression has been found to be associated with single base changes in *lac* by Dickson et al. (1975) and Gilbert (1976).

Physical Mapping of the *ara* Regulatory Region

Studies by Schleif and coworkers using electron microscopy have disclosed visible complexes on a fragment of *ara* DNA containing the regulatory region (Hirsh and Schleif 1976). This DNA fragment of approximately 1100 base pairs was obtained by forming heteroduplex molecules between two *ara* transducing phages carrying, in common, a region of *ara* DNA which included the entire regulatory region plus portions of *araB* and *araC* genes. All DNA outside this region was removed by a combination of S_1 nuclease digestion and electrophoretic separation on acrylamide gel slabs (Lis and Schleif 1975a,b). One such visible complex was observed when the DNA fragment was incubated with RNA polymerase, *araC* and CGA proteins, plus L-arabinose and cAMP. It was shown that the position of this complex corresponded to the promoter for the *araBAD* operon.

In addition, a second complex centered at about 100 base pairs to the right (towards *araC*) was formed when D-fucose was substituted for L-arabinose during the preincubation. This was termed a "repression complex," functionally equivalent to the complex between *araC* and *araO* (Hirsh and Schleif 1976).

In a later report, Hirsh and Schleif (1977) obtained a shorter DNA fragment, 440 base pairs long, which contained shorter segments of *araB* and *araC* genes than the fragment employed in the previous study. This 440-base-pair fragment was obtained after digestion with the restriction endonuclease *Hae*III. Since there is a known restriction site for *Hae*III (G-G-C-C-) from position +43 to +47 on *araBAD* messenger RNA (Lee and Carbon 1977), this provides a point of reference for this restriction fragment. Two RNA species were synthesized when this restriction fragment was used as the template DNA in in vitro RNA synthesis. The smaller species of 45 nucleotides was believed to be the *araBAD* RNA. One major species was an RNA fragment of 250 base pairs, believed to be *araC* messenger. These length measurements would then place the start site of *araC* transcription 150 base pairs to the right of the start site for *araBAD* transcription, very near the position of the repression complex previously described (Hirsh and Schleif 1976). Incubation of RNA polymerase with DNA under the conditions used in transcription gave rise to a visible complex under the electron microscope, and the position of the complex corresponded to the start site of *araC* transcription. The relation between this site and the site of the repression complex remained unclear.

THE *araC* GENE

Purification of *araC* Protein

The *araC* gene codes for a protein that has been isolated by a combination of affinity column and DNA-cellulose chromatography (Wilcox et al. 1971b; Wilcox 1972; Wilcox et al. 1974a; Wilcox and Clementson 1974). This procedure took advantage of the specific binding of *araC* protein to the anti-inducer D-fucose. The affinity column contained 4-[4-(4-aminophenyl-)butanamido-]phenyl-β-D-fucopyranoside linked to Sepharose 4B through the 4-amino group of the phenyl moiety. Two passages through a small (1.5×10 cm) column containing 5–10 substituents per milliliter bed volume effected a 300-fold purification of *araC* protein over the crude extract, prepared from 15 g of cells from a strain diploid in *araC* gene (Wilcox and Clementson 1974). Chromatography of an eluate from the affinity column on salmon sperm DNA–cellulose resulted in its further purification to near homogeneity (Wilcox et al. 1974a). This material had a subunit molecular weight of 28,000 daltons, based on the migration rate of the principal band in sodium dodecyl sulfate (SDS)-acrylamide gel electrophoresis. The quantity of protein capable of binding *araO* DNA was estimated to be only 1% of the total in this preparation (Wilcox et al. 1974a). This may partly be due to the lability of *araC* protein under the conditions of its purification, which employed neither L-arabinose nor D-fucose in the buffers.

A more promising approach toward the isolation of *araC* protein of high biological activity appears to involve modification of the buffers to include the protease inhibitor phenylmethylsulfonyl fluoride and the ligand L-arabinose (Yang and Zubay 1973; Wilcox and Meuris 1976). Utilizing the ability of *araC* activator to stimulate enzyme synthesis in vitro (Greenblatt and Schleif 1971; Yang and Zubay 1973; Wilcox et al. 1974c), the purification of *araC* protein can be monitored without complications due to the presence of L-arabinose in the buffers. A combination of ammonium-sulfate fractionation, DNA-cellulose chromatography, and glycerol-gradient centrifugation has yielded *araC* protein highly active in promoting transcription of the *araBAD* operon in vitro (Lee et al. 1974). This material, however, was only about 50% pure, as judged by the quantity of the 28,000-dalton molecular-weight species in gel electrophoresis. The activator activity of partially purified *araC* protein appears to be more stable at slightly acid pH, and there is an increase in the thermal lability of the protein with purification (Wilcox and Meuris 1976).

The coupled assay for *araC* activity has been used to characterize this protein in the absence of extensive purification. It was found that *araC* protein sedimented in linear 5–20% glycerol gradients in the Spinco SW 65 rotor with a rate midway between those of bovine serum albumin (m.w. 67,000) and ovalbumin (m.w. 45,000), corresponding to a sedimentation coefficient of 4S and a molecular weight of about 60,000 daltons (Wilcox and Meuris 1976). No alteration in the sedimentation profile was detected when D-fucose was substituted for L-arabinose in the gradient, indicating either that the expected conformational change did not occur under these conditions or that the change was not associated with a discernible change in the sedimentation rate.

Difficulty with the isolation of *araC* in a homogeneous, highly active state, and in large quantity, has hindered its structural characterization. The presence of a band of 28,000-dalton molecular weight upon electrophoresis in SDS-acrylamide gels in all fractions containing *araC* activity, taken in conjunction with the sedimentation properties of the native protein, suggests that the native protein consists of two polypeptides of equal size (Wilcox and Meuris 1976).

Regulation of *araC*

Recently, Casadaban (1976) investigated the regulation of *araC*. Creating a region of homology by inserting mu phage genomes into *araC* and into a lambda transducing phage carrying a *lacZ* gene fused to the *trp* operon, Casadaban succeeded in inserting the *lacZ* gene near *araC* by a crossover within the prophage mu, ending with *lacZ* and *araC* oriented in the same direction. The presence of a heat-sensitive repressor gene on the mu phage permitted the selection of mu phage deletions, some of which had fused the *lacZ* gene to the *araC* promoter. Three independently isolated *araC-lacZ* fusion strains, recognized on the basis that they produced low constitutive levels of β-galactosidase, were employed in the study of *araC* regulation. Into these strains, which lacked a functional *araC* gene, were introduced episomes carrying various alleles of *araC*, and the measurement of β-galactosidase activity provided a convenient assay for *araC* expression. The finding that a *trans* C^+ allele repressed the level of β-galactosidase tenfold suggested an autogenous regulation of *araC* expression by its own product. A mutational allele (either C^-_{amber} or C^c) in the *trans* position either diminished or abolished the repression, indicating that this epistatic effect on β-galactosidase synthesis was associated with the *araC* gene product itself.

At present it is not known whether this effect of *araC* protein on its own synthesis is exerted at the level of transcription through a repressor-operator type of interaction. Addition of L-arabinose to *araC* protein produces a shift in its conformation toward the activator form (Wilcox 1974). Although this shift has a pronounced effect on *araBAD* operon expression, it does not appear to affect the expression of the *araC* gene (Casabadan 1976). It was suggested that the putative operator for *araC* binds both P1 and P2 forms of *araC* protein and that this operator might have been the site which bound *araC* protein in the nitrocellulose assay (Wilcox et al. 1974a; Casabadan 1976). Alternatively, that which binds the putative *araC* operator may be a derivative of the *araC* protein, formed by the complexing of *araC* to an as yet undefined component, and as such does not dissociate from its operator in the presence of L-arabinose. In vitro experiments (Hirsh and Schleif 1977) indicate that the induction of *araBAD* somehow interferes with the initiation of *araC* transcription; thus, in the presence of L-arabinose, derepression of *araC* may be offset by an inhibition of its transcription by the activation of *araBAD cis* to the *araC* gene.

The above study (Casadaban 1976) also demonstrated that the expression of *araC* was sensitive to catabolite repression. A threefold reduction in *araC* is observed in vivo when the strain is *crp cya*. A similar reduction is observed in vitro when the CGA protein is omitted from the synthesis mixture (Hirsh and Schleif 1977).

The *Cⁱ* and *Cʰ* Alleles

Two classes of *araC* mutations have been isolated recently. One class, termed C^i, was detected by Heffernan et al. (1976) in Ara⁺ revertants of a *cya crp* strain which contained wild-type *ara* genes. By plating on minimal 0.2% L-arabinose agar plates—conditions which required the entire *ara* regulon to be induced in the absence of cAMP and CGA protein—47 spontaneous and mutagen-induced revertants were isolated. Eleven of these mutations, all 2-aminopurine-induced, were shown to be located in *araC* by their map position and their ability to confer catabolite insensitivity to *trans araBAD* genes. One of these mutations, *araC^i1*, was analyzed in detail. It produced a higher basal level of *araBAD* enzymes in the absence of L-arabinose, about ten times that of the wild type. The differential rates of isomerase and permease synthesis in minimal glucose and minimal glycerol media were both higher than those of the wild type in minimal glycerol. In an in vitro DNA-dependent protein-synthesis system (Heffernan and Wilcox 1976), when an extract of *araC^i1* was used as a source of *araC* protein to activate isomerase synthesis, it was found that the extract could activate isomerase synthesis, without added cAMP in the system, to 50% of the +cAMP level. When the quantities of isomerase synthesized as a function of the concentration of added cAMP were compared between *araC^i1* and the wild-type extracts, it was found that the maximal level of isomerase synthesis with the *araC^i1* extract was attained at much lower concentrations of cAMP (100-fold lower than in the case of the wild type). The *araC^i1* protein also appeared to be more thermolabile than the wild-type product, suggesting a structural modification in *araC*.

A second class of mutations in *araC*, designated *araC^h*, was detected by Gendron and Sheppard (Gendron and Sheppard 1974; Sheppard and Eleuterio 1976). Strains with the *araD* mutation *araD139* were sensitive to L-arabinose in its growth medium due to the defective 4-epimerase gene (Englesberg et al. 1962; Boyer et al. 1962). Direct selection for strains with secondary mutations which are resistant to arabinose in the presence of glucose but remain sensitive to arabinose in the absence of glucose yielded two mutants which showed an increased sensitivity to catabolite repression of *araBAD*. This increased sensitivity was specific for *ara*; the *lac* operon was not affected. These mutations occurred in the *araC* gene or its controlling sites, since they confer catabolite hypersensitivity to *trans araBAD* genes.

The finding that mutations in *araC* could alter the sensitivity of *araBAD* operon to catabolite repression raised questions concerning the functions of these two positive regulators and how they are interrelated. In *lac* and *gal* operons, it has been postulated that the binding of CGA protein to DNA facilitates local denaturation of the DNA helix by RNA polymerase (Dickson et al. 1975; Musso et al. 1977). The initiator region of *araBAD* differs from the *lac* and *gal* promoters in that the presence of CGA protein is not sufficient to effect a productive interaction between RNA polymerase and DNA. This might conceivably be due to the following: (1) A CGA binding site is unavailable unless *araC* activator is bound to a neighboring site. (2) A binding site similar to the CGA binding site exists in *ara* which could only bind a complex of *araC* activator and CGA protein. (3) Two discrete binding sites on *ara* DNA (for CGA and *araC* proteins) must both be occupied to effect interaction between RNA polymerase and DNA. (4) The binding of *araC* activator to either RNA polymerase or DNA is required for the recognition of a promoter site which has been activated by CGA protein. (5) The binding of *araC* to either RNA polymerase or DNA is required for continued RNA synthesis beyond a termination signal. The distinction between schemes 1 and 3 is that *araC* does not affect the telestability of *ara* DNA directly in scheme 1. In schemes 4 and 5, the structural modification resulting from the *araC^i* mutation would alter the interaction with RNA polymerase or DNA in such a way that the requirement for CGA activation was bypassed. These and other more complex schemes may be postulated, but all require experimental support.

ACKNOWLEDGMENTS

The author is grateful to Drs. R. Schleif and G. Wilcox for communicating unpublished DNA sequence data. This work is supported by grant GM-14652 from the U.S. Public Health Service.

REFERENCES

Bachman, B. J., B. K. Low, and A. L. Taylor. 1976. Recalibrated linkage map of *Escherichia coli* K12. *Bact. Rev.* **40**:116.

Bass, R., L. Heffernan, K. Sweadner, and E. Englesberg. 1977. The site for catabolite deactivation in the L-arabinose BAD operon in *Escherichia coli* B/r. *Arch. Microbiol.* **110**:135.

Beverin, S., D. E. Sheppard, and S. S. Park. 1971. D-Fucose as a gratuitous inducer of the L-arabinose operon in strains of *Escherichia coli* B/r mutant in gene *araC*. *J. Bacteriol.* **107**:79.

Boyer, H., E. Englesberg, and R. Weinberg. 1962. Direct selection of L-arabinose negative mutants of *Escherichia coli* strain B/r. *Genetics* **45**:412.

Boulter, J. and N. Lee. 1975. Isolation of specialized transducing bacteriophage lambda carrying genes of the L-arabinose operon of *Escherichia coli* B/r. *J. Bacteriol.* **123**:1043.

Brown, C. E. and R. Hogg. 1972. A second transport system for L-arabinose in *Escherichia coli* B/r controlled by the *araC* gene. *J. Bacteriol.* **111**:606.

Casadaban, M. 1976. Regulation of the regulatory gene for the arabinose pathway, *araC*. *J. Mol. Biol.* **104**:557.

Clarke, L. and J. Carbon. 1975. Biochemical construction and selection of hybrid plasmids containing specific segments of the *Escherichia coli* genome. *Proc. Natl. Acad. Sci.* **72**:4361.

Colomè, J., G. Wilcox, and E. Englesberg. 1977. Constitutive mutations in the controlling site region of the *araBAD* operon of *Escherichia coli* B/r that decrease sensitivity to catabolite repression. *J. Bacteriol.* **129**:948.

Dickson, R., J. Abelson, W. Barnes, and W. Reznikoff. 1975. Genetic regulation: The *lac* control region. *Science* **187**:27.

Doyle, M. E., C. Brown, R. Hogg, and R. B. Helling. 1972. Induction of the *ara* operon of *Escherichia coli* B/r. *J. Bacteriol.* **110**:56.

Eleuterio, M., B. Griffin, and D. E. Sheppard. 1972. Characterization of strong polar mutations in a region immediately adjacent to the L-arabinose operator in *Escherichia coli* B/r. *J. Bacteriol.* **11**:373.

Englesberg, E. 1961. Enzymatic characterization of 17 arabinose negative mutants of *Escherichia coli*. *J. Bacteriol.* **81**:996.

————. 1971. Regulation in the L-arabinose system. In *Metabolic pathways: Metabolic regulation* (ed. H. J. Vogel), vol. 1, p. 257. Academic Press. New York.

Englesberg, E. and G. Wilcox. 1974. Regulation: Positive control. *Annu. Rev. Genet.* **8**:219.

Englesberg, E., C. Squires, and F. Moronk. 1969. The L-arabinose operon in *Escherichia coli* B/r: A genetic demonstration of two functional states of the product of a regulatory gene. *Proc. Natl. Acad. Sci.* **62**:1100.

Englesberg, E., J. Irr, J. Power, and N. Lee. 1965. Positive control of enzyme synthesis by gene *C* in the L-arabinose system. *J. Bacteriol.* **90**:946.

Englesberg, E., R. L. Anderson, R. Weinberg, N. Lee, P. Hoffee, G. Huttenhauer, and H. Boyer. 1962. L-Arabinose sensitive, L-ribulose 5-phosphate 4-epimerase deficient mutants of *Escherichia coli* B/r. *J. Bacteriol.* **84**:137.

Gendron, R. P. and D. E. Sheppard. 1974. Mutations in the L-arabinose operon of *Escherichia coli* B/r that result in hypersensitivity to catabolite repression. *J. Bacteriol.* **117**:417.

Gielow, L., M. Largen, and E. Englesberg. 1971. Initiator constituting mutants of the L-arabinose operon (OIBAD) of *Escherichia coli* B/r. *Genetics* **69**:289.

Gilbert, W. 1976. Starting and stopping sequences for the RNA polymerase. In *RNA polymerase* (ed. R. Losick and M. Chamberlin), p. 193. Cold Spring Harbor Laboratory, Cold Spring Harbor, New York.

Gottesman, S. 1971. A generalizable method for isolation of regulatory protein. Ph.D. thesis, Harvard University, Cambridge, Massachusetts.

Gottesman, S. and J. R. Beckwith. 1969. Directed transposition of the L-arabinose operon: A technique for the isolation of specialized transducing bacteriophages for any *Escherichia coli* gene. *J. Mol. Biol.* **44**:117.

Greenblatt, J. and R. Schleif. 1971. Arabinose C protein—Regulation of the arabinose operon *in vitro*. *Nat. New Biol.* **233**:166.

Gross, J. and E. Englesberg. 1959. Determination of the order of mutational sites governing L-arabinose utilization in *Escherichia coli* B/r by transduction with phage P1bt. *Virology* **9**:314.

Heffernan, L. and G. Wilcox. 1976. Effect of *araC* product on catabolite repression in the L-arabinose regulon. *J. Bacteriol.* **126**:1132.

Heffernan, L., R. Bass, and E. Englesberg. 1976. Mutations affecting catabolite repression of the L-arabinose regulon in *Escherichia coli* B/r. *J. Bacteriol.* **126**:1119.

Helling, R. B. and R. Weinberg. 1963. Complementation studies of L-arabinose genes in *Escherichia coli*. *Genetics* **48**:1397.

Hirsh, J. and R. Schleif. 1976. Electron microscopy of gene regulation: The L-arabinose operon. *Proc. Natl. Acad. Sci.* **73**:1518.

————. 1977. The *araC* promoter: Transcription mapping and interaction with *araBAD* promoter. *Cell* **11**:545.

Hogg, R. and E. Englesberg. 1969. L-Arabinose binding protein from *Escherichia coli* B/r. *J. Bacteriol.* **100**:423.

Irr, J. and E. Englesberg. 1971. Control of expression of the L-arabinose operon in temperature sensitive mutants of gene *araC* in *Escherichia coli* B/r. *J. Bacteriol.* **105**:136.

Kaplan, D. A., L. Greenfield, T. Boone, and G. Wilcox. 1978. Hybrid plasmids containing the *araBAD* genes of *Escherichia coli*. Gene (in press).

Katz, L. 1970. Selection of *araB* and *araC* mutants of *Escherichia coli* B/r by resistance to ribitol. *J. Bacteriol* **102**:593.

Katz, L. and E. Englesberg. 1971. Hyperinducibility as a result of mutation in structural genes and self-catabolite repression in the *ara* operon. *J. Bacteriol.* **107**:34.

Kessler, D. P. and E. Englesberg. 1969. Arabinose-leucine deletion mutants of *Escherichia coli* B/r. *J. Bacteriol.* **98**:1159.

Lee, N. and I. Bendet. 1967. Crystalline L-ribulokinase from *Escherichia coli*. *J. Biol. Chem.* **242**:2043.

Lee, N. and J. A. Carbon. 1977. Nucleotide sequence of the 5' end of *araBAD* operon messenger RNA in *Escherichia coli* B/r. *Proc. Natl. Acad. Sci.* **74**:49.

Lee, N. and E. Englesberg. 1962. Dual effect of structural genes in *Escherichia coli*. *Proc. Natl. Acad. Sci.* **48**:335.

Lee, N. and J. W. Patrick. 1970. Subunit structure of L-ribulokinase from *Escherichia coli*. *J. Biol. Chem.* **245**:1357.

Lee, N., J. W. Patrick, and M. Mason. 1968. Crystalline L-ribulose 5-phosphate 4-epimerase from *Escherichia coli*. *J. Biol. Chem.* **243**:4700.

Lee, N., G. Wilcox, W. Gielow, J. Arnold, P. Cleary, and E. Englesberg. 1974. *In vitro* activation of the transcription of *araBAD* operon by *araC* activator. *Proc. Natl. Acad. Sci.* **71**:634.

Lis, J. T. and R. Schleif. 1973. The isolation and characterization of plaque-forming arabinose transducing bacteriophage λ. *J. Mol. Biol.* **95**:395.

————. 1975. The regulatory region of the L-arabinose operon. Its isolation on a 1000-base-pair fragment from DNA heteroduplexes. *J. Mol. Biol.* **95**:409.

Maxam, A. M. and W. Gilbert. 1977. A new method for sequencing DNA. *Proc. Natl. Acad. Sci.* **74**:560.

Musso, R., R. DiLauro, M. E. Rosenberg, and B. de Crombrugghe. 1977. Nucleotide sequence of the operator-promoter region of the galactose operon of *Escherichia coli*. *Proc. Natl. Acad. Sci.* **74**:106.

Nathanson, N. M. and R. Schleif. 1975. Paucity of sites mutable to constitutivity in the *araC* activator gene of the L-arabinose operon of *Escherichia coli*. *J. Mol. Biol.* **96**:185.

Novotny, C. and E. Englesberg. 1966. The L-arabinose permease system in *Escherichia coli* B/r. *Biochim. Biophys. Acta* **117**:217.

Parsons, R. and R. Hogg. 1974. Crystallization and characterization of the L-arabinose binding protein of *Escherichia coli* B/r. *J. Biol. Chem.* **249**:3602.

Patrick, J. W. and N. Lee. 1968. Purification and properties of an L-arabinose isomerase from *Escherichia coli*. *J. Biol. Chem.* **243**:4312.

————. 1969. Subunit structure of L-arabinose isomerase from *Escherichia coli*. *J. Biol. Chem.* **244**:4277.

Power, J. and J. Irr. 1973. Regulatory gene control of transcription of the L-arabinose operon in *Escherichia coli. J. Biol. Chem.* **248:**7806.

Pribnow, D. 1975. Nucleotide sequence of an RNA polymerase binding site at an early T7 promoter. *Proc. Natl. Acad. Sci.* **72:**784.

Schleif, R., 1972. Fine structure deletion map of the *Escherichia coli* L-arabinose operon. *Proc. Natl. Acad. Sci.* **69:**3479.

Schleif, R. 1969. An arabinose binding protein and arabinose permeation in *Escherichia coli. J. Mol. Biol.* **46:**185.

Schleif, R. and J. T. Lis. 1975. The regulatory region of the L-arabinose operon: A physical, genetic and physiological study. *J. Mol. Biol.* **95:**417.

Schleif, R., J. Greenblatt, and R. Davis. 1971. Dual control of arabinose genes on transducing phage λd*ara. J. Mol. Biol.* **59:**127.

Sheppard, D. E. and M. Eleuterio. 1976. Hypersensitivity to catabolite repression in the L-arabinose operon of *Escherichia coli* B/r is *trans* acting. *J. Bacteriol.* **126:**1014.

Sheppard, D. E. and E. Englesberg. 1967a. Positive control in the L-arabinose gene-enzyme complex of *Escherichia coli* B/r as exhibited with stable merodiploids. *Cold Spring Harbor Symp. Quant. Biol.* **31:**345.

———. 1967b. Further evidence for positive control of the L-arabinose system by gene *araC. J. Mol. Biol.* **25:**443.

Shimada, K., R. Weisberg, and M. E. Gottesman. 1972. Prophage lambda at unusual chromosmal locations. I. Location of the secondary attachment sites and the properties of the lysogens. *J. Mol. Biol.* **63:**483.

Squires, C., F. Lee, K. Bertrand, C. L. Squires, M. J. Bronson, and C. Yanofsky. 1976. Nucleotide sequence of the 5' end of tryptophan messenger RNA of *Escherichia coli. J. Mol. Biol.* **103:**351.

Steitz, J. A. and K. Jakes. 1975. How ribosomes select initiator regions in mRNA: Base pair formation between the 3' terminals of 16S rRNA and the mRNA during initiation of protein synthesis in *Escherichia coli. Proc. Natl. Acad. Sci.* **74:**49.

Wilcox, G. 1972. "*AraC* protein from *Escherichia coli.*" Ph.D. thesis, University of California, Santa Barbara.

———. 1974. The interaction of L-arabinose and D-fucose with *araC* protein. *J. Biol. Chem.* **249:**6892.

Wilcox, G. and K. J. Clementson. 1974. AraC protein. *Methods Enzymol.* **34:**368.

Wilcox, G. and P. Meuris. 1976. Stabilization and size of *araC* protein. *Mol. Gen. Genet.* **145:**97.

Wilcox, G., J. Boulter, and N. Lee. 1974a. Direction of transcription of the regulatory gene *araC* in *Escherichia coli* B/r. *Proc. Natl. Acad. Sci.* **71:**3635.

Wilcox, G., J. Singer, and L. Heffernan. 1971a. Deoxyribonucleic acid-ribonucleic acid hybridization studies on the L-arabinose operon of *Escherichia coli* B/r. *J. Bacteriol.* **108:**1.

Wilcox, G., K. J. Clementson, P. Cleary, and E. Englesberg. 1974b. Interaction of the regulatory gene product with the operator site in the L-arabinose operon of *Escherichia coli. J. Mol. Biol.* **85:**589.

Wilcox, G., K. J. Clementson, D. Santé, and E. Englesberg. 1971b. Purification of the *araC* protein. *Proc. Natl. Acad. Sci.* **68:**2145.

Wilcox, G., P. Meuris, R. Bass, and E. Englesberg. 1974c. Regulation of the L-arabinose operon *BAD in vitro. J. Biol. Chem.* **249**:2946.

Yang, H.-L. and G. Zubay. 1973. Synthesis of the arabinose operon regulator protein in a cell-free system. *Mol. Gen. Genet.* **122**:131.

Zubay, G., L. Gielow, and E. Englesberg. 1971. Cell free studies on the regulation of the arabinose operon. *Nat. New Biol.* **223**:164.

Zubay, G., D. Schwartz, and J. Beckwith. 1970. Mechanism of activation of catabolite-sensitive genes: A positive control system. *Proc. Natl. Acad. Sci.* **66**:104.

The Mechanism of Phase Variation

Janine Zieg, Michael Silverman, Marcia Hilmen,
and Melvin I. Simon
Department of Biology
University of California, San Diego
La Jolla, California 92093

INTRODUCTION

Studies of the properties of the *lac* operon have formed the basis for our understanding of a number of regulatory mechanisms. The *lac* operon model focuses attention on systems that involve the binding of repressor or activator proteins to sites adjacent to structural genes, leading to enhanced expression or to repression of gene activity. There are, however, many observations involving the regulation of gene activity which cannot be explained by mechanisms analogous to the *lac* operon. For example in yeast, the interconversion of mating types (Hicks et al. 1977) is best explained by a model involving site-specific recombination, i.e., gene expression requires the transposition of genetic material from one chromosomal locus to another. In the *Zea mays* genetic system, McClintock (1957) recognized and identified transposable chromosomal elements that control the functions of a variety of genes. Many other observations in genetic systems as varied as *Drosophila* (Green 1977), *Paramecium* (Sonnenborn 1977), and *Escherichia coli* (Starlinger and Saedler 1972) are most readily explained by invoking a specific recombination event, e.g., an inversion or transposition, or some other kind of modification that changes the state of the gene and thus affects its expression. However, very little is known about the exact molecular events that occur in any of these systems.

Just as the development of genetic systems in *E. coli* allowed an analysis of the mechanism of regulation of the *lac* operon, so the introduction of gene cloning techniques allows a direct examination of DNA that might be involved in site-specific recombinational events that affect regulation. Using these techniques to study the phase-variation system in *Salmonella*, we have been able to demonstrate a change at the DNA level that correlates with gene expression. *Salmonella* strains have two genes that determine the structure of the flagellar filament subunit protein, flagellin. These genes are located on opposite sides of the *Salmonella* genome and they are expressed alternatively (Iino 1977; Silverman and Simon 1977a). Thus, a strain of *Salmonella* which is in phase 1 assembles its flagellum using the product of the *H1* gene, and a cell expressing phase 2 uses the *H2*-gene product. Strains can switch from one phase to the other at frequencies on the order of 10^{-3} to 10^{-5} per cell/per generation. Lederberg and Iino (1956) showed that the ability to switch from one gene to the other is controlled by a genetic element linked to the *H2* gene and that the state of this element can be transduced. They suggested, therefore, that the phase transition involves a change in the structure of the genetic material.

To determine the nature of the structural change in the DNA, we prepared hybrid DNA molecules which carried the *Salmonella H2* gene and other molecules carrying the *Salmonella H1* gene (Zieg et al. 1977a,b). It has been shown that the *Salmonella* phase-variation genes can be transferred on exogenetic elements into *E. coli* (Makela 1964; Pearce and Stocker 1967; Enomoto and Stocker 1975) and still be fully functional with respect to expression of *H1* and *H2* activities and the ability to show phase variation. Therefore, we, studied the expression of these genes after transformation of an *E. coli* mutant that lacked the structural gene for flagellin (*hag*). There was nothing anomalous about the expression of the *H1* gene. However, cells carrying the *H2* gene showed the same pattern of transient expression observed in the parent *Salmonella* strain, i.e., transition from the ability to make *H2* flagella to the inability to form flagella. The DNA carrying the *H1* gene was examined by electron microscopy both before and after denaturation and renaturation, and no anomalous structures were found. However, when the DNA carrying the *H2* gene was examined after denaturation and renaturation, a fraction of the molecules showed an anomalous "bubble" structure. The DNA carrying the *H2* gene was also cloned onto a bacteriophage lambda vehicle. We could separate two kinds of bacteriophages in all of the clones. Both carried the *H2* gene; however, one gave low levels of abortive transduction and was assumed to be in the "off" state, and the other gave high levels of transduction and was assumed to be in the "on" state. When DNA extracted from each of these virus populations was denatured and renatured with itself, a very low frequency of molecules with the anomalous structure was observed by electron microscopy. However, when the DNA from the two different virus populations was heteroduplexed, a very high frequency of molecules carrying the anomaly was observed (Zieg et al. 1977a). These results lead us to conclude that the mechanism illustrated in Figure 1 is involved in regulating the expression of the *H2* gene.

We have suggested that the region involved in the bubble structure is the genetic element that regulates *H2*-gene expression. It presumably carries a promoter and includes specific sites which are recognized by an enzyme that can catalyze the inversion of the element. When the region is in one orientation, the promoter is coupled to the *H2* gene; this results in *H2*-gene expression. When the sequence is inverted, the promoter and the *H2* gene are uncoupled, thus eliminating *H2*-gene expression. This model makes the following predictions: (1) The DNA that codes for the

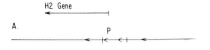

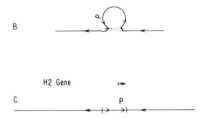

Figure 1 Model for the phase transition. (*A*) Promoter initiates transcription which proceeds through the *H2* gene. (*B*) Specific sites are recognized and a cross-over occurs at these sites. (*C*) In the resulting structure, the region is inverted and the promoter can no longer initiate *H2* transcription.

H2-gene product is adjacent to or overlaps the region that is observed as the bubble structure. (2) The bubble structure is formed as a result of a specific inversion. (3) There are specific sites at which this inversion occurs, presumably at the end of the 800-base-pair (bp) region that forms the bubble structure. (4) An *H2*-specific promoter is included in the inversion region. In this chapter, we present evidence that supports the first two predictions and clearly shows that the observed anomaly is the result of a specific, *recA*-independent inversion.

MATERIALS AND METHODS

Hybrid Molecules

Hybrid plasmids were obtained by two independent methods: (1) *Salmonella* DNA was treated with *Eco*RI endonuclease and these fragments were introduced into the *Eco*RI site on colicinogenic factor E1 as previously described (Zieg et al. 1977a). The DNA that carried the *H2*-gene activity (pJZ1) was treated with *Sal*I endonuclease and an abbreviated fragment, pJZ60, was isolated (Fig. 2). (2) *Salmonella* DNA was sheared, and the fragments were introduced into the *Pst*I endonuclease site on the plasmid by the method of Otsuka (1978), which involves the addition of polydeoxycytidine and polydeoxyguanine "tails" onto the insert and the plasmid. This approach has been described (Zieg et al. 1977b). The technique allows subsequent treatment of the hybrid with *Pst*I endonuclease to remove the insert. The plasmid pJZ100 was formed in this way. The endonuclease map of the plasmid was derived from analyses of double digestion with restriction enzymes followed by agarose gel electrophoresis (Zieg et al. 1977b). Fragments of pJZ100 were further cloned after pJZ100 was treated with *Pst*I using the plasmid pBR322 (Bolivar et al. 1977) as vehicle. After transformation clones carrying an insert were selected and individual clones were grown up, DNA was

H2 gene

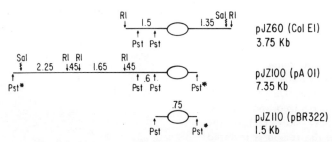

Figure 2   Restriction maps of inserted *Salmonella* DNA. pJZ60 was derived from pJZ1 by restriction of the plasmid with *Sal*I followed by ligation. The pJZ100 fragment was obtained after random shearing of the *Salmonella* DNA. The *Pst*I sites are created in the process of attaching the insert to the vehicle (Otsuka 1978). pJZ110 was derived from pJZ100 by restriction with *Pst*I. The lengths of the segments, given in kilobase pairs, were determined by electron microscopy and by agarose gel electrophoresis.

isolated and analyzed by restriction and agarose gel electrophoresis. In this way, the plasmid carrying pJZ110 (Fig. 2) was obtained.

The insert DNA was prepared as follows. The whole plasmid was treated with restriction enzyme, and the products separated by agarose gel electrophoresis. The band corresponding to the insert DNA was then cut out of the gel. To extract the DNA, the agarose was crushed and the supernatant liquid containing the fragment was removed. Electroelution was also used to extract the DNA. The fragment was precipitated at −20°C with 2.5 volumes of ethanol after the addition of sodium acetate to a final concentration of 0.3 M.

The large-scale preparation of plasmid DNA and the conditions for endonuclease restriction, DNA ligation, transformation, and agarose gel electrophoresis were the same as those described by Bolivar et al. (1977).

Restriction enzymes and other enzymes were purchased from BRL (Bethesda, Maryland).

Bacterial Strains

The strains used to test the effects of the *recA* gene on the frequency of inversion were HB101 (*pro, leu, thi, lacY, str*, r_k^-, m_k^-, *recA*) and MS987 (*leu, thi, thr, hag, recA67*). The primary recipient strain that was used to test for the presence of the *H2* gene was a derivative of C600 (r_k^-, m_k^-, *hag*⁻), previously described (Zieg et al. 1977a). *Salmonella* DNA was extracted from SL4213 obtained from B. Stocker. The strain used to test for *trp*-gene activity was JMB9, a derivative of C600 that carries a *trpB*-*E* deletion (Selker et al. 1977). The pJZ60 fragment was mixed with *Eco* RI-treated pES9 (Selker et al. 1977) and ligated. The resulting mixture was used to transform JMB9, and C600 *hag*, kanamycin-resistant clones were selected. These were grown and spread onto rich plates; individual clones were picked and stabbed into minimal plates and into minimal plates containing indole or into motility plates.

RESULTS

The *H2* Gene Is Adjacent to the Bubble Structure

Figure 2 shows the restriction maps of the DNA that were obtained from clones carrying *H2*-gene activity. It is clear that the region adjacent to the bubble structure, on the left-hand side, is responsible for the *H2*-gene activity. Deletions removing that part of the DNA also eliminate *H2*-gene activity, whereas deletions removing material from the right-hand side of the bubble structure have no effect on *H2*-gene activity or on the formation of the bubble structure. Thus, for example, in pJZ100, only a 300-bp portion of DNA remains on the right side of the bubble; however, the pJZ100 plasmid completely maintains *H2*-gene activity. On the other hand, removal of material from the left side (e.g., pJZ110) leads to a complete loss of *H2*-gene activity. The *H2*-gene product, flagellin, is composed of about 500 amino acids (Kondoh and Hotani 1974) and would require a gene which includes at least 1500 bp. The *H2*-gene region on pJZ60 (Fig. 2) contains 1.5 kilobase pairs (kbp). Thus the gene must be adjacent to or partly contained within the bubble region.

Mutations in the *recA* gene had little or no effect on the formation of the bubble structure in pJZ60, pJZ100, and pJZ110. All of these plasmids were transformed into strain HB101 which carries *recA* and into strain MS987 which carries the *recA67* allele. A number of clones were picked, and the DNA isolated and examined by electron microscopy. After denaturation and renaturation, the bubble structures appeared with approximately the same frequency in both the *recA* and the wild-type cells. Therefore, the event that forms the bubble is not dependent on the *recA* system of the host cell.

The Bubble Is the Result of a Specific Inversion

The simplest interpretation of the bubble structure is that it results from a specific inversion. To determine if such an inversion is indeed involved, two kinds of experiments were done. First, we used heteroduplex formation and electron microscopy to find structures that are diagnostic of inversions. Second, we used a series of restriction enzymes to look for a distinctive pattern which could only result from sequence inversion.

Heteroduplex Analysis

The inversion model predicts that, during heteroduplex formation, some of the molecules should associate through the sequences in the inverted region. This would result in the formation of structures where the inverted region is paired and the regions outside the inversions are single-stranded (Hsu and Davidson 1974). Figure 3A shows such a structure, derived from heteroduplexes formed with pJZ110 DNA. Even more diagnostic structures were obtained when pJZ110 DNA was heteroduplexed with pJZ60 DNA. In this structure, shown in Figure 3B, the double-stranded region corresponds in length to the bubble and the single-stranded arms correspond to the length of the arms of pJZ60 and pJZ110. Finally, one would expect that if many of the structures shown in Figure 3B were formed, they occasionally could interact with each other. In such cases, the single-stranded arms would be able to pair, and then a complex structure composed of double-stranded DNA would be formed. Such structures are shown in Figure 3C. In this case, each side of the

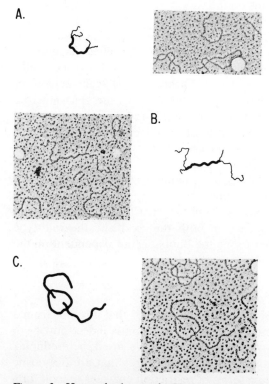

A.

B.

C.

Figure 3 Heteroduplexes of pJZ60 and pJZ110. (*A*) An example of a structure found after denaturation and renaturation of pJZ110. The dark region indicates the region that is thought to be composed of double-stranded DNA. (*B*) An example of a structure found after denaturation and renaturation of equal amounts of pJZ60 and pJZ110. (*C*) Another kind of structure found after hybridization of pJZ60 and pJZ110.

bubble is made ɪp of double-stranded DNA; the arms are double-stranded and correspond in length to the arms of pJZ60 and pJZ110, respectively. Therefore, these structures indicate that the bubble observed in heteroduplexes of DNA carrying the *H2* gene is the result of the inversion of a specific sequence of approximately 800 bp.

Restriction Enzyme Analysis

To further determine if the region involved in the bubble structure resulted from an inversion, we prepared DNA from the plasmid pJZ110. After treatment with endonuclease *Pst*I and agarose gel electrophoresis, a small, 1500-bp fragment of DNA could be isolated. This DNA appeared as a single band and it was extracted from the gel. The DNA was treated with restriction enzyme, and Figure 4 shows the results of *Hae*II

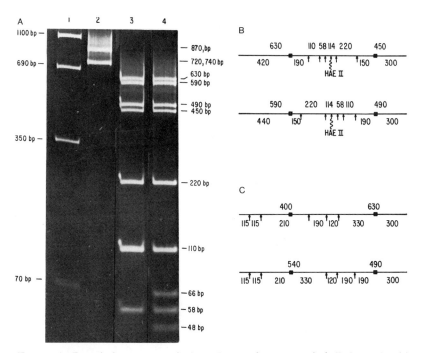

Figure 4 Restriction maps of the pJZ110 fragment. (*A*) Polyacrylamide gel electrophoresis of endonuclease digests of the 1.5-kbp pJZ110 fragment. The numbers at the left indicate the relative sizes of the marker DNA bands. (1) *Hae*II digest of *Eco*RI marker DNA; (2) *Hae*II digestion products of pJZ110; (3) *Hae*III digestion products; (4) *Hae*III and *Hae*II double digestion. (*B*) Map of the *Hae*III and *Hae*II sites. (*C*) Map of the *Hpa*II sites. The numbers above the line in the segment with the black box represent the bands actually found on the agarose gel. The numbers below the line are inferred, as is the position of the small black box on the line, which represents the region in which the inversion occurs.

digestion. There appears to be a single *Hae*II site approximately in the middle of the molecule. However, the situation is a bit more complicated because, when the agarose gel was run for a longer time, each of the single bands appeared to split into two different bands. The lower band appears to include 720- and 740-bp fragments, and the upper band appears to be composed of 840- and 880-bp components. This complexity is seen more clearly in the *Hae*III digestion of the 1500-bp DNA fragment. The DNA was digested with *Hae*II and *Hae*III. The double digestion resulted in the appearance of two new bands corresponding to DNA fragments of 66 bp and 48 bp. These must be derived from a 114-bp fragment which coelectrophoresed with the 110-bp fragment in the *Hae*III digestion. Since the *Hae*II restriction site appears to be in the middle of the 1.5-kbp molecule, the 114-bp *Hae*III fragment must also be in the middle of the molecule. If all of the fragments resolved by electrophoresis of the *Hae*III digest of the 1.5-kbp molecule are added up, the total is 2600 bp—almost twice as much as the initial fragment. This suggests that the initial fragment was heterogeneous with respect to its sequence and that, although the *Hae*II restriction site is in the middle of the molecule, some of the *Hae*III sites are located asymmetrically with respect to the DNA region that undergoes inversion. This could account for the additional fragments. Figure 4B shows the restriction map derived from partial digests with *Hae*III and from double digests with the enzyme *Hpa*II. The map is consistent with the presence of a specific inversion. The doublets observed at the top of agarose gels of the *Hae*III digest are the result of the asymmetric position of the *Hae*III cuts within the region that inverts. Digestion at one of these sites generates two alternative fragments, one from each of the orientations of the inverted sequence. A similar pattern was found in digests of the 1500-bp molecule by *Hpa*II. DNA fragments with molecular weights corresponding to 630 bp and 540 bp, 490 bp and 400 bp, as well as digestion products corresponding to 190 bp and 120 bp, were all found in the limit digest. Each of these fragments was labeled at the 5′ terminus by [γ-^{32}P]ATP and polynucleotide kinase (Maxam and Gilbert 1977). When the end-labeled *Hpa*II fragments were digested with *Hae*III and the products analyzed by polyacrylamide gel electrophoresis, all of the fragments found were consistent with the map shown in Figure 4B and C. We conclude, therefore, that the restriction enzyme data indicate the presence of an 800-bp inversion in the central part of the 1500-bp fragment.

The *H2* Promoter

One effective way to examine the properties of the *lac* promoter has been to fuse it to other genes, putting a variety of gene activities under *lac* control. If the *H2* promoter resides within the inversion region and the

H2 gene is on the left-hand side of the cloned fragment (Fig. 2), then transcription should proceed through the *H2* gene. It should be possible to insert the *Eco*RI fragment from pJZ60 into another vehicle so that genes that do not have their own promoters would be adjacent to the *H2*-gene region. This could result in the added genes showing the properties of phase variation. We have been able to prepare a number of such hybrids. The pJZ60 fragment was inserted into an *Eco*RI site at the beginning of the *trpB* gene (Selker et al. 1977). Before insertion of the fragment, there was no apparent *trpB* activity, i.e., the introduction of the plasmid into a *trpB* deletion strain did not allow it to grow on indole. However, after insertion of the *H2*-gene fragment, colonies, that carried the new plasmid were selected and found to be heterogeneous. Some were able to grow normally on indole and others formed very small colonies. When the clones that were able to grow on indole were picked, restreaked, and tested, they were again heterogeneous with respect to their ability to grow on indole-containing plates. This behavior was exactly analogous to the observations of *H2*-gene expression in the Hag⁻ mutant strain and suggests that the *trpB* gene has been put under *H2* control. When the plasmid DNA was isolated and analyzed by restriction with *Eco*RI and *Sal*I endonucleases, the *trpB* gene and the *H2* fragment were found to be contiguous. We can interpret the results as indicating that transcription proceeds through the *H2* gene and into the *trpB* gene. This would be consistent with the notion that the inversion region contained the *H2* promoter.

A similar construction was made with specific λ phage that carried the *che* genes. We were able to insert the pJZ60 fragment in an *Eco*RI site adjacent to the *cheW* gene (Silverman and Simon 1977b), and we could show that *H2* and *cheW* were expressed coordinately and that both behaved as if they were undergoing phase variation. We conclude, therefore, that the fragment carrying the inversion region also carries an element, presumably a promoter, that is able to extend phase-variation-like regulation to contiguous genes oriented so that they can be cotranscribed along with the *H2* gene.

DISCUSSION

An examination of the cloned DNA molecules carrying the phase-variation determinants clearly revealed that the DNA that codes for the *H2*-gene product is adjacent to an 800-bp sequence which is able to undergo inversion. The specific inversion event does not appear to be dependent upon the *recA* system of the host. Nothing is known about the mechanism responsible for the inversion. Presumably, there are specific sequences flanking the 800-bp region that are recognized by an enzyme that catalyzes the inversion. This could be a protein that has some other function in the cell and fortuitously recognizes the phase-variation sequence, or the enzyme could be a product of the DNA included in the inversion. There is sufficient coding capacity in this region to account for a polypeptide with a molecular weight of 25,000.

The inversion region also includes a promoter and a regulatory site that are specific for *H2*-gene expression. Eventually, studies of mutations that map in this region and analysis of the base sequence of the region will allow us to make assignments of particular sequences to each of these functions. These data will be necessary in order to understand the variation in the frequency of inversion. For example, the rate of phase variation is not the same in both directions, i.e., transition from phase 2 to phase 1 can be ten times more frequent than the reverse transition (Makela 1964). It also varies with the nature of the specific strain tested. In some strains, the frequency may be as high as 10^{-2} per cell/per generation (Stocker 1949), in other strains, it may be almost indistinguishable from the frequency of mutation. There are also stabilized strains (*vH2⁻*) where the transition is not detected (Iino 1969). However, if the *H2* gene, along with the stabilized region, is introduced into the chromosome of a different strain (Enomoto and Stocker 1975), phase transition is again observed. Therefore, the frequency of phase transition may be affected by the position of the phase-determining element on the chromosome. Furthermore, it is possible that there may be physiological or environmental effects that induce changes in the frequency of *Salmonella* flagellar phase variation. There are reports of mechanisms similar to phase variation that regulate pili formation (Ottow 1975; Swaney et al. 1977), and in these systems the frequency of transition appears to change in response to growth conditions. It is not difficult to imagine how the transition could be regulated. The formation of a site-specific recombination enzyme or the availability of the inversion sequences provides two points at which control could be exercised. However, physiological regulation has not yet been observed in the flagellar phase-variation system.

The general properties of the phase-variation system are different from those of other regulatory systems. Phase variation introduces a relatively stable change in gene expression into a small fraction of the population and therefore maintains heterogeneity in the population. For *Salmonella*, the ability to express an alternate flagellar antigen might ensure survival of a fraction of the population after the host organism mounts an immune response to the primary flagellar antigen. In contrast to the *lac* operon system, phase variation appears to increase the probability of survival of the clone but has, on average, only a marginal effect on the survival of all the individual organisms in the population.

The phase-variation mechanism does not appear to be restricted to the flagellar system in *Salmonella*. There are many observations suggesting phase-variation-like regulation in other systems. Among the prokaryotes, these include (1) fimbriae formation in *E. coli*, i.e., the variation in the ability to form pili (Ottow 1975; Swaney et al. 1977); (2) the K-dark variants of *B. harveyi* that alternate between bioluminescent and nonluminescent forms (Hastings and Nealson 1977); and (3) the transition between strains of *Haemophilus influenzae* that are able to restrict and modify bacteriophage S2 and the type that is nonrestrictive (Gromkova et al. 1973). There are other examples of transition between two phenotypes at frequencies that cannot be easily rationalized as the result of mutational changes. There are, of course, other explanations for some of these observations, and changes at the DNA level have not yet been observed in any of these systems. In the bacteriophage mu system, on the other hand, a change at the DNA level has been observed. When mu lysogens are induced, a specific region (the G-loop) undergoes inversion (Chow and Bukhari 1977). A homologous inversion region was found in bacteriophage P1. However, the role of these specific inversions in the life cycle of the phages is not known.

The flagellar phase transition in *Salmonella* controls the expression of both a structural gene activity and a regulatory gene product. Iino and his coworkers (Fujita and Yamaguchi 1973; Iino 1977) have shown that there is another gene coordinately expressed with *H2*—the *rhl* gene. This gene codes for the synthesis of a repressor of the phase-1 gene. When *H2* is "on," the *rhl* product is also synthesized and *H1* gene expression is repressed. Thus, the phase transition may have pleiotropic effects and could be involved in complicated regulatory circuits. In fact, some *Salmonella* strains show transition between four different alternate flagellar phases, implying an elaborate interaction among alternate forms of a gene (Edwards et al. 1962).

The relative stability of the phase-induced changes and the possibility that they could initiate a series of regulatory events that would result in the expression of a complex phenotype have led to the suggestion that similar mechanisms could be involved in development and in differentiation. If phase transitions exist during the early stages of embryogenesis, they might be "fixed" at some point during development. If, for example, the enzyme that catalyzed the rearrangement were no longer formed, cells would be trapped in one phase or the other. Furthermore, it is possible that there are as yet undiscovered inducing events that could coordinate the timing and direction of gene rearrangements. The idea that specific inversions and translocations are involved in differentiation has been developed by McClintock (1967) based on her work with the *Zea mays* genetic system. Recent advances in DNA technology will allow a clear test of these ideas. Evidence that a DNA rearrangement is involved in gene expression in eukaryotes has been reported by Tonegawa and coworkers (1977). Their work suggests that the formation of the immunoglobulin gene in mice involves a large translocation that puts the two portions of the gene together so that they can be expressed in the mature differentiated cell. Intensive work on phase-variation-like mechanisms in both the eukaryotic and the prokaryotic systems in the next few years will indicate whether they represent a general form of regulation that is involved in cell differentiation or whether they are exceptional mechanisms that have evolved to regulate specialized gene products.

SUMMARY

Phase variation, the alternative expression of genes regulating bacterial flagella formation, is regulated by a specific inversion which is located adjacent to one of the flagellar genes. Heteroduplex and restriction analyses indicate that the region is capable of inversion and that the inversion event is independent of the *recA* system of the host. The inversion region may contain a promoter that initiates transcription of the *H2* gene only when the inversion is in one orientation. It is suggested that DNA rearrangement, e.g., inversion and translocations, may be involved in a variety of regulatory events in both prokaryotes and eukaryotes.

ACKNOWLEDGMENTS

This work was supported by grants from the National Science Foundation (PCM-76-17197) and the National Institutes of Health (USPHS AI-13008-02).

REFERENCES

Bolivar, F., R. Rodriguez, M. Betlach, and H. Boyer. 1977. Construction and characterization of new cloning vehicles. *Gene* (in press).

Chow, L. and A. I. Bukhari. 1977. Bacteriophage mu genome: Structural studies on mu DNA and mu mutants carrying insertions. In *DNA insertion elements, plasmids, and episomes* (ed. A. I. Bukhari et al.), p. 295. Cold Spring Harbor Laboratory, Cold Spring Harbor, New York.

Edwards, P., R. Sakasaki, and I. Kato. 1962. Natural occurrence of four reversible flagellar phases. *J. Bacteriol.* **82**:99.

Enomoto, M. and B. A. D. Stocker. 1975. Integration of *hag* or elsewhere of *H2* genes transduced from *Salmonella* to *Escherichia coli. Genetics* **82**:595.

Fujita, H. and S. Yamaguchi. 1973. Studies on H-O variants in *Salmonella* in relation to phase variation. *J. Gen. Microbiol.* **76**:127.

Green, M. M. 1977. The case for DNA insertion mutations in *Drosophila*. In *DNA insertion elements, plasmids, and episomes* (ed. A. I. Bukhari et al.), p. 437. Cold Spring Harbor Laboratory, Cold Spring Harbor, New York.

Gromkova, R., J. Bindter, and S. Goodgal. 1973. Restriction and modification of bacteriophage S2 in *Haemophilus influenzae. J. Bacteriol.* **114**:1151.

Hastings, J. W. and K. M. Nealson. 1977. Bacterial bioluminescence. *Ann. Rev. Microbiol.* **31**:549.

Hicks, J., J. Strathern, and I. Herskowitz. 1977. The cassette model of mating-type interconversion. In *DNA insertion elements, plasmids, and episomes* (ed. A. I. Bukhari et al.), p. 457. Cold Spring Harbor Laboratory, Cold Spring Harbor, New York.

Hsu, M.-T. and N. Davidson. 1974. Electron microscope heteroduplex study of the heterogeneity of mu phage and prophage DNA. *Virology* **58:** 229.

Iino, T. 1969. Genetics and chemistry of bacterial flagella. *Bacteriol. Rev.* **33:** 454.

———. 1977. Genetics of structure and function of bacterial flagella. *Annu. Rev. Genet.* **11:** 161.

Kondoh, H. and H. Hotani. 1974. Flagellin from *E. coli* 12: Polymerization and molecular weight in comparison with *Salmonella* flagellins. *Biochim. Biophys. Acta* **336:** 117.

Lederberg, J. and T. Iino. 1956. Phase variation in *Salmonella*. *Genetics* **46:** 1475.

Makela, P. H. 1964. Flagellar homologies between *E. coli* and *Salmonella*. *J. Gen. Microbiol.* **35:** 503.

Maxam, A. and W. Gilbert. 1977. A new method for sequencing DNA. *Proc. Natl. Acad. Sci.* **74:** 560.

McClintock, B. 1957. Controlling elements and the gene. *Cold Spring Harbor Symp. Quant. Biol.* **21:** 197.

———. 1967. The role of the nucleus. Genetic systems regulating gene expression during development. *Devel. Biol.* (Suppl.) **1:** 84.

Otsuka, A. 1978. Insertion and excision of DNA fragments from *Pst* I endonuclease sites. *Gene* (in press).

Ottow, J. C. 1975. Ecology, physiology and genetics of fimbriae and pili. *Annu. Rev. Microbiol.* **29:** 79.

Pearce, N. and B. A. D. Stocker. 1967. Phase variation of flagellar antigens. *J. Gen. Microbiol.* **49:** 335.

Selker, A., K. Brown, and C. Yanofsky. 1977. Mitomycin C-induced expression of *trpA* of *Salmonella typhimurium* inserted into the plasmid Col E1. *J. Bacteriol.* **129:** 388.

Silverman, M. and M. Simon. 1977a. Bacterial flagella. *Annu. Rev. Microbiol.* **31:** 397.

———. 1977b. Identification of polypeptides necessary for chemotaxis in *E. coli*. *J. Bacteriol.* **130:** 1317.

Sonnenborn, T. M. 1977. Genetics of cellular differentiation: Stable nuclear differentiation in eukaryotic unicells. *Annu. Rev. Genet.* **11:** 349.

Starlinger, P. and H. Saedler. 1972. Insertion mutations in microorganisms. *Biochimie* **54:** 177.

Stocker, B. A. D. 1949. Measurements of rate of mutation of flagellar antigen phase in *Salmonella typhimurium*. *J. Hyg.* **47:** 398.

Swaney, L., Y.-P. Liu, C.-M. To, C.-C. To, K. Ippen-Ihler, and C. Brinton, Jr. 1977. Type 1 pilus mutants and phase variants. *J. Bacteriol.* **130:** 495.

Tonegawa, S., N. Hozumi, G. Matthyssens, and R. Schuller. 1977. Somatic changes in the content and context of immunoglobulin genes. *Cold Spring Harbor Symp. Quant. Biol.* **41:** 877.

Zieg, J., M. Silverman, M. Hilmen, and M. Simon. 1977a. Recombinational switch for gene expression. *Science* **196:** 170.

———. 1977b. The mechanism of phase variation. *ICN-UCLA Symp. Mol. Cell. Biol.* **8:** 25.

Reference Index

Numbers in *italics* refer to pages on which the complete references are listed: **boldface** type designates where author's article is located in this volume.

Subject Index